Herpetic Eye Diseases

Documenta Ophthalmologica
Proceedings Series volume 44

Editor H. E. Henkes

Herpetic Eye Diseases

Proceedings of the International Symposium
at the Katholieke Universiteit Leuven,
Leuven, Belgium, May 17–19, 1984

P.C. Maudgal and L. Missotten (Editors)

1985 **DR W. JUNK PUBLISHERS**
a member of the KLUWER ACADEMIC PUBLISHERS GROUP
DORDRECHT / BOSTON / LANCASTER

Distributors

for the United States and Canada: Kluwer Academic Publishers, 190 Old
Derby Street, Hingham, MA 02043, USA
for the UK and Ireland: Kluwer Academic Publishers, MTP Press Limited,
Falcon House, Queen Square, Lancaster LA1 1RN, UK
for all other countries: Kluwer Academic Publishers Group, Distribution
Center, P.O. Box 322, 3300 AH Dordrecht, The Netherlands

Library of Congress Cataloging in Publication Data

Main entry under title:

Herpetic eye diseases.

   (Documenta ophthalmologica. Proceedings series ;
v. 44)
   1. Keratitis--Congresses. 2. Herpes simplex virus--
Congresses. I. Maudgal, P. C. II. Missotten, Luc.
[DNLM: 1. Keratitis, Dendritic--congresses.
2. Herpesvirus Hominis--pathogenicity--congresses.
W3 DO637 v.44 / WW 220 H563 1984]
RE338.H47 1985   617.7'19   85-4734

ISBN-13: 978-94-010-8935-7   e-ISBN-13: 978-94-009-5518-9
DOI: 10.1007/978-94-009-5518-9

Copyright

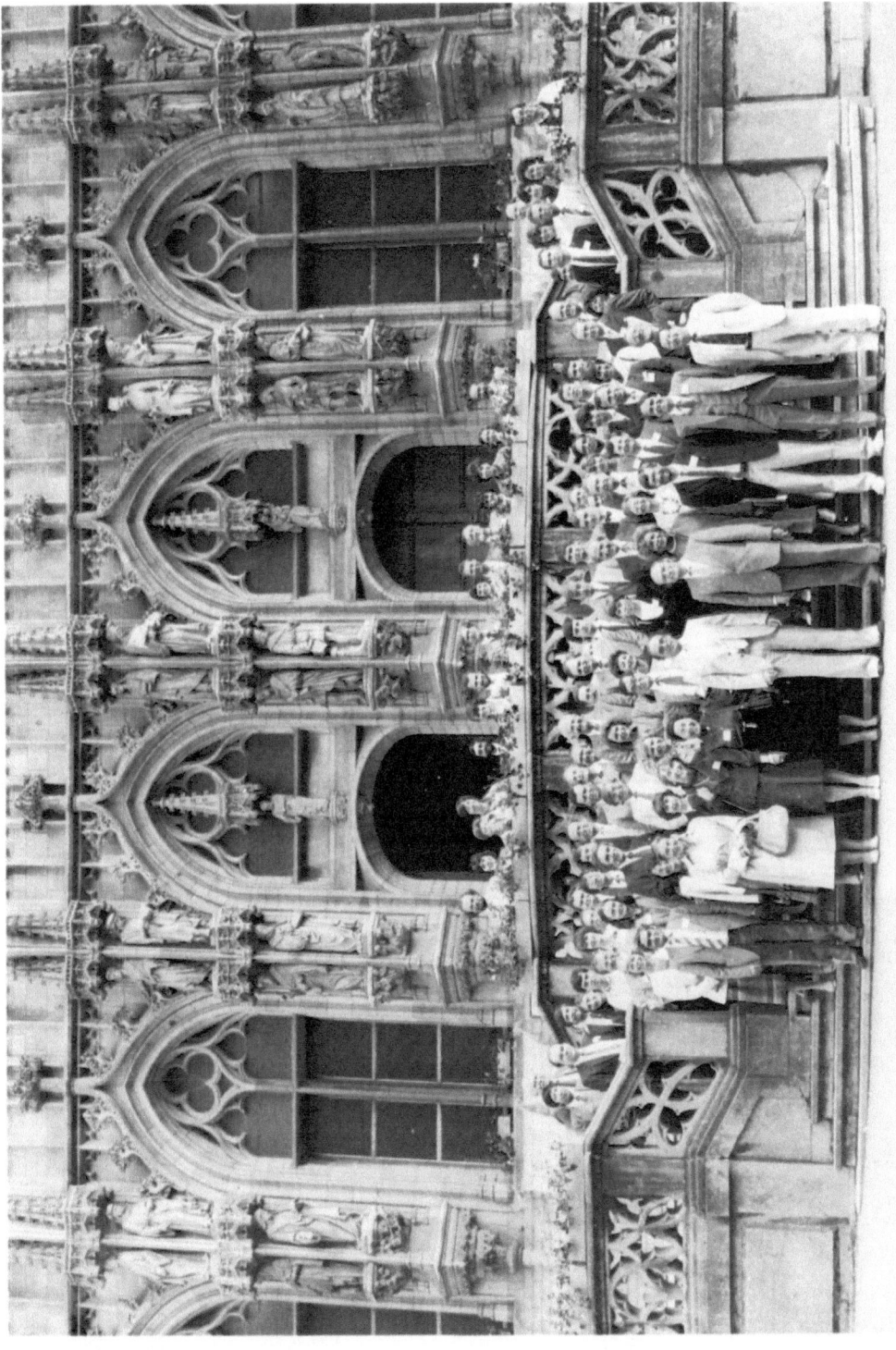

CONTENTS

Welcome address
    P.De Somer   XIII

SESSION I : Virology, Pathogenesis
Chairman : D.L.Easty (Bristol)

Pathogenesis of herpes virus infections
    H.J.Field   1

Herpes simplex virus infection of corneal cells
    in vitro
    C.Carter, H.Dyson and D.L.Easty   9

Cytopathogenic effects of herpes simplex virus
    on corneal epithelium
    P.C.Maudgal and L.Missotten   17

Superior cervical ganglion in experimental
    herpes simplex virus eye disease
    C.R.Dawson, W.-h.Zhang and O.Briones   23

Recurrent and non-recurrent HSV-1 strains :
    Effect of temperature
    Y.Centifanto-Fitzgerald   27

Herpes simplex virus cycle : Model of mechanism
    of acute disease, latency and reactivation
    A.Romano and D.Gamus   33

SESSION II : Pathology, Immunology
Chairman : C.R.Dawson (San Francisco)

Spread of herpes simplex virus to the eye
    following cutaneous inoculation in the
    snout of the mouse
    C.Shimeld, D.L.Easty, A.B.Tullo, W.A.Blyth and T.J.Hill   39

Light microscopic evaluation of rabbit corneal nerves:
    Comparison of the normal with dendritic herpetic
    keratitis
    P.A.Asbell and R.Beuerman   49

Isolation of herpes simplex virus from corneal discs of
    patients with chronic stromal keratitis
    A.B.Tullo, D.L.Easty, C.Shimeld, P.E.Stirling
    and J.M.Darville   57

Genetic influence from chromosome 12 on murine
    susceptibility to herpes simplex
    C.S.Foster, R.Wetzig, D.Knipe and M.I.Greene   67

Systemic immune responses after ocular antigen
    encounter
    C.S.Foster   77

The role of virus-infected mononuclear leukocytes
    in the pathogenesis of herpetic chorioretinitis
    of newborn rabbits
    Y.Ohashi, J.O.Oh and K.-H. Tung-ou   91

                SESSION III : Immunology,Vaccination
                Chairman : C. S. Foster (Boston)

The influence of prednisolone on external eye disease,
    virus proliferation and latent infection in an
    animal model of herpes simplex keratitis
    D.L.Easty, A.B.Tullo, C.Shimeld, T.J.Hill and W.A.Blyth   95

Suppressive effect of cyclosporine on the induction
    of secondary herpes simplex uveitis
    J.O.Oh, P.Minasi, G.Grabner and Y.Ohasi   99

T-cell subsets in herpes zoster cyclitis
    T.M.Radda, J.Funder, U.M.Klemen and U.Köller   103

Experimental and clinical preliminary study of immuno-
    modulators in the treatment of ocular herpes
    J.Denis, T.Hoang-Xuan, J.F.Bonissent, K.Dogbe, C.Clay,
    D.Viza, F.Rosenfeld, J.Phillips and J.M.Vich   111

Subunit vaccine compared with infection as protection
    against experimental herpes simplex keratitis
    B.A.Harney, D.L.Easty and G.R.B.Skinner   119

Immunological aspects and thymic hormone therapy of
    herpetic keratitis
    P.Pivetti-Pezzi, P.De Liso, W.Calcatelli,M.C.Sirianni,
    M.Fiorilli, I.Mezzaroma and L.Palmisano   129

                SESSION IV : Clinical Disease
                Chairman : P.Wright (London)

Primary ocular HSV infections in adults
    C.Ameye, P.C.Maudgal and L.Missotten   133

A case of bilateral herpes simplex eye disease
    of long duration
    A.A.Tye   141

Differential diagnosis of herpetic keratitis by
means of a new electronic optical aesthesiometer
J.Draeger, R.Winter and G.Krolzig 147

Lacrimal secretion after herpetic keratitis
J.G.Orsoni, M.Bonacini, A.Piccioni and M.C.Tomba 155

A computer-based method to provide subspecialist expertise
on the management of herpes simplex infections of the eye
C.R.Dawson, J.Kastner, S.Weiss and C.Kulikowski 163

SESSION V : Antiviral Agents-I
Chairman : L.M.T.Collum (Dublin)

New antiviral drugs for the treatment of herpesvirus
infections
E.De Clercq 169

Ocular herpesvirus infections and the development of
virus-drug resistance
H.J.Field 179·

Relevance of viral thymidine kinase for clinical
resistance to antiviral drugs when treating
herpes simplex eye infections
A.R.Karlström, C.F.R.Källander, J.S.Gronowitz
and P.J.Wistrand 187

A rapid micromethod for evaluating the sensitivity of
ocular herpes simplex strains to antiviral drugs
M.Langlois, J.Denis, J.Ph.Allard and M.Aymard 193

A review of acyclovir in the management of herpes simplex
infections of the eye
P.J.Rees 197

A comparison of the antiherpes activities in vitro and
in vivo of foscarnet and mono- and dihydroxybutylguanine
R.Datema,A.-C.Ericson, A.Larsson, K.Stenberg, A.Nyqvist-
Mayer, F.Y.Aoki, N.-G.Johansson and B.Öberg 207

SESSION VI : Antiviral Agents-II
Chairman : O.P.van Bijsterveld (Utrecht)

Acyclovir treatment in stromal herpetic keratitis
R.van Ganswijk, J.A.Oosterhuis and J.Versteeg 213

Antiviral treatment of herpes simplex stromal disease
J.I.McGill 217

Treatment of herpetic kerato-uveitis : Comparative
    action of vidarabine,trifluorothymidine and
    acyclovir in combination with corticoids
    J.Colin, D.Mazet and C.Chastel   227

Oral acyclovir (Zovirax^R) in herpetic keratitis
    L.M.T.Collum, P.MacGerrtick, J.Akhtar and P.J.Rees   233

A double-blind, dual-centre comparative trial of
    acyclovir (Zovirax^R) and adenine arabinoside
    in the treatment of herpes simplex amoeboid ulcers
    S.O.Hung, A.Patterson, L.M.T.Collum,P.Logan and
    P.Rees   241

                    SESSION VII : Antiviral Agents-III
                    Chairman : E.De Clercq (Leuven)

Topical bromovinyldeoxyuridine treatment of herpes
    simplex keratitis
    P.C.Maudgal, M.Dieltiens, E.De Clercq and L.Missotten   247

Permeability of the cornea to (^{125}I)IVDU, an analogue of
    bromovinyldeoxyuridine
    A.M.Verbruggen, E.De Clercq, P.C.Maudgal, C.Ameye,
    R.Busson, R.Bernaerts, M.De Roo and L.Missotten   257

Use of ara-A in herpetic eye diseases : A review
    C.Ameye   263

Trifluridine induced corneal epithelium dysplasia
    P.C.Maudgal, B.Van Damme and L.Missotten   279

Steroid addiction : A complication of use and abuse of
    steroids in herpes simplex keratitis
    I.S.Jain, A.Gupta and M.R.Dogra   287

Management of herpetic keratitis by instillation of
    citreous honey
    M.H.Emarah   293

                    SESSION VIII : Keratoplasty
                    Chairman : H.-J.Thiel (Tübingen)

Severe herpes simplex keratitis, frequency of
    complicating cataract, results of corneal grafting
    M.Rydberg   297

Penetrating keratoplasty in herpetic corneal diseases
    with perforation or severe stromal keratitis
    E.G.Weidle, H.-J.Thiel and W.Lish   303

Keratoplasty in herpetic corneal disease
    H.Knöbel, E.N.Hinzpeter and G.O.H.Naumann   311

Prevention and treatment of herpes recurrence
   in the corneal graft with acyclovir
   C.C.Kok-van Alphen and H.J.M.Völker-Dieben   319

The influence of prospective HLA-A and -B matching
   in 288 penetrating keratoplasties for herpes
   simplex keratitis
   H.J.Völker-Dieben, C.C.Kok-van Alphen,
   J.D'Amaro and P.De Lange   329

                    SESSION IX : Interferon
                    Chairman : J. Colin (Brest)

Interferon treatment of herpetic keratitis
   G.Smolin   339

Lymphoblast and fibroblast-interferon in a
   combination therapy of keratitis dendritica
   Chr.Fellinger, M.E.Reich and H.Hofmann   343

Beta interferon cream therapy in periocular
   herpetic infections
   A.Romano, M.Revel and T.Doerner   349

Human leukocyte interferon plus trifluorothymidin
   versus recombinant alpha 2 arg interferon plus
   trifluorothymidin for therapy of dendritic
   keratitis. A controlled clinical study
   R.Sundmacher, D.Neumann-Haefelin, A.Mattes,
   W.Merk, G.Adolf and K.Cantell   359

Acyclovir and recombinant human alpha 2 arg interferon
   treatment for dendritic keratitis
   P.J.Meurs and O.P.van Bijsterveld   367

             SESSION X : Herpes Zoster, Cytomegalovirus
                    Chairman : R.Sundmacher (Freiburg)

The acute retinal necrosis syndrome and retinal necrosis
   associated with encephalitis
   A.Leys, B.De Cnodder and L.Missotten   377

Clinical comparison between herpes simplex and herpes
   zoster ocular infections
   R.Ahonen and A.Vannas   389

Corneal complications of herpes zoster ophthalmicus
   T.J.Liesegang   395

Oral bromovinyldeoxyuridine treatment of herpes zoster
   ophthalmicus
   P.C.Maudgal, M.Dieltiens, E.De Clercq and L.Missotten   403

Herpes zoster treatment
   J.I.McGill   413

SESSION XI : General Discussion
Chairman : R.Sundmacher (Freiburg)

General discussion on the management of
   herpetic eye diseases
   P.C.Maudgal   425

Closing remarks
   P.C.Maudgal   439

List of participants   XV

WELCOME ADDRESS

Ladies and Gentlemen,

I feel honoured and proud that you came from so many countries to our university to exchange your clinical and laboratory experience on herpes virus. This is a mixed meeting of ophthalmologists and virologists, clinicians asking questions and learning from people working in the laboratory, and laboratory people looking to the problems expressed by the clinicians - an example of mutual fecundation of applied and fundamental medical science.

We owe this meeting to an enthousiastic young man, Dr. Maudgal, who for the first time brought together the Department of Ophthalmology of Dr. Missotten and the Laboratory of Virology of Dr. De Clercq in a collaborative study of herpes infections and who organised this gathering as an extension of this intiative. He is entitled to your gratitude and also to your criticism.

Our university will be your host for these few days you will spend with us. We have no luxury to offer you in this medieval city, I hope you will be able to adapt to its quiet atmosphere and its poor accomodations, that you will relax, far from your own laboratories and clinics, in this old university where for more than 5 centuries scholars from all countries gathered together, just like you, to find inspiration to solve their problems.

I wish to all of you that your stay with us will be interesting and pleasant. The progress of science is based on the communication of knowledge and communication depends on good relations between people. The contribution of this meeting to a better knowledge of what herpes virus is and does, will depend as much on the friendship that you will develop from living together for three days, as on the quality of the work that will be presented.

I hope that you will be successful in realising both and that Leuven will remain an important date for your future work. As a virologist myself, I got lost in university administration. I regret very much that I cannot stay with you to learn about the latest news in herpes research, it would be more exciting than to run a university.

My best wishes for a successful meeting !

Professor P. DE SOMER,
Rector K.U.Leuven.

PATHOGENESIS OF HERPES VIRUS INFECTIONS.

H.J. Field, Dept. Clinical Veterinary Medicine, University of Cambridge,
U.K.

Towards a Molecular Understanding of Herpes Pathogenesis

My original intention was to relate some of the recent developments in
the molecular understanding of the herpes virus to its diverse pathogenicity, paying special attention to the ocular manifestations of
disease. Of the large family of herpes viruses only the neurotropic
human herpes viruses will be considered - especially herpes simplex. In
the event even this restricted survey proves to be a difficult task and
emphasizes the gulf which still exists between the molecular detail
(much of the genome has now been sequenced) and the disease processes.

One difficulty is the large and complex nature of the virion. The virus
is relatively "intelligent", having a genome molecular weight of approximately 100×10^6 Daltons; this being coding potential for about 100 polypeptides. In fact, over 80 virus-induced products have been detected in
infected cells, so it is going to be very difficult to relate any particular aspects of the pathogenic process to a particular gene product of
the virus. The genome itself is a linear, double-stranded molecule made
up of unique and repeated sequences. A long and a short unique sequence
of nucleotides (that is, they occur only once in the genome) is each
flanked by repeated sequences which occur at the termini and internally
in the genome. A hinge point exists between the internal repeated
sequences such that each unique sequence can flip-flop relative to the
other, generating 4 possible isomeric forms of the complete DNA molecule
- this point will be relevant to the consideration of 'latency', below.

Herpesvirus Interactions with Differentiated Cells

Among the range of products encoded by the herpes genome about half are
structural components of the virus particle; of these, six or more are
glycoproteins. The glycoproteins may be especially important in pathogenesis since they become incorporated in the envelope of the virus and
are involved in the first interactions between the virus and the cells
which it can infect and with the host's immune system.

About half the virus-polypeptides are not structural components of the
virion but are involved in the replication process within the infected
cells and among these are at least six virus-induced enzymes. Two of
these - the deoxypyrimidine kinase (usually known as thymidine kinase)
and DNA-polymerase will be referred to often in this volume because they
have a vital rôle in the modes of action of several successful antiviral
compounds which are active against herpes.

One of the problems with understanding the strategy of the herpes virus

Maudgal, P.C. and Missotten, L., (eds.) Herpetic Eye Diseases.
© *1985, Dr W. Junk Publishers, Dordrecht/Boston/Lancaster. ISBN 978-94-010-8935-7*

is that most of our biochemical information has necessarily been obtained from the study of productively infected replicating cells, challenged at high multiplicity with herpes simplex virus. Of course, in the real case things are very much more complex. The typical sequence of events in a herpes simplex infection is well known: epidermal cells, often at a mucocutaneous junction are the first cells to be encountered and undergo a productive infection. But things become more mysterious when the virus finds its way into the sensory nerve endings and travels to the cell bodies of those neurons probably by retrograde transport within the axons. The recent work of Lycke et al. (1984) (using cultured neural cells) suggests that virus travels up the axon as unenveloped particles - while virus travelling centrifugally, at least from productively infected neurons seem to be in the enveloped, mature form. The virus can cause a productive infection in neurons (killing the cells) but it may (perhaps usually) establish a stable relationship with the neurons giving rise to a latent infection; the state of the virus and the controlling events which govern latency and reactivation have yet to be elucidated.

Something that one often forgets is that there are many cells, other than neurons, in the nervous system with which the virus can interact. We are extremely ignorant about the nature of virus interactions with glial cells, for example the schwann cells in the peripheral nerve or the satellite cells which engulf the ganglion neurons, or with the supporting cells in the CNS. In some cases the virus seems to infect these cells in an abortive fashion such that no morphologically mature virus particles are released. Whether glial cells can sometimes survive such inter- actions is doubtful but unclear. In any case these cells may have an important rôle in insulating a focus of infected neurons from the other uninfected, susceptible tissue?

Factors Involved in Herpes Tissue Specificity

To emphasize our ignorance we will consider a few of the many different factors which may influence the virus interactions with these highly differentiated cells. Much interest has been directed towards the glyco- proteins. Among these are the receptors which may determine the kind of cells to which the virus can adsorb to initiate the infection. They also cause a number of interesting biological effects; they give rise to "Fc- receptors" on infected cells which can bind to the Fc portion of immuno- globulin molecules and yet another feature is to bring about the fusion between adjacent cells. We are very uncertain about the relevance and importance of these interesting observations. Apart from the glyco- protein receptors, other virus features that may be important in deter- mining the outcome of the infection of a particular tissue may be found among the non-structural polypeptides. Examples of this type are the enzyme activities which occur in the herpes-infected cells. The fact that both herpes simplex and varicella-zoster can make their own thymi- dine kinase may make them better able to infect cells, such as neurons, which are normally not prepared for DNA replication to occur. The DNA- polymerase complex itself may involve cellular components and these inter- actions would be likely to vary in different kinds of cells. Yet other enzymes, about which we know less, may also have a rôle to play? Once the cells are infected we know that there are sequences in the herpes DNA which are regulatory sequences or "signposts" which help to control the expression of the virus genome. These regulatory sequences may interact with cellular proteins which contribute a regulatory function and these proteins may vary among different kinds of cells. So we begin to build

3

Establishment of Latency Giving Ocular Recurrence of Virus

1) <u>Primary infection of the eye</u> (several animal models with ocular
shedding on trigeminal stimuli)

2) <u>Secondary Infection</u>

a) Spread within ganglion   (occurs in mice)

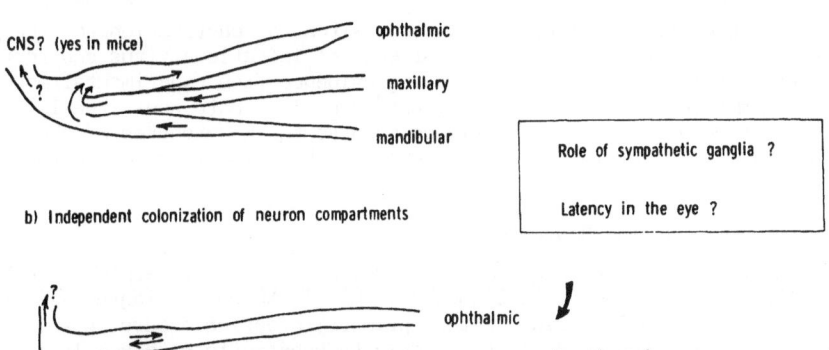

b) Independent colonization of neuron compartments

Role of sympathetic ganglia ?

Latency in the eye ?

Fig.1. A Schematic Diagram to Illustrate the General Possibilities for
the Establishment of Recurrent Ocular Herpes Infections in Man.

4

up an extremely complex picture of the virus in its interactions with differentiated cells, and still more so with the intact host, its active non-specific defence systems and specific immune responses to the presence of the parasite.

Developments in Understanding Herpes Latency

There has recently been an important development in this field with the discovery that the virus DNA detected in "latently-infected" mice was in a form dissimilar from normal replicating DNA. Rock & Fraser (1983) reported that residual herpes virus DNA could be detected in the trigeminal ganglia or brainstems of experimentally infected mice (several weeks after the acute disease) by means of Southern blot hybridization analysis. When the digested infected mouse brain DNA was hybridized to a probe comprizing a short sequence of herpes DNA, obtained from the junction region, the anticipated terminal fragments were absent (the internal junction sequences are repeated at the termini and are thus "recognized" by this probe) while the junction itself was clearly visible. The most likely explanation for this result seems to be that the DNA molecules are present in circular form. However, even if this does turn out to be a crucial feature of the latent genome (and it is still possible that a small minority of genomes are present in a different form, for example integrated into the host DNA) it is still uncertain which virus sequences or gene products regulate latency and switch to reactivation and the sequence of events leading to recurrence of infectious virus and recrudescence. Moreover, there is increasing evidence from experimental models and in man that virus latency may not be exclusive to neural cells but may also occur in non-neural tissue such as the keratocytes of the corneal stroma (A. Tullo, this volume) or the skin of the mouse footpad (Al-Saadi et al., 1983).

Herpes in Recurrent Ocular Disease

There seem to be two general ways in which a recurrent herpes infection of the eye can become established and this is shown in diagrammatic form Fig. 1. The simplest case is that primary infection occurs in the eye and there are good experimental models to substantiate this. It is notable that in these models (for example rabbits or mice infected with herpes simplex by applying virus to the scarified cornea) virus establishes latency in the trigeminal ganglia from where it can be reactivated by the appropriate stimuli to the eye or to the ganglion itself resulting in virus shedding. Another feature of these models is that virus finds its way centrally into the brainstem, though whether this kind of translocation occurs in man (either regularly or rarely) is unknown.

The second general possibility for the establishment of ocular herpes is that the disease arises as a secondary infection following the spread of virus from a primary infection at another site such as the lip. Virus may either be transmitted exogenously from a skin lesion to the eye, or more likely virus spreads within the trigeminal ganglion to the compartment containing the neurons of the ophthalmic branch. The virus then may spread centrifugally to reach the eye. Our own studies show that this sequence of events can occur in intra-nasally infected mice (Anderson & Field, 1983) and it was shown earlier by Tullo et al. (1982)

in a model involving lip inoculation of mice. Again virus spread into the CNS can be demonstrated in these models. Similar events can probably occur in man during a primary oral infection, however, it seems likely that the nervous systems of the experimental animals are much more permissive to the translocation of virus than is the case in man where the infection may be better insulated from related tissue? A particularly interesting study which bears on this is that of Tullo et al. (1983) who divided the left and right trigeminal ganglia explanted from human cadavers into the three compartments - maxillary, mandibular, and ophthalmic and tested each for the presence of reactivatable virus. In a necessarily small number of cases none were found to contain virus in the ophthalmic compartment while the other parts yielded positive isolations - however, a very much larger number of ganglia would need to be examined to include herpes keratitis sufferers since this manifestation occurs in as few as 1% of the total herpes cases.

Before leaving the question of the events leading to recurrent ocular herpes we should not close our minds to other possibilities that may be important. It has been shown in mice (Price et al., 1975 and C. Dawson, this volume) and in man (Warren et al., 1978) that the autonomic ganglia can harbour latent herpes and indeed the eye itself seems to be another possibility either in the retinal neurons as suggested by Openshaw (1983) or perhaps more likely in sympathetic neurons or even keratocytes (A.Tullo, this volume). However, whether these other possibilities have a rôle in human disease, perhaps making the troublesome complications or frequent recurrences more or less likely, we do not yet know; one suspects that among the total human ocular herpes all these possibilities have a part to play.

Animal Models for the Study of Ocular Herpes

The advantages and problems of the different available models will not be discussed here except with regard to one very general point - to plead caution about extrapolating too far from animal data. It is attractive to consider that the different kinds of ocular herpes seen in different individuals may relate, at least in part, to the particular strain of virus that has been encountered. Indeed, if a dozen different isolates of herpes simplex are inoculated into a standard animal model then several quite distinct disease patterns will become apparent. However, these features such as the production of encephalitis by one strain but not another may have little or no relevance to the natural infection in man. Because of the complexity of the cellular interactions mentioned above it is highly unlikely that any particular manifestation such as the production of deep stromal disease will be mapped to a particular gene product such as a glycoprotein. It will surely turn out that particular constellations of many gene products will act in concert to produce a particular effect in certain individuals. Having thus cautioned against over-interpreting the pathogenicity data obtained from animal models, my concluding paragraphs will discuss two types of eye disease which can be produced in mice using a herpes simplex virus; they are examples where internal translocations of virus result in two quite different manifestations of ocular herpes.

Translocation of Virus to the Eye in Experimentally Infected Mice

1. Intra-cerebral Inoculation

When virus was inoculated into BALB/c mice by the intra-cerebral route virus spread via the optic nerve to involve the retina. Normally there was a concurrent and overwhelming encephalitis which resulted in death. If the lethal encephalitis was prevented by chemotherapy or by using an attentuated mutant then a florid infection of the retina and nerve head occurred in surviving mice. It was notable that the anterior eye was invariably spared. The mice given this type of infection recovered to look overtly normal but the ocular damage (which in the acute phase, 3-12 days after infection, involved virus titres of up to 10^9 pfu in the eye) was reflected in the development of cataracts (Anderson & Field, 1982; Field et al., 1982). The lens of the mouse is almost spherical and no doubt extremely susceptible to any nutritional deprivation or other disturbance of the lens epithelium (which itself did not appear to become infected). This then may be a useful model to study the retinitis which occurs in man particularly in neonates with generalized herpes and in the terminal phase of herpes encephalitis. Both these conditions are likely to become more frequent in those surviving these serious manifestations of herpes as a result of effective chemotherapy. Cataracts form in these mice very reproducibly, thus this may also represent a useful model to study the genesis of cataracts which result from non-virus stimuli such as the use of silicone in treatment of detached retina.

2. Intra-nasal Inoculation

The second model to be described involves the inoculation of similar mice but by means of introducing virus into the nares. The infection was initiated in the neurons of the olfactory mucosa and spread up the unmyel-inated olfactory nerve into the olfactory bulbs. However, virus infection occurred concurrently in the more anterior mucosa and spread via the 5th nerve to the trigeminal ganglion where virus antigen could be detected 3-5 days after inoculation. The interesting feature of this infection was that virus then spread centrifugally and infected the anterior eye by means of the sensory route (Anderson & Field, 1984). The iris and cilliary body were often involved and in some cases corneal ulcers were also present. It was notable that while the cilliary body sometimes con-tained a florid mass of virus antigen-containing cells, the neighbouring retina was always spared, for in this model the retina was never involved and cataracts did not develop. Perhaps this emphasizes the importance of the particular route by which virus arrives to infect the cells of an organ as well as the potential the virus has to infect different cell types. Clearly, the mouse retinal neurons are exquisitely sensitive to herpes simplex and may even be infected with mutants which are highly attenuated, but possibly the infection needs to be initiated via the axonal route?

This reference to two specific examples of ocular pathogenesis in mice completes my rather superficial survey of the molecular events underlying herpes infections. There has not been time to devote attention to those aspects of the disease which involve host inflammatory and immunological responses. Several genetically engineered vaccines are well forward in development and these will shortly be under evaluation. Results in animals are very encouraging but again we may find that it is much easier to protect against or influence the pathogenicity in the animal infections than turns out to be the case in the natural infection where things are beautifully balanced between host and parasite and this probably also applies to the testing of chemotherapy. However, the use of vaccines and effective chemotherapy in man should modify some aspects of the patho-genesis of herpes and this will complement the data from animal studies

and in turn should help to bridge the gulf between our molecular understanding of the workings of the herpes genome and the range of diseases
this virus can produce.

REFERENCES

Al-Saadi, S.A., Clements, G.B. & Subak-Sharpe, J.H. (1983) Viral genes
modify herpes simplex virus latency both in mouse footpad and sensory
ganglia. J. Gen. Virol., 64, 1175-1179.

Anderson, J.R. & Field, H.J. (1982) The development of retinitis in mice
with non-fatal herpes simplex encephalitis. Neuropath. & Appl. Neurol.
8, 277-287.

Anderson, J.R. & Field, H.J. (1983) The distribution of herpes simplex
type 1 antigen in mouse central nervous system after different routes of
inoculation. J. Neurol. Sci., 60, 181-195.

Anderson, J.R. & Field, H.J. (1984) An animal model of ocular herpes
keratitis, retinitis, and cataract in the mouse. B. J. Exp. Path. in
press.

Field, H.J., Anderson, J.R. & Wildy, P. (1982) Atypical patterns of
neural infection produced in mice by drug-resistant strains of herpes
simplex virus. J. Gen. Virol., 59, 91-99.

Lycke, E., Kristensson, K., Svennerholm, B., Vahlne, A. & Ziegler, R.
(1984) Uptake and transport of herpes simplex virus in neurites of rat
dorsal root ganglia cells in culture. J. Gen. Virol. 65, 55-64.

Openshaw, H. (1983) Latency of herpes simplex virus in ocular tissue of
mice. Inf. Immun., 39, 960-962.

Price, R.W., Katz, B.J. & Notkins, A.L. (1975) Latent infection of the
peripheral autonomic nervous system with herpes simplex virus. Nature,
London, 257, 686-688.

Rock, D.L. & Fraser, N.W. (1983) Detection of HSV-1 genome in central
nervous system of latently infected mice. Nature, London, 302, 523-525.

Tullo, A.B., Easty, D.L., Hill, T.J. & Blyth, W.A. (1982) Ocular herpes
simplex and the establishment of latent infection. Trans. Ophthal. Soc.
U.K., 102, 151-18.

Tullo, A.B., Shimeld, C., Easty, D.L. & Darville, J.M. (1983) Distribution of latent herpes simplex virus infection in human trigeminal ganglion.
Lancet, I, 353.

Warren, K.G., Brown, S.M., Wroblewska, Z., Gilden, D., Koprowski, H. &
Subak-Sharpe, J.H. (1978) Isolation of latent herpes simplex virus from
the superior cervical and vagus ganglions of human beings. N.Eng. J.
Med., 289, 1068-1069.

DISCUSSION :

Y. Centifanto (New Orleans) : You showed the joint regions of
   the HSV genome of the isolated virus by Southern blot, but
   you didn't show the termini. I would like to know when, in
   the infection cycle, the brain stem and ganglia were removed ?
   All I see is the virus in the brain stem, and none in the
   ganglia.

H.J. Field (Cambridge) : We have not been able to detect the virus in the ganglia, but Rock and Fraser have; it just seems
   to be a question of the level of sensitivity. The brain stems
   were obtained 5 weeks after inoculation.

HERPES SIMPLEX VIRUS INFECTION OF CORNEAL CELLS <u>IN VITRO</u>

C. CARTER, H. DYSON, D.L. EASTY
Department of Ophthalmology, University of Bristol, U.K.

SUMMARY

Methods have been developed for obtaining confluent secondary cultures of corneal epithelium, keratocytes and endothelium, in sufficient numbers for virological or other studies requiring a number of data points and replicates.

Virus growth curves following infection of these cultures with herpes simplex virus (HSV) at 0.1 - 0.2 PFU/cell showed that HSV replicated in each cell type, but that different amounts of infectious virus were produced by the 3 types of corneal cell cultures. Corneal epithelium (and Vero cells) produced the highest levels of virus, keratocytes (and skin fibroblast-like cells) less, and corneal endothelium least.

1. INTRODUCTION

An interest in herpetic disease in the cornea at the cellular level has led us to examine herpes simplex virus (HSV) infection in cultured corneal cells. <u>In vitro</u> the cell types from the three tissue layers of the cornea can be separated and HSV infection can be studied in detail. This approach has previously been used to compare the susceptibilities of corneal epithelial, keratocyte and endothelial cultures to infection by HSV types 1 and 2 (1); to examine the ability of antibody plus complement or leukocytes to kill HSV-infected keratocytes (2,3); and to test the effect of prednisolone on infection and antibody-dependent cell-mediated killing of keratocytes (4).

The main aim of the experiments reported below was to compare the production of infectious HSV in corneal epithelial, keratocyte and endothelial cultures. Firstly, however, methods were developed for growing sufficient numbers of cultures under comparable conditions.

Maudgal, P.C. and Missotten, L., (eds.) Herpetic Eye Diseases.
© *1985, Dr W. Junk Publishers, Dordrecht/Boston/Lancaster. ISBN 978-94-010-8935-7*

Secondary cultures of rabbit cells were used to allow for some cell proliferation _in vitro_ but to avoid the specific culture requirements of more extensively passaged corneal cells. A number of split ratios and serum concentrations were tested to select those to be used to obtain confluent secondary cultures of each cell type. Vero cells (a serially-passaged monkey kidney-derived cell line commonly used as a sensitive indicator of HSV) and skin fibroblast-like cells (skin fibroblasts) were infected in addition to the corneal cell types, for comparison.

2. METHODS
2.1.Cell Culture

Primary cultures of each corneal cell type were set up using a single set of corneas (5). Eight corneas were removed within the limbus from excised New Zealand White rabbit eyes, and each cornea separated into anterior and posterior halves. The anterior halves were treated with Dispase to detach the epithelial sheets (6) which were then dissociated with trypsin-EDTA (0.05% and 0.02%) in phosphate buffered saline (PBS). Meanwhile the posterior halves of the corneas were incubated with trypsin-EDTA (0.025% and 0.01%) in PBS on the endothelial surfaces for 10 minutes at 37° C, excess medium was added and the endothelial cells were detached mechanically. After removal of Descemet's membrane, the posterior stromas were cut into segments and explanted to allow outgrowth of keratocytes. Skin fibroblasts were cultured from explants of rabbit dermis.

The primary cultures were grown in medium 199 with Earle's salts, 0.22% $NaHCO_3$, antibiotics, and 10% foetal calf serum, on tissue culture plastic at 37ºC and in a humidified incubator with 5% CO_2. The primary cultures were split when confluent. Split ratios of 1:2,1:4 and 1:8 and serum concentrations of 2% to 18% were tested, and percent confluency in the resulting secondary cultures was estimated visually at intervals. Secondary cultures for infection experiments were grown in 4 cm² plastic wells, in medium containing 10% serum. Confluent cultures were maintained in medium containing 2% serum for 1 or more days before inoculation of HSV.

2.2. Virology

HSV type 1, strain SC16, was used throughout. Cultures were infected with 0.1 ml. of virus suspension containing 0.1-0.2 plaque-forming units (PFU; titrated on Vero cells) per cell, in medium containing 2% serum. 1 ml. medium containing 2% serum was added 1 hour later. At intervals, media from triplicate wells were removed and centrifuged. The pellets and 1 ml. aliquots of medium were pooled with the cells remaining in the respective wells ('cell-associated virus'). These samples and the supernatants ('cell-free virus') were stored at -70 °C. The cell-associated fractions were frozen and thawed 3 times to release intracellular virus. Virus suspension was also introduced into empty wells for determination of the decay of virus inoculum during the experiment. Samples were titrated by plaque assay on Vero cells and the results corrected to PFU per 10^5 cells.

RESULTS.

3.1. Cell Culture

The capacity for growth to confluency differed markedly in the 3 corneal cell types (Fig. 1). Under the conditions used, cultured corneal epithelium proliferated little and consequently required a low split ratio from primary to secondary cultures, even in the presence of

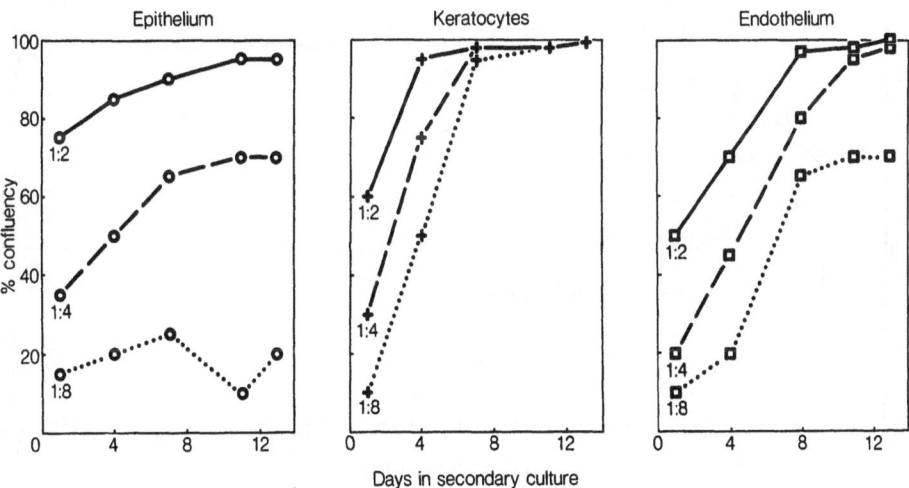

FIGURE 1. Growth to confluence in secondary cultures of corneal cells. 1:2, 4, 8 : split ratio. Data for 10% serum.

high serum concentrations. By contrast keratocytes proliferated rapidly and were capable of becoming confluent from sparse cultures or in low serum concentrations. Corneal endothelium required a split ratio of no more than 1:4 and serum concentrations of at least 10% to produce confluent secondary cultures.

3.2 Virology

HSV replicated in all 3 types of corneal cell culture (Fig. 2). However, it was reproducibly observed that there was a gradation in the amounts of total virus produced. Corneal epithelial cultures produced as much infectious virus as did Vero cells, on a per cell basis: the maximum levels being 1.4×10^6 and 1.6×10^6 per 10^5 cells, respectively. Approximately 1 log. less virus per 10^5 cells was detected in both keratocyte and skin fibroblast cultures. The amounts of HSV were further decreased by approximately 1 log. in the endothelial cultures. These differences between the cell types showed no apparent

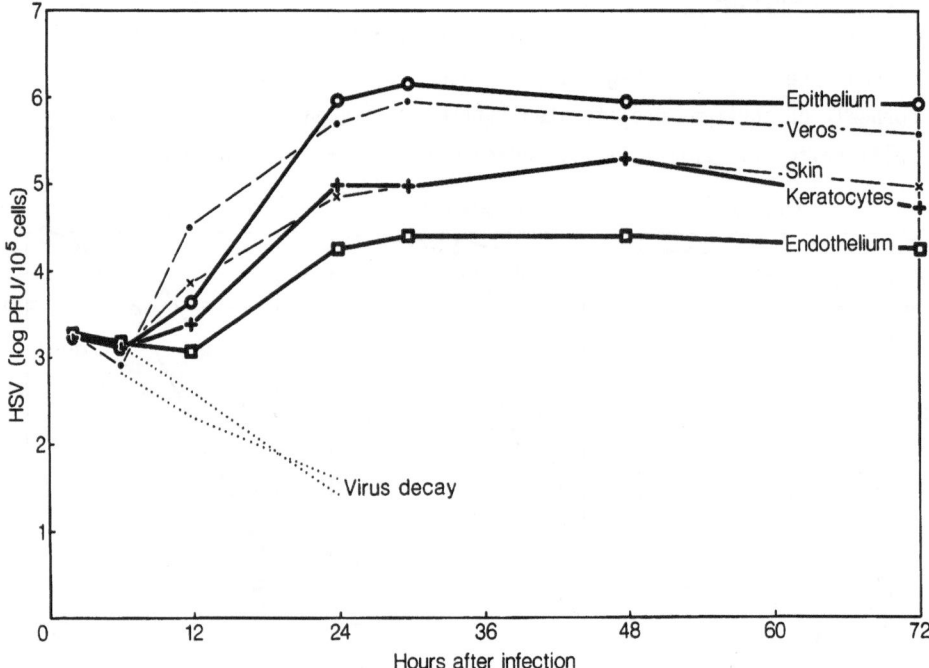

FIGURE 2. Growth of HSV in corneal in vitro: total virus (cell-associated and cell-free). Means of triplicate cultures.

relation to the minor differences in multiplicity of infection and cell density. The timecourses of infection following inoculation at low multiplicity appeared to be broadly similar in the various cell types. Virus levels reached their maximum at about 24 hours and then remained approximately constant until 72 hours. When cell-associated and cell-free virus were considered separately, the same gradation in amounts of virus produced by epithelial, keratocyte and endothelial cultures was observed. Up to 48 hours after infection, most of the virus was in the cell-associated fraction. By 72 hours the majority of the total virus detected was in the cell-free fraction. The proportion of total virus released into the medium was similar in all cell types, except endothelial cultures in which it tended to be relatively low.

4. DISCUSSION.

In this study confluent secondary cultures of rabbit corneal epithelium, keratocytes and endothelium have been obtained from small numbers of animals, using the same standard tissue culture conditions for all 3 cell types. Such cultures can be employed in further virological studies, and in a range of other investigations requiring a number of data points and replicates.

In vitro systems have the disadvantage that the environment and probably the physiology of the cells differ from those in vivo and these differences may affect the course of HSV infection. For this reason, the results of in vitro infection cannot be used to draw confident conclusions about in vivo pathogenesis. However, they do permit direct comparison of HSV infection in different cell types, and indicate definite possibilities for the behaviour of the cells in infection in vivo

The results of in vitro infection at low multiplicity suggest that differences in infectious virus production by corneal epithelial, stromal and endothelial cell populations should be anticipated in vivo. Such differences may contribute to the characteristics of disease in the 3 layers of the cornea. Further investigation is needed to determine the stage in the infection of individual cells at which the variations between the cell types occur.

It is interesting to note that cultured rabbit corneal epithelium has a high capacity for virus production, similar to that of Vero cells. This may be due to the higher susceptibility to infection of cultured corneal epithelium compared to keratocytes or endothelium which have similar susceptibilities (1). The similarity between virus production in keratocytes and in skin fibroblasts, which are similar morphologically, should also be remarked. The demonstration of the production and release of infectious HSV by cultured corneal endothelium is consistent with recent proposals that endotheliitis is a significant factor in ocular herpetic disease (7). If the low levels of virus produced and especially released by endothelial cultures reflect *in vivo* circumstances, they may help to explain the less than obvious nature of endothelial involvement.

REFERENCES

1. Oh, J.O. 1976. Type 1 and type 2 herpes simplex virus in corneal cell cultures. Surv. Ophthalmol. 21, 160-164
2. Sheppard, A.M., Smith, J.W. 1981. Antibody-mediated destruction of keratocytes infected with herpes simplex virus. Current Eye Res. 7, 397-402
3. Smith, J.W., Sheppard, A.M. 1982. Activity of rabbit monocytes, macrophages and neutrophils in antibody-dependent cellular cytotoxicity of herpes simplex virus infected corneal cells. Infect. Immun. 36, 685-690
4. Cooper, J.A.D., Daniels, C.A., Trofatter, K.F. 1978. The effect of prednisolone on antibody-dependent cell-mediated cytotoxicity and the growth of type 1 herpes simplex virus in human cells. Invest. Ophthalmol. Vis. Sci. 17, 381-385
5. Carter, C., Easty, D.L. (In press) Corneal cell culture. In 'External Eye Disease' ed. Easty, D.L., Smolin G., pub. Butterworths
6. Gipson, I.K. and Grill, S.M. 1982. A technique for obtaining sheets of intact rabbit corneal epithelium. Invest. Ophthal. Vis. Sci. 23, 269-273
7. Sundmacher, R. 1981. A clinico-virologic classification of herpetic anterior segment diseases with special reference to intraocular herpes. In 'Herpetic Eye Diseases' ed. Sundmacher, R., pub. Bergman-Verlag.

DISCUSSION :

G.O. Waring (Atlanta) : David, have you been able to isolate or identify, in your other work, viral genomes or viral particles in the endothelium ?

D.L. Easty (Bristol) : I don't think so, if you are referring to human cornea.

G.O. Waring (Atlanta) : Human organ culture.

D.L. Easty (Bristol) : We are referring to the corneal discs. We have not looked very hard. We have not come across it, put it that way.

G. Smolin (San Francisco) : Does the age of the cell line determine how fast a virus will grow in that cell line ?

C. Carter (Bristol) : We just use secondary cultures. So that is a possibility, sure.

J.O. Oh (San Francisco) : In vivo, the cornea temperature is lower than 36° or 37°C. Now, your experiments were done at 36° or 37° ?

C. Carter (Bristol) : Yes.

J.O. Oh (San Francisco) : Do you know what would happen if you studied it at 32°C which is the temperature of the cornea in vivo when the eye is open ?

C. Carter (Bristol) : No, I don't know. Didn't you look at 30°C ?

J.O. Oh (San Francisco) : Yes, that is why I am asking.

C. Carter (Bristol) : Did you find much difference, though, wasn't it at 40° that you saw a difference ?

J.O. Oh (San Francisco) : What we were looking for was the difference between type 1 and type 2 HSV. We could not find any difference whatsoever. I am just wondering if you can pick up any differences by varying the temperature.

C. Carter (Bristol) : That is one of the range of things that it would be nice to look at with this system.

C.S. Foster (Boston) : Recently at the ARVO meeting Doyle Stulting from Emory and his group reported on studies in some respect similar to these, using a variety of congenic mouse strains. They showed a marked difference in permissivity of the keratocytes in allowing replication of HSV. Did you look at this system or other strains of rabbits ?

C. Carter (Bristol) : No, we haven't. I think one would need
to use mice to get the differentiation between strains probably.

C. Claoué (Southampton) : Have you looked at virus replication
in keratocytes derived from the anterior stroma ? I think your
discs were derived from the posterior part.

C. Carter (Bristol) : No, we haven't compared the two. I used
the posterior part because I felt it was easier to make sure
you had no endothelium. You know, with the anterior part,
it would be more difficult to make sure that you have no epithelial cells contaminating the preparation. Do you think there
might be a difference ?

C. Claoué (Southampton) : I don't know, but the anterior stroma
is histologically distinct, and most scarring from herpetic epithelial disease is very superficial.

CYTOPATHOGENIC EFFECTS OF HERPES SIMPLEX VIRUS ON CORNEAL
EPITHELIUM.

P.C. MAUDGAL and L. MISSOTTEN

1. Corneal Replica technique

Histopathological and cytological changes in the experimental
herpes simplex virus (HSV-1) keratitis and dendritic corneal ulcers
in patients was studied by using the in vivo corneal replica technique[1-3]. To make a corneal replica a topical anesthetic is instilled thrice into the eye at five minutes intervals. The eyelids are
separated by an ocular speculum. Corneal surface is dried by
blowing air for about one minute. An airpump used in fish-tanks
is suitable for this purpose. Collodion solution in amyl acetate
(2.12 to 4%, depending upon the quality of collodion) is painted
on the cornea with a soft painter's brush. The painted solution on
the cornea is dried again for about two minutes. Amyl acetate
evaporates quickly and a thin membrane of collodion is formed on
the cornea. This membrane, which is a replica of the cornea, is
peeled off by using a fine curved foreceps. Diseased epithelium
cells are easily removed with the replica. It is mounted in 0.1%
albumin or gelatin with the epithelium side down. After drying,
the replica can be examined by phase contrast or oblique illumination microscopy. The replica can be dissolved in acetone to study
the attached epithelium cells after staining.

2. Cytology of experimental herpes simplex keratitis

We have previously reported on the cytology and re-

Maudgal, P.C. and Missotten, L., (eds.) Herpetic Eye Diseases.
© *1985, Dr W. Junk Publishers, Dordrecht/Boston/Lancaster. ISBN 978-94-010-8935-7*

plication stages of the herpes virus in experimental HSV-1 keratitis in rabbits[1,3-5]. In the replication cycle of the virus, the first cytological change is the enlargement of nucleolus which develops into the "A type" inclusion or "A body". In the "A bodies" "A granules" appear which are the replicating and maturing virus particles. The "A granules" are released by ballooning of nuclear membrane and extend in long chains of rounded inclusion bodies interconnected by thin filamentous structures. The thin filaments ultimately disappear to leave free rounded inclusions. The rounded inclusions show an internal ring structure and may be found in the cell or out of the cells. Sometimes rearrangement of "A granules" into rounded inclusion bodies occurs inside the nucleus. These are extruded out of the cell at a later stage. The rounded inclusions probably float freely in the tearfilm and thus help in the transport of the virus from its site of replication.

Replication of the virus is accompanied by an increase in the RNA content of the cytoplasm. C-mitotic lesions or colchicin-like effect produces multinucleate giant cells. Other cells may become rounded and swollen, and stain intensely with different histochemical stains. Their number gradually increases and some of them form variable sized syncytia by fusion. Thin pseudo-podia-like processes extend from syncytia to other cells. Rounded ghost cells, having an eosinophillic cytoplasm and a basphillic central mass, appear after two weeks of infection. Some cells are devoid of central basophillic mass. Their significance is not known. No inflammatory cells have been observed during these studies.

3. Dendritic corneal ulcers

Dendritic corneal ulcers and herpetic punctate keratitis show a typical histological picture by the replica technique[3,6,7]. Both types of lesions contain rounded epithelium cells which fuse to form different sized syncytia. Pseudopodia-like processes extend from the syncytia to peripheral cells, or between two punctate lesions. The peripheral cells that come in contact with the pseudopodia-like process become rounded, swollen and start fusing. In this way a dendritic figure develops.Partly fused cells are present at the border of syncytia, that are surrounded by a few rows of elongated cells forming an arcuate pattern. The elongated cells represent the areas of cell palisading observed by biomicroscopy. The partly fused cells and elongated cells contain intranuclear inclusions, "A granules", and rarely cytoplasmic inclusions. In a corneal replica from a dendritic ulcer, without associated epithelial or stromal edema, cytological lesions may be observed upto 4 mm away from the dendrite.

REFERENCES
1. MAUDGAL PC. 1976. The epithelial response in keratitis sicca and keratitis herpetica (an experimental and clinical study). Doctoral Thesis, University of Leuven. Doc. Ophthalmologica 45, 223-327, 1978.
2. MISSOTTEN L and MAUDGAL PC. 1977. The replica technique used to study superficial corneal epithelium in vivo. Amer J Ophthalmol 84, 104-111.
3. MAUDGAL PC. and MISSOTTEN L. 1980. Superficial keratitis Monographs in Ophthalmology I. The Hague, W. Junk bv Publishers.
4. MAUDGAL PC. and MISSOTTEN L. 1977. Development of disseminating inclusion bodies in primary experimental herpes simplex keratitis. Bull Soc belge Ophtalmol. 179, 25-36.

5. MAUDGAL PC. and MISSOTTEN L. 1979. Histopathology and histo-
   chemistry of the superficial corneal epithelium in experimental
   herpes simplex keratitis. Alb v Graefes Arch Exp Klin Ophthalmol. 209, 239–248.

6. MAUDGAL PC. and MISSOTTEN L. 1978. Histopathology of the
   human superficial herpes simplex keratitis. Brit J Ophthalmol. 62, 46–52.

7. MAUDGAL PC. and MISSOTTEN L. 1979. Histopathological study of the human herpes simplex dendritic and punctate keratitis by replica technique. Doc Ophthalmol Proc Series 20,
   211–219.

DISCUSSION :

D.L. Easty (Bristol) : What was your technique for getting these pictures ?

P.C. Maudgal (Leuven) : A few years ago, we developed the in vivo corneal replica technique for the histopathological study of superficial corneal lesions. The technique has been described in the poster. Since not many people had a chance to see the poster yet, I shall briefly describe the technique. Collodion in amyl acetate solution is prepared in a 2% to 4% concentration. Sometimes you don't get a transparent solution. It depends upon the quality of collodion. One needs a transparent solution. After topical anesthesia, the corneal surface is dried, we paint the solution and dry again. Amyl acetate evaporates quickly and collodion forms a membrane on the corneal surface. This membrane, which is the replica of the corneal surface, is peeled off. You can mount it on glass slides and examine by phase contrast or oblique illumination microscopy. Diseased cells are easily removed with the membrane. You can stain them to study the cytology or cytopathology.

D.L. Easty (Bristol) : So these photographs are by light microscopy.

P.C. Maudgal (Leuven) : Yes.

D.L. Easty (Bristol) : Can you use them with scanning E.M. for example ?

P.C. Maudgal (Leuven) : I tried it. The results were not that good. Collodion burns under the electron beam, especially at high magnification.

C. Carter (Bristol) : Around the periphery of the dendrite, are the epithelial cells flowing in, migrating in, towards the lesion ?

P.C. Maudgal (Leuven) : That is a good question. I thought they are compressed, they are certainly not migrating. These elongated cells around the lesion are probably pushed aside by the edematous, swollen, large cells in the ulcer. In the edematous cells you see syncytia formation. Clinically, if you detect such an arrangement of peripheral elongated cells around

a lesion, you can be sure it is herpes simplex infection. We
have examined a large number of other epithelium lesions, and
no where else we find such an arrangement of cells around
the ulcer.

D.L. Easty (Bristol) : Have you tried any study on animal corneas ?

P.C. Maudgal (Leuven) : Yes we did. It was done to investigate
the cytopathology and replication of the virus in vivo. You
can study the virus replication very well with this technique.

C.P. Herbort (Lausanne) : Did you study the toxicity of the solvent you use, amyl acetate ?

P.C. Maudgal (Leuven) : Yes, we did it to investigate any toxic
effects of the solution upon repeated application. We made
corneal replicas in rabbits, once a week, for 10 consecutive
weeks. Clinical and histological examination of these eyes
did not reveal any damage to the cornea. We have made corneal replicas in more than 200 patients. There have been
no complications. It is a very safe method.

C.P. Herbort (Lausanne) : Can you tell me what happens to Bowman's membrane ?

P.C. Maudgal (Leuven) : It is not damaged. I may add here
that if you make a replica of a dendritic ulcer, or any other
superficial localised epithelial lesion, it has an excellent therapeutic effect. The epithelium defect produced by the replica
heals in about 3 to 5 days.

SUPERIOR CERVICAL GANGLION IN EXPERIMENTAL
HERPES SIMPLEX VIRUS EYE DISEASE

Chandler R. Dawson, M.D., Wen-hua Zhang, M.D. and Odeon Briones, B.A.,
F.I. Proctor Foundation, University of California, San Francisco, San
Francisco, CA 94143, USA.*

The present animal models of recurrent herpes simplex virus (HSV)
eye infections include mechanical and electrical stimulation of the
trigeminal ganglia (TG) and treatment of the external eye with adrenergic drugs (1, 2). Because adrenergic drugs (epinephrine and 6-
hydroxydopamine or 6-OHDA) are so effective for inducing HSV shedding
in the eye, we are studying the role of the superior cervical ganglion
(SCG) in this process.

Our present experiments are based on the hypothesis that stimulation of HSV shedding in the eye by adrenergic drugs is due to stimulation of the SCG neurons at the pre-synaptic junction.

Effect of pre-treatment with 6-OHDA on HSV infection of TG and SCG

In previously uninfected New Zealand white rabbits, iontophoresis
was applied two days before and on the day of inoculation with McKrae
strain HSV. Treatment with 1% 6-OHDA was given to 11 rabbits and
saline to 12.

Immediately after the second iontophoresis, both eyes were
infected with McKrae strain HSV. Established HSV infection of the eye
was confirmed by culture for all animals on days 3 and 7 postinfection. On day 7 the animals were sacrificed and homogenates of TG

* Supported by EY.03917 and Cecilia Vaughan Fellowship.

Maudgal, P.C. and Missotten, L., (eds.) Herpetic Eye Diseases.
© *1985, Dr W. Junk Publishers, Dordrecht/Boston/Lancaster. ISBN 978-94-010-8935-7*

and SCG were tested separately for virus by reisolation in cell culture.

TG and SCG were infected with both treatments. It was apparent that 6-OHDA had no effect on the virus infection in TG but did appear to reduce significantly the total number of SCG infected. Among those ganglia infected, moreover, the 6-OHDA treatment reduced the titer of virus substantially in the SCG of treated animals, but not in TG.

This reduction of SCG infection following treatment of the external eye with 6-OHDA is in direct contrast to the work of Price, who found that systemic 6-OHDA potentiated acute HSV infection of SCG in mice who received intraocular HSV challenge (3). We propose, however, that 6-OHDA, when given by iontophoresis, has a destructive effect on nerve terminals in the eye; this effect of 6-OHDA has been noted by Traenzer and Thoenen (4) and by Flach et al. when topical epinephrine was administered to the eye (5). It is probable that the destruction of these nerve terminals prevented uptake of the virus from the infected external tissues or otherwise interfered with viral replication in the autonomic neurons (SCG) but not sensory neurons (TG).

Ocular shedding of HSV after surgical extirpation of SCG

To further elucidate the role of the SCG, we removed both SCG from young NZW rabbits and infected the eyes five days after surgery by topical application of 25 microliters of McKrae strain HSV. Control animals were sham operated but the ganglia were not removed.

From six to eight weeks after surgery and infection, the eyes were treated with 6-OHDA by iontophoresis and epinephrine drops (2).

Conjunctival swabs for virus isolations were taken before iontophoresis and for five days after the stimulation. The rate of HSV shedding was compared in the sham operated and ganglionectomized animals before and after adrenergic stimulation.

Virus was detected in eye swabs in both control and ganglion-ectomized animals. Shedding occurred from all the animals at least once.

The presence of virus after removal of SCG may have several causes, among which are :

- Persistent sympathetic fibers
- A direct effect of 6-OHDA and epinephrine on trigeminal axon terminals
- Local trauma from iontophoresis

The action of adrenergic mediators on stimulation of HSV shedding does not depend entirely on stimulation of the pre-synaptic neurons of the SCG but the possibility of non-SCG adrenergic neurons must also be considered (6). Because the receptor for the actions of these drugs is not known, our group is examining this problem in more detail.

References

1.   Green, M.T. et al.: Inf. & Immun. 34:69, 1981.

2.   Shimomura, Y. et al.: Invest. Ophthalmol. 24:1588, 1984.

3.   Price, R.W.: Science 205:518, 1979.

4.   Traenzer, J.P. and Thoenen, H.: Experienta 24:155-156, 1968.

5.   Flach, A.J. et al.: Experimental eye research 32:389, 1981.

6.   Palumbo, L.T.: Ann. Ophthalmol. 84:947, 1976.

DISCUSSION :

G. Smolin (San Francisco) : I have done some work with iontophoresis, and I know how much it destroys the corneal epithelium.
Using it causes very large erosions. Do you have any control
groups where you just had the iontophoresis without 6-hydroxy-
dopamine ?

C.R. Dawson (San Francisco) : Yes, we always have control groups.
With our earlier animals we did get corneal erosions with both
6-hydroxydopamine (6-HD) and with the normal saline used
in the iontophoresis apparatus. We are not now getting these
corneal erosions as we did before. The pH of the 6-HD is carefully adjusted to 6.5 and we limit the iontophoresis to three
to four minutes and are careful in the application of the corneal cup used with the apparatus.

D.L. Easty (Bristol) : Were there any correlates in your studies ?
I saw recently a patient who had carotid vascular surgery
and came with the first attack of herpetic ocular disease. Have
you seen anything like that which might correlate with the
laboratory models, such as the one you have described ?

C.R. Dawson (San Francisco) : We have not seen obvious correla-
tions with these laboratory models, for example people on topical epinepherine therapy with frequent recurrences. There
is always the possibility, however, that herpes simplex recurrences during emotional crises and other kinds of stress may
be mediated by release of epinepherine or other mediators.

RECURRENT AND NON-RECURRENT HSV-1 STRAINS: EFFECT OF TEMPERATURE

Ysolina Centifanto-Fitzgerald, Ph.D. (Louisiana State University Eye Center, New Orleans, Louisiana, U.S.A.)

1. INTRODUCTION

Infection of the rabbit cornea with HSV-1 results in ocular disease and the establishment of latency in the trigeminal ganglia. Work from our laboratory has shown that the type of disease, as well as the severity and duration, is a characteristic attributable to the infecting strain and is not dependent on the inoculum size (1-3). We have also demonstrated that the disease manifestations are determined by a specific region of the viral DNA, located within 0.70 to 0.83 map units of the HSV-1 DNA (4). That the inherent characteristics of the viral strain are a determinant in the outcome of the disease process was also clearly demonstrated. Based on the results of these studies, we focused our attention on the events in the trigeminal ganglia. We observed that ocular infections with different HSV strains lead to the establishment of latency with similar efficiency (80-90%), but patterns of shedding or recurrent disease were not the same. In a recent report, it was shown that in a single animal infected in each eye with a different virus, the pattern of shedding and recurrences for each eye was particular to the infecting strain (5).

In other words, it appears that whether or not the latent virus is reactivated to the infectious state, and thus the pattern of shedding or recurrent disease, may be characteristic of the virus strain itself, although host or external stimuli may influence the frequency of reactivation.

Maudgal, P.C. and Missotten, L., (eds.) Herpetic Eye Diseases.
© *1985, Dr W. Junk Publishers, Dordrecht/Boston/Lancaster. ISBN 978-94-010-8935-7*

28

thymidine (0.5 µCi/ml) was added. The plates were incubated
for an additional 4-6 hours, at which time they were fixed,
stained, and photographed.   The dried plates were then
placed in contact with X-ray film.   Incorporation of the
radiolabel was seen around the edges of plaques produced by
virus with thymidine kinase. No incorporation of label was
seen in plaques produced by TK⁻ viruses (6).

3. RESULTS

Initially we determined the optimal growth temperature
for the parent strain.   The virus grew well at 33°C; at
39°C, 48% of the plaques developed.

At 30 days postinfection, 50% of the rabbits infected
with this virus stock were dead.   Some of the remaining
rabbits were sacrificed and the virus recovered from the
explanted cornea.   Virus isolates were obtained from three
types of animals: rabbits with a low frequency of recurrent
episodes; rabbits with no recurrent episodes; and rabbits
with neither recurrences nor shedding.   All three kinds of
isolates were examined for optimal growth temperature,
correlated with the number of recurrent episodes (Table 1).

Table 1. HSV Isolates from rabbits infected with McKrae
strain HSV-1

Virus strain	No. plaques at 33°C	39°C	Recurrent episodes	TK Phenotype
M 4611	188	405	1	+
M 4606	350	328	dead	+
M 4591	129	259	3	+
M 4574	244	304	5	+
M 1711	95	152	0	+
M 1300	90	182	0	+

We interpret our results as follows. The McKrae strain
of HSV-1 has a high frequency of recurrences, as well as

To evaluate this possibility, we studied the McKrae strain of HSV-1, which is our prototype of recurrent disease. Infection of the rabbit eye with this strain results in severe ocular disease, 50% mortality, and the establishment of latency in the surviving animals.

Some McKrae-infected animals have recurrent episodes and some do not. We compared recurrent, non-recurrent, and the parent strain in terms of growth at 33°C and 39°C and thymidine kinase phenotype (6). Because these two factors appear to influence the ability of the virus to replicate in the ganglion, they may be related to the likelihood and frequency of shedding and recurrent disease (7-10).

2. PROCEDURE

2.1 Methods

2.1.1. Temperature studies. Confluent monolayer cultures of Vero cells were infected with the appropriate PFU of HSV-1 adsorbed at 37°C for 30 min. The excess unadsorbed virus was washed out and the plates incubated at 33° or 39°C. The plates were stained with crystal violet at the same time and the plaques were counted on an illuminator.

2.1.2. Animal studies. Rabbits were infected by the corneal route with 10^5 PFU of the McKrae strain. At 30 days postinfection, the mortality rate was recorded and the surviving rabbits were examined by slit lamp for recurrent episodes three times a week for 60 days. Swab cultures of the conjunctiva were taken and the recovered isolates were examined for optimal growth temperature, as described above.

2.1.3. Thymidine kinase phenotype. Confluent monolayers of Vero cells were infected with 100 PFU of the HSV isolates. The virus was adsorbed at 37°C for 30 minutes with gentle rocking of the plates to ensure even distribution of plaques. At the end of the adsorption period, maintenance medium (2% calf serum, glutamine, and antibiotics) was added at 48 hours, upon the appearance of discrete plaques. The medium was decanted and fresh medium containing [^{14}C]-

shedding episodes. It is a heterogeneous stock; the ganglia are colonized by any of the virions. Reactivation of the virus, as evidenced by either shedding or recurrent episodes, is frequent.

In some cases, the isolates obtained during the shedding period (latency) grew better at the reactivation temperature of the rabbit (39°C) than at the corneal temperature. There was also some suggestion that frequent recurrent episodes of disease could be correlated with the ability of the virus strain to grow at 33°C, but the number of isolates was small and a positive statement is not possible at this time.

In contrast, virus recovered from animals with neither recurrence nor shedding grew better at 39°C than at the corneal temperature (33°C).

We examined the optimal growth temperature of clinical isolates from patients with multiple or sporadic recurrent episodes of disease. We found that those strains isolated from patients with high frequency recurrence (several per year) showed an optimal growth temperature of 33°C (epithelial temperature), and those strains from patients with low frequency recurrence (one episode every two or three years) grew equally well at 33°C and 39°C.

These data suggest that the ability to grow at the host core temperature is a factor in the frequency of reactivation and shedding, while the ability to grow at the external temperature of 33°C is a factor in the development of clinical episodes of disease.

4. DISCUSSION

The ability to establish latency after primary infection is a well-established property of HSV. The latent period can be divided in three phases: the establishment of latency, which varies with the strain; the maintenance of latency; and the reactivation stage. It is known that in latently infected animals, as well as humans, virus shedding occurs in the absence of disease, and that the frequency of recurrent episodes varies among individuals. These observations then suggest that both phenomena may have different regulatory mechanisms. Reactivation at the ganglionic site may be related to the characteristics of the virus strain and that recurrent episodes of clinical disease may be partially determined by host factors.

We think that the optimal temperature of growth does have an effect on the frequency of lesions, and the ability of the virus to grow at 33°C may increase the number of disease episodes. We also believe that host factors, such as local and systemic immunity and interferon induction, may be important.

Our animal studies showed that viruses that cause no recurrences or apparent shedding grow better at 39°C and very poorly at 33°C. These findings are in agreement with the studies from clinical isolates.

It is not clear whether viruses with different optimal temperatures have the same reactivation rates as these studies deal only with isolates from the McKrae strain. Studies with other non-recurrent strains are now in progress.

ACKNOWLEDGEMENT

This work was supported in part by PHS grants EY02389 and EY02377 from the National Eye Institute, National Institutes of Health, Bethesda, Maryland.

REFERENCES

1. Wander AH, Centifanto YM, Kaufman HE. 1980. Strain specificity of clinical isolates of herpes simplex virus. Arch Ophthalmol 98, 1458-1461.
2. Centifanto-Fitzgerald YM, Fenger T, Kaufman HE. 1982. Virus proteins in herpetic keratitis. Exp Eye Res 35, 425-441.

3. Smeraglia R, Hochadel J, Varnell ED, Kaufman HE, Centifanto-Fitzgerald YM. 1982. The role of herpes simplex virus secreted glycoproteins in herpetic keratitis. J Exp Med 35, 443-459.

4. Centifanto-Fitzgerald YM, Yamaguchi T, Kaufman HE, Tognon M, Roizman B. 1982. Ocular disease pattern induced by herpes simplex virus is genetically determined by a specific region of viral DNA. J Exp Med 155, 475-489.

5. Gerdes JC, Smith DS. 1983. Recurrence phenotypes and establishment of latency following rabbit keratitis produced by multiple herpes simplex virus strains. J Gen Virol 64, 2441-2454.

6. Tenser RB, Jones JC, Ressel SJ, Fralish FA. 1983. Thymidine plaque autoradiography of thymidine kinase-positive and thymidine kinase-negative herpesviruses. J Clin Microbiol 17, 122-127.

7. Ben-Hur T, Hadar J, Shtram Y, Gilden DH, Becker Y. 1983. Neurovirulence of herpes simplex virus type 1 depends on age in mice and thymidine kinase expression. Arch Virol 78, 303-308.

8. Field HJ, Wildy P. 1978. The pathogenicity of thymidine kinase-deficient mutants of herpes simplex virus in mice. J Hygiene 81, 267-277.

9. Tenser RB, Dunstan ME. 1979. Herpes simplex virus thymidine kinase expression in infection of the trigeminal ganglion. Virology 99, 417-422.

10. Rubenstein R, Price RW. 1983. Replication of thymidine kinase deficient herpes simplex virus type 1 in neuronal cell culture: infection of the PC 12 cell. Arch Virol 78, 49-64.

HERPES SIMPLEX VIRUS CYCLE: MODEL OF MECHANISM OF ACUTE DISEASE,
LATENCY AND REACTIVATION

A. ROMANO, D. GAMUS

Maurice & Gabriela Goldschleger Eye Institute, Tel-Aviv University
Sackler School of Medicine, Chaim Sheba Medical Center, Tel Hashomer,
52621, Israel.

INTRODUCTION

The amazing secret of HSV survival for thousands of years and its
adjustment to human organism still remain a mystery, and probably are
due to the complex and almost perfect mechanism of latency and reactivations
of the disease.

During past years, a model of ganglionic latency was widely accepted.
According to it, after the primary disease (whether with clinical manifestations or not) HSV enters sensory nerve endings and propagetes through
axoplasma towards the corresponding ganglia[1]. Neuronal latency is
apparently established 2-3 weeks after the onset of primary disease, and
latent herpetic reservoir in the ganglia becomes the source of the recurrent infection.

Fig. No. 1

Therefore, we are discussing two phases of Herpetic disease: 1. internal
cycle in which the virus has no direct contact with immunologic defense
system, or external world, and can remain in latent state because of the
low metabolic rate in neurons, which are non-dividing cells. There is a
possibility that during recurrent local infection, viral spread to other
ganglia is limited by $INF^{(2)}$ and $I_gG^{(3)}$, which are among the principle
components of immune system that can reach CNS-through blood-brain-barrier.

Clinical appearance of reactivation occurs in target organ, where epithelial cells meet amyelinated nerve fibers of the affected ganglia. HSV
enters now its external cycle. In this part of virus life cycle reproductive
viral replication takes place, in close interaction with immunologic defence
system.

Manifestations of recurrent diseases is usually presented in mucocutaneous
organs - eyes, nose, mouth (HSV-1) genital and anal areas (HSV-2). Those
regions are very special in several aspects: they are invaginations of the
external world into internal mucosas, are hormone sensitive organs, get

Maudgal, P.C. and Missotten, L., (eds.) Herpetic Eye Diseases.
© *1985, Dr W. Junk Publishers, Dordrecht/Boston/Lancaster. ISBN 978-94-010-8935-7*

34

Fig No. 1

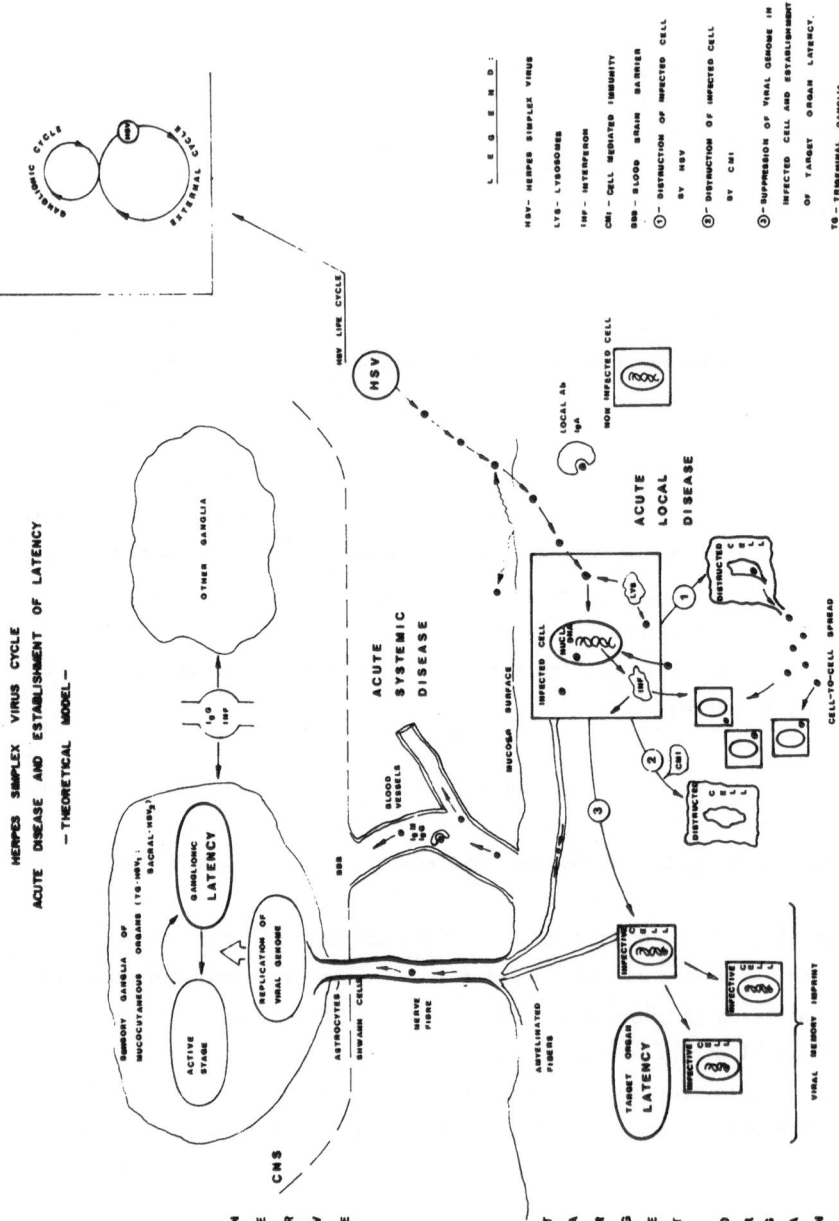

HERPES SIMPLEX VIRUS CYCLE
ACUTE DISEASE AND ESTABLISHMENT OF LATENCY
- THEORETICAL MODEL -

LEGEND:

HSV- HERPES SIMPLEX VIRUS
LYS- LYSOSOMES
INF- INTERFERON
CMI- CELL MEDIATED IMMUNITY
BBB- BLOOD BRAIN BARRIER
①- DESTRUCTION OF INFECTED CELL
       BY HSV
②- DESTRUCTION OF INFECTED CELL
       BY CMI
③- SUPPRESSION OF VIRAL GENOME IN
       INFECTED CELL AND ESTABLISHMENT
       OF TARGET ORGAN LATENCY.
TG- TRIGEMINAL GANGLIA.

rich blood supply (except for the cornea which is practically avascularized) and rich innervation by the somatic sensory nerves to mucosal surfaces: trigeminal (HSV-1) and Sacral (HSV-2) ganglia. (The other internal mucosas are supplied by autonomic nervous system). Both TG and Sacral ganglia are among the largest in the human body, and besides neural cell there are fibroblasts in TG ganglion, which can facilitate viral spread inside the ganglion.

Although other areas of skin and internal organs can be involved in acute herpetic disease, predisposing factors such as damage to mechanical barrier (Herpes gladiatorum, eczema herpeticum) or severe immunosuppression are usually present.

Upon its entry into mucosal surface, HSV meets mechanical and immunologic defence systems: local antibodies - secretory I_gA, I_gG CMI in addition to INF and lysosomal enzymes secretion. We think that there is a possibility that HSV is not completely eliminated from periferal tissues after recovery from acute disease, but stays in non-infective form as viral memory imprint in dose connection with host cell DNA. Cells that carry such an imprint (basal cells) can get a rise to a new generation of cells with new genetic composition.

Fig. No. 2

Under influence of certain triggers, that disturb this delicate balance, reactivation of the disease in ganglia or in target organ takes place. There is a wide variety of factors capable of affecting recurrence rate in human and can act both on neural and periferal tissues. The influence of these factors is through several levels: hormonal, cellular and viral activity level. The role of steroids on the course of the natural history of herpetic disease is well known[4]. A large group of systemic triggers known to induce recurrent disease can cause to an elevation of endogenous steroid hormones (whether directly or through hypothalamus - hypophisis axis), and steroid preparations given in certain diseases lead to a rise of exogenous steroids in the body.

Besides its collagenolytic activity, stabilization of lysosomes and immune suppression, steroids can change metabolic activity of the cell - by binding to specific cytosol receptor entering as a complex to the nucleus binding to chromatin to cause start of host cell DNA transcription (whether in ganglia or in the target organ). There are evidences that steroids have direct effect on HSV spread[5].

36

Fig. No. 2

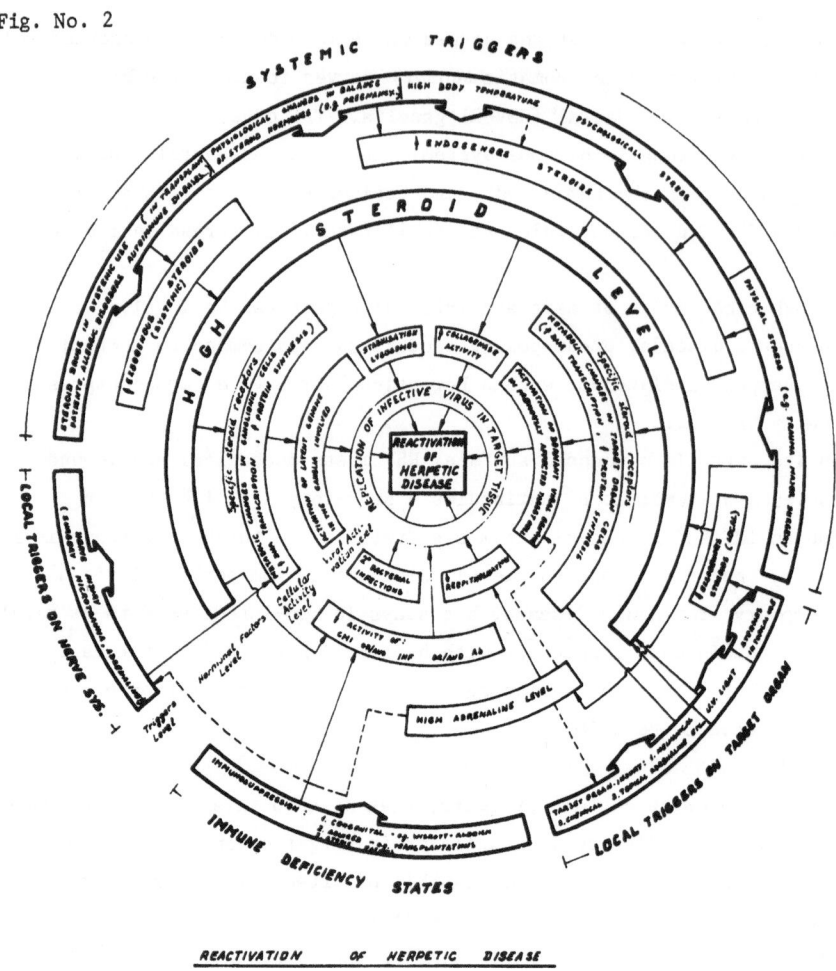

REACTIVATION OF HERPETIC DISEASE

Local triggers on nervous system (microtraumas and probably-adrenaline[6])
and local triggers on target organ probably cause to the same metabolic
cellular changes in neuronal and target tissues respectively.

If viral genome is incorporated or is in close contact with host cell
DNA (whether in the ganglia of in target organ), such metabolic changes
can cause to activation of viral genome.

Immune deficiency states are not triggers as such, but can aggravate the
damage when present.

REFERENCES

1. Barringer R. 1981. Latency in Neuronal Tissues of Herpes Simplex and in Varicella Zoster Virus: in Herpetic Eye Diseases. R. Sundmacher (ed.) J.F. Bergmann Verlag Munchen pp. 27-32.
2. Sokawa Y, Ando T, Shihara Y. 1980. Induction of 2'5' - Oligoadenylate Synthetase and Interferon in Mouse Trigeminal Ganglia. Infect. Immun. 28: 719-723.
3. Stevens JG, Cook ML. 1974. Maintenance of Latent Herpetic Infection: An Apparent Role for Anti-Viral I G. J. Immun. 113: 1685-1693.
4. Thygeson P. 1976. Historical Observations on Herpetic Keratitis. Surv. Ophthalmol. 21: 82-90.
5. Weistein BI, Schwartz J, Gordon GG, Dominiques MO, Varma S, Dunn MW, Southern L. 1982. Characterization of Glucocorticoid Receptor and the Direct Effect of Dexamethazone on Herpes Simplex Virus Infection of Rabbit Corneal Cells in Culture. Invest. Ophthalmol. Vis. Sci. 23: 651-659.
6. Flach AJ, Peterson S. 1979. Epinephrine Nerve Terminal Degeneration. ARVO Abstracts, p. 40.

SPREAD OF HERPES SIMPLEX VIRUS TO THE EYE FOLLOWING CUTANEOUS
INOCULATION IN THE SKIN OF THE SNOUT OF THE MOUSE

C. Shimeld[1], D.L. Easty[1], A.B. Tullo[1*], W.A. Blyth[2], T.J. Hill[2]
Department of Ophthalmology[1] and Microbiology[2], University of Bristol, U.K.

* Present address; Manchester Royal Eye Hospital

SUMMARY

Mice were inoculated in the skin of the snout with the virulent HSV1
strain SC16 or the avirulent strain KOS. Both viruses caused clinical
disease of the ocular surface and the deep tissue of the eye, virus was
shed in eye secretions and latent infection was established in all 3
parts of the trigeminal ganglion and the superior cervical ganglion.

INTRODUCTION

In man primary ocular infection with HSV is rare and it has been
argued from experimental studies in animals (1) that the virus might
establish latent infection in neurons serving the eye after cutaneous
infection around the mouth. We now show that in the mouse cutaneous
infection in the snout can spread to cause eye disease and latent
infection in neurons of the ophthalmic, maxillary and mandibular parts
of the trigeminal ganglion. With the relatively virulent strain HSV1
SC16 permanent ocular damage often resulted but with less virulent
strain KOS, the eye usually recovered.

MATERIALS AND METHODS

Virus

HSV1 strain SC16 (2) and the relatively avirulent HSV1 strain KOS
(kindly supplied by Prof. B. Roizman) were grown in Vero cells.

Animals

Mice were 8 week old male outbred Bristol /2 (3). Methods of
selection and anaesthesia have been described (4)

Inoculation of Mice

Mice were anaesthetised and the skin of the left tip of the snout
was shaved. Whilst viewing with a binocular dissecting microscope, 5µl.
of the virus suspension was placed onto the shaved area and using a 25
gauge needle 50 stabs were made in an area of 3 mm^2 into the skin
through the inoculum. The doses for strains SC16 and KOS were 1x10[5] pfu

Maudgal, P.C. and Missotten, L., (eds.) Herpetic Eye Diseases.
© *1985, Dr W. Junk Publishers, Dordrecht/Boston/Lancaster. ISBN 978-94-010-8935-7*

and 8×10^6 pfu respectively.

Isolation of virus from eyewashings

Has been described (5).

Examination of the eyes and skin of the snout

Both eyes of anaesthetised mice were examined daily using a Zeiss 10SL slit lamp microscope. Rose Bengal stain was used when appropriate to enhance any suspected epithelial deficits in the cornea. The skin of the snout, forehead, cheek and lower jaw of both sides of the head were also examined for signs of disease using the slit lamp microscope.

Detection of latent infection in the trigeminal ganglia and the superior cervical ganglion

Animals were killed by intra-peritoneal injection of sodium pentobarbitone and exsanguinated by evisceration. The left trigeminal ganglion (T.G.) was divided in situ into three parts, ophthalmic (I), maxillary (II) and mandibular (III) using separate sterile instruments for each part (4). The right T.G. was dissected out whole and the left superior cervical ganglion (S.C.G.) was removed.

Each sample of tissue was placed in 0.5 ml. G.M. and incubated for 5 days at $36^{\circ}C$ in 5% CO_2. Tissues were then ground in sterile glass grinders and 0.1 ml. of the suspension was placed onto monolayers of Vero cells for isolation of virus.

RESULTS

Eye Washings

Virus was isolated from the eyewashings of 11 of the 25 mice inoculated with strain SC16, from 6 of these animals virus was isolated on more than one occasion. Virus was first isolated 4 days after inoculation and the peak incidence of isolations was 8/25 (32%) on day 6 (Fig. 1). Virus was isolated from the eyewashings of 12 of the 25 mice inoculated with strain KOS, from 5 of these animals virus was isolated on more than one occasion. Virus was first isolated 3 days after inoculation and the peak incidence of isolation was 9/25 (36%) on day 5 (Fig. 1).

Eye Disease

In mice inoculated with strain SC16 signs of disease of the ocular surface namely corneal ulceration and/or lid margin disease were first observed 4 days after inoculation and reached a peak incidence of 56% on day 6 (Fig. 2). Signs of deeper eye disease namely iris hyperaemia and

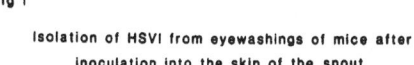

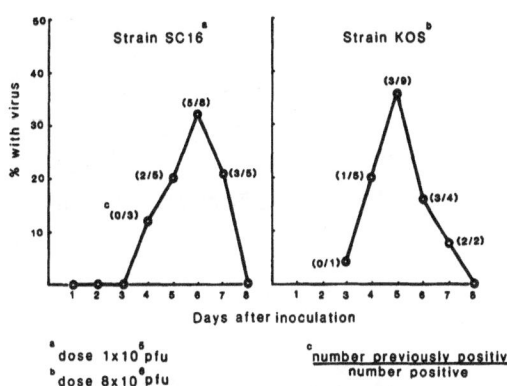

Fig 1

Isolation of HSVI from eyewashings of mice after inoculation into the skin of the snout

Days after inoculation

[a] dose 1x10[5] pfu
[b] dose 8x10[6] pfu
[c] number previously positive / number positive

Fig 2

Disease of the ocular surface and skin lesions in mice after inoculation with HSV1 into the skin of the snout

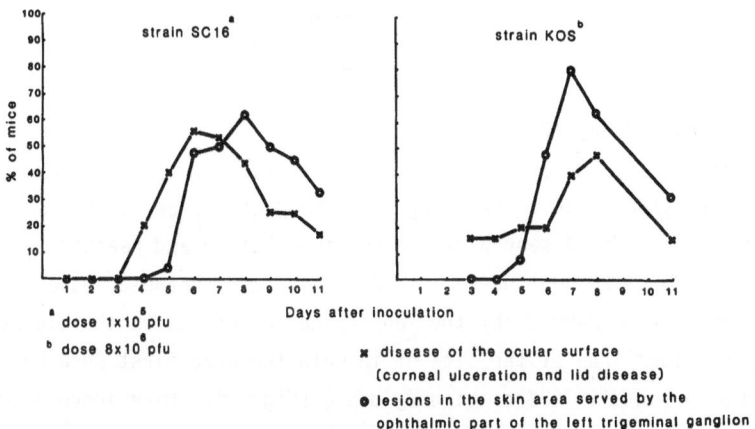

Days after inoculation

[a] dose 1x10[5] pfu
[b] dose 8x10[6] pfu

× disease of the ocular surface (corneal ulceration and lid disease)
● lesions in the skin area served by the ophthalmic part of the left trigeminal ganglion

mydriasis were first noted 5 days after inoculation, stromal opacity was first observed 6 days after inoculation and hypopyon on day 9. Stromal opacification and corneal vascularisation persisted in 40% and 29% of mice respectively until at least day 45 (Fig. 3). With strain KOS, disease of the ocular surface was seen on the first day of examination 3 days after inoculation, by day 7 48% of mice showed corneal ulceration and/or lid margin disease (Fig. 2). Other signs of eye disease occurred in very few animals (Fig. 3) and corneal vascularisation was present in

Fig 3

**Eye disease in mice after inoculation of HSV1
into the skin of the snout**

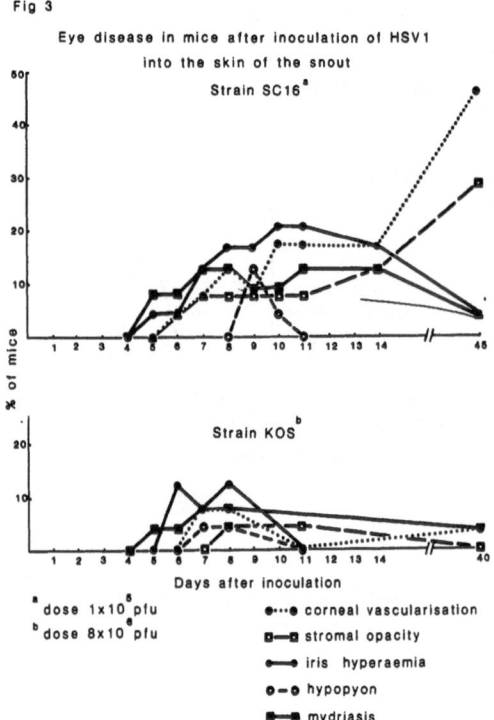

a dose 1×10^6 pfu
b dose 8×10^6 pfu

●···● corneal vascularisation
☐—☐ stromal opacity
●—● iris hyperaemia
○—○ hypopyon
■—■ mydriasis

only 1 mouse at day 40.

Skin disease

With strain SC16 swelling of the left side of the snout and forehead was first seen 3 days after inoculation and reached a maximum incidence of 32% on day 5. Pustules and scabbed lesions in the cutaneous area served by the sensory nerves of the ophthalmic part of the T.G. other than at the site of inoculation were first seen on day 5. These were found in 62% of mice by day 8 (Fig. 2). Mice inoculated with strain KOS first developed such swelling on day 3 and skin lesions on day 5, by day 7 80% of mice had skin lesions (Fig. 2).

Signs of eye disease and isolation of virus from eyewashings

Strain SC16

Virus was isolated from 5 mice on one occasion each. One of these eyes never showed signs of disease, 4 had transient corneal and/or lid margin ulceration lasting 1 or 2 days. Of the 6 mice whose eye washings

Table I

Incidence of latent infection in mice[a] after inoculation of HSV1 strain KOS or
SC16 into the skin of the snout.

Tissues tested

Strain of HSV1 Dose	LTG1[b]		LTG2		LTG3		LSCG[c]		RTG[d]	
SC16 1 x 10^5 p.f.u.	21/24[e]	(88)	8/24	(33)	5/24	(21)	8/24	(33)	5/24	(21)
KOS 8 x 10^6 p.f.u.	22/25	(88)	10/25	(40)	2/25	(8)	6/25	(24)	8/25	(32)

a   outbred 8 weeks old at the time of inoculation.

b   LTG1 ophthalmic part of left trigeminal ganglion,
LTG2 maxillary part, LTG3 mandibular part.

c   LSG   left superior cervical ganglion

d   RTG   right trigeminal ganglion

e   Virus isolated (%) / total tested

yielded virus on more than one occasion, 5 had severe disease with 2 or more of the following signs: corneal ulceration, stromal opacity, iris hyperaemia, mydriasis, lid disease and corneal vascularisation and all but one eye still showed corneal vascularisation on day 45. Of the 14 mice from whose eye washings virus was not isolated only 1 had signs of such severe disease, 5 had transient corneal ulceration lasting 1-2 days and 5 never had signs of eye disease.

Strain KOS

Of the 12 mice from whose eye washings virus was isolated, 2 eyes never showed signs of disease. The other 10 had lid ulceration which lasted for 1-16 days and 2 of these had corneal ulceration lasting 1 day only. Eleven of the 12 eyes were normal 40 days after inoculation and 1 had a small lid ulcer. Of the 13 mice from whose eye washings virus was not isolated, 8 never had signs of eye disease and 2 had lid disease lasting 5-7 days. One mouse had severe eye disease but the eye was normal at day 40, one mouse had a mydriasis at day 40 which was present from day 5 after inoculation and one mouse had corneal vascularisation at day 40, which was not present on day 11.

Latent infection

Forty five days after inoculation with strain SC16 and 40 days after inoculation with strain KOS the mice were killed and the tissues were examined for the presence of latent HSV infection (Table1). Latent infection was detected in part I of the left T.G. in the majority of mice (88%) inoculated with either strain of virus. Both strains were also detected in the non-ophthalmic parts of this ganglion, in the right T.G. (removed whole) and in the left S.C.G.

DISCUSSION

At present there is no mouse model of recurrent herpetic keratitis and the development of such a model would help investigation of mechanisms underlying control and recrudescence of the disease. Inoculation of HSV1 by scarification of the cornea or conjunctiva of mice results in a high proportion of animals with latent infection of the ophthalmic part of the ipsilateral trigeminal ganglion but with a relatively virulent strain such as SC16 the inoculated eye is often severely and irreversibly damaged during the acute disease (4,5). With a less virulent strain such as KOS permanent ocular damage can be avoided but in the skin of the mouse this strain (unlike SC16) has not so far produced recrudescent disease (3). Mice protected by previous HSV infection in the skin suffer relatively mild eye disease after corneal inoculation with strain SC16 but the incidence of latent infection is also decreased (4,5) so that the chance of recrudescent disease is again diminished.

The tip of the snout lies in the cutaneous field of the ophthalmic part of the trigeminal ganglion so that, with inoculation of this site zosteriform spread (3,6) might provide ocular infection without scarification of the cornea and with the possibility of avoiding permanent damage to the eye. The distribution and timing of development of lesions on the skin, the eye disease and the timing of isolation of virus from the eye washings suggests that such spread of infection does result from zosteriform spread of virus from the snout. The routes by which virus spreads from the site of inoculation have been discussed previously (6), the frequent latent infection of the superior cervical ganglion again shows that the virus can spread by sympathetic as well as sensory nerves.

With the doses of either strain of virus used here disease of the eye with shedding of virus from the ocular surfaces develops in about half the mice inoculated into the skin of the snout and there was a clear correlation between clinical signs of eye disease, isolation of virus from eye washings and length of time for which such isolation was made. With both viruses some eyes, after the acute infection, appeared normal by slit-lamp examination though the proportion was far greater with strain KOS. In both groups a high proportion of animals was latently infected in the ophthalmic part of the trigeminal ganglion with a lower incidence of such infection in the other 2 parts of this ganglion, the ipsilateral superior cervical ganglion and the contralateral trigeminal ganglion. Inoculation of mice in a non-ocular site to produce reversible herpetic eye disease and latent infection may thus prove useful in investigating recurrent ocular disease. It may also be valuable in testing the effects of therapy on HSV infection in the eye.

REFERENCES

1. Tullo, A.B., Easty, D.L., Hill, T.J. and Blyth, W.A. 1982
   Ocular herpes simplex and the establishment of latent infection.
   Trans. Ophthalmol. Soc. U.K. 102, 15-18

2. Hill, T.J., Field, H.J. and Blyth, W.A. 1975. Acute and recurrent
   infection with herpes simplex virus in the mouse: A model for
   studying latency and recurrent disease.
   J. gen. Virol. 28, 341-353

3. Blyth, W.A., Hill, T.J. and Harbour, D.A. In Press

4. Tullo, A.B., Shimeld, C., Blyth, W.A., Hill, T.J. and Easty, D.L.
   1982. Spread of virus and distribution of latent infection following ocular herpes simplex in the non-immune and immune mouse.
   J. gen. Virol. 63, 95-101

5. Tullo, A.B., Shimeld, C., Blyth, W.A., Hill, T.J. and Easty, D.L.
   1983. Ocular infection with herpes simplex virus in non-immune
   and immune mice.
   Arch. Ophthalmol. 101, 961-964

6. Hill, T.J. 1983. Herpes viruses in the central nervous system in
   'Viruses and Demyelinating Diseases' ed. C. Mims, Academic Press
   29-45

DISCUSSION :

C.S. Foster (Boston) : David, I think that others have shown that inoculation in the auricula, for example, can result in the establishment of ganglionic latency in the trigeminal ganglion. I think that a great many people have presumed that in human herpes keratitis, the primary site for virus entery is not the eye, but infact probably the respiratory, nasal or oral mucosa, and not the skin. I wonder what you have done, in your mouse model system, to eliminate the possibility that the virus found in the eye and the virus causing keratopathy was not infact transferred by the animals paw or surroundings on the cage directly from the site of inoculation from snout to the eye, and not from neuronal spread ?

D.L. Easty (Bristol) : Well, we have done work evaluating productive virus. And sequential studies at daily intervals following eye inoculation show that the productive virus can be found in the first division on approximately day 3 or day 4. Then by day 4 to 5 you can find it in brain stem. And then if you take the 2nd part or 3rd part you find it in that part at day 5, 6 or 7. So you can actually track it along these routes. You can also find it in the opposite trigeminal ganglion and the superior cervical ganglion. So I think when you follow productive virus in that way, it is evident that it is via the CNS rather than by auto-inoculation. Other studies by Hill and Blyth have shown that in their zosteriform spread experiments, if you cut nerves supplying other parts of the particular dermatome, prior to inoculation, virus does not spread to that part of the dermatome. So I think there is very solid evidence that indicates that you are looking at neuronal spread rather than surface spread.

C.S. Foster (Boston) : That was the reason of the question. I just wondred whether nerve transections have been done in your model yet.

D.L. Easty (Bristol) : We have not done that in our model. We have difficulty identifying where the nasociliary is. Perhaps we should look into that.

C.R. Dawson (San Francisco) : Did the other eye become infected ?

D.L. Easty (Bristol) : I am not sure if cultures were done. I don't think it was infected. We did not look very closely at that.

H.J. Field (Cambridge) : I would just like to comment in relation to a previous question : our own observations in a similar mouse model, in which virus was inoculated intranasally, are totally supportive of Professor Easty's analysis. Everything is consistent with the sequential spread of virus up through the maxillary and mandibular divisions of the fifth nerve, and then centrifugally via the ophthalmic division to the eye. Then one can see antigen in the ciliary nerves. The temporal appearence of virus antigen in our experience was thus consistent with the route of spread proposed by Professor Easty.

C.R. Dawson (San Francisco) : Have you considered that virus may be spread to other divisions of the trigeminal ganglion through connections in the mid-brain ? Your supposition has been that all the spread occurs by contiguous infection within the ganglion itself, not through the connections in the mid-brain.

D.L. Easty (Bristol) : If you take productive virus, which indeed we did, we cultured midbrains and found productive virus. Although we could not establish latency in the midbrain itself. So it only seems to pass through it, but it does not leave any messages behind.

LIGHT MICROSCOPIC EVALUATION OF RABBIT CORNEAL NERVES:
COMPARISON OF THE NORMAL WITH DENDRITIC HERPETIC KERATITIS.

PENNY A. ASBELL, MOUNT SINAI MEDICAL CENTER, NEW YORK, NY
ROGER W. BEUERMAN, LSU EYE CENTER, NEW ORLEANS, LA

1. INTRODUCTION

Although some researchers have noted degeneration and edema of corneal stromal nerves in HSV-1 keratitis, such changes have not been described in detail or quantified.[1,2] Work by Tullo et al. demonstrated a decrease in corneal sensitivity as well as levels of corneal substance P in a herpes simplex keratitis model in the mouse, using a radioimmuno assay for substance P.[3] Metcalf et al. used a histochemical method for acetylcholine esterase, but failed to show loss of nerves in the stroma although a significant decrease in corneal sensitivity was found.[4] These results suggest that changes in corneal sensitivity could be due to an altered function of corneal nerves, rather than to a decrease in corneal nerve density. However, recently Rozsa and Beuerman showed a parallel between corneal nerve density and psychophysical thresholds for corneal stimulation.[5]

We compared the organization of the corneal innervation at both the intraepithelial and stromal levels in normal rabbits and following the development of herpetic dendritic keratitis.

2. MATERIALS AND METHODS

2.1 Animals: New Zealand albino rabbits (1.5 - 2.0 kg).

2.2 Virus: RE strain of HSV-1 (kindly supplied by Dr. Centifanto-Fitzgerald) was used. Virus stock was grown on Vero cells, and the titre of each viral stock was determined on monolayer cultures. Innoculum size per eye was approximately 0.100 ml of 10^6 PFU/ml.

Partially funded by NEI # EYO4681 and # EYO1867 and by the National Society to Prevent Blindness # EYO9074.

Maudgal, P.C. and Missotten, L., (eds.) Herpetic Eye Diseases.
© *1985, Dr W. Junk Publishers, Dordrecht/Boston/Lancaster. ISBN 978-94-010-8935-7*

2.3 <u>Innoculation of rabbit cornea</u>: Innoculation was performed so as to minimize damage to the corneal epithelium and to the corneal nerves. Sterile paper strips (Schirmer tear test strips, Cooper Vision Pharmaceuticals, Inc, San Germain, PR) soaked in the viral suspension, was placed on the rabbit cornea after achieving anaesthesia with two drops of proparacaine 0.5% solution. The lids were then pulled closed and gently rubbed for 30 seconds, after which the Schirmer paper was removed. Control eyes were handled identically, except that the Schirmer paper was soaked in tissue culture media without virus.

2.4. <u>Nerve staining</u>. Rabbits were sacrificed by intravenous injection of sodium pentobarbitol. For orientation purposes, a small incision was made at the 12:00 o'clock position of the cornea at the limbus. Both corneas were incised and processed in parallel by a modified gold chloride technique. [5] Briefly, the tissue was immersed in 1.0% gold chloride solution for 12 to 15 minutes, followed by incubation in acidulated water for 14 to 15 hours, at which time the solution was replaced with 70% alcohol to stop further staining. The tissue was dissected into 4-6 lamellae in the frontal plane before dehydration and mounted flat on slides for observation and photography. Some specimens were not dissected, but were imbedded in paraffin and then used to make 15 μ cross-sections.

2.5 <u>Histology</u>: Selected rabbit corneas were also evaluated for routine histology by fixation of the tissue in normal buffered formalin and then 5 μ cross-sections were stained by hemotoxin and eosin.

2.6 <u>Procedure</u>: After viral corneal innoculation, rabbits were followed by slit lamp examination. Photographs, with and without fluorescein, and viral cultures were made at periodic intervals. At selected times, animals were sacrificed for histological evaluation.

3.0 RESULTS

3.1 <u>Normal innervation</u>: The cornea is innervated by 12 to 16 large nerves which enter in the mid-stroma at the limbus. Some 2 to 3mm within the cornea, these nerves contain both myelinated and unmyelinated axons. The deep stromal nerves cross towards the middle of the cornea, giving off collateral branches which in turn form the ramifying subepithelial plexus. At this level of organization, the nerves are preterminal. Terminals then extend upward into the epithelium from the plexus. These terminals appear to be unspecialized and continue forward as terminal leashes or can simply break into random nerve endings. Gold chloride impregnation of the nerves in the central cornea in normal rabbits demonstrated nerves within the stroma as well as the subepithelial plexus. Terminal endings within the epithelial cell layer were also evident in all cases.

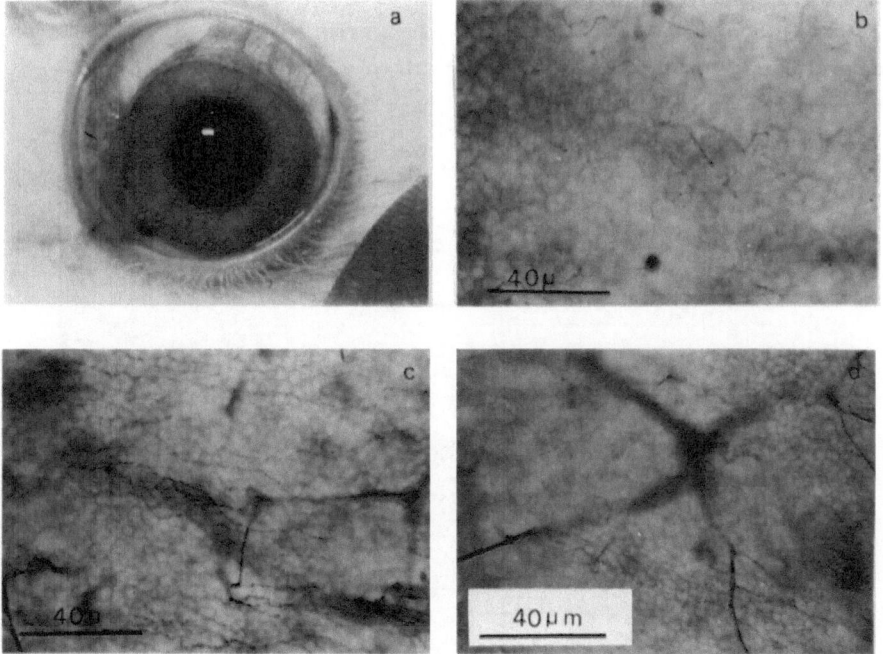

Figure 1. Normal, control cornea: (a) Limbal markings. Flat mounts (gold chloride): (b) Intraepithelial nerve endings; (c) Intraepithelial leashes; (d) Subepithelial plexus. Note that nerves are located at all layers.

52

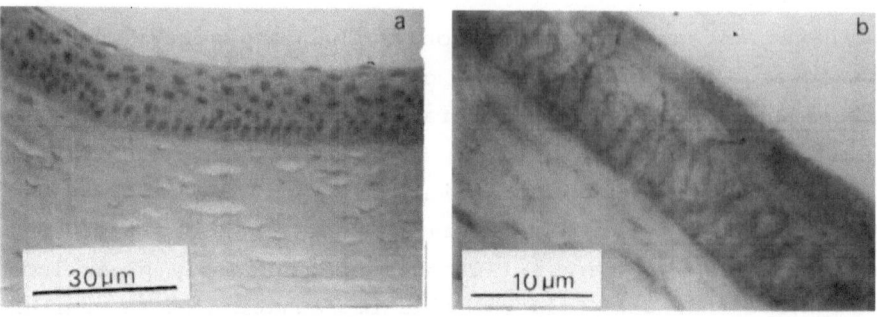

Figure 2. Normal, control cornea: (a) H & E; (b) gold chloride: abundant intraepithelial terminals noted.

3.2 <u>Herpetic dendritic keratitis</u>: Evaluation of corneas 3 to 5 days post innoculation showed striking differences, including a marked decrease in intraepithelial nerve endings. This was particularly observed around the dendritic lesions. There was no evidence of wound response in terms of leash formation. There was also marked plexus degeneration, particularly directly under the ulcer bed.

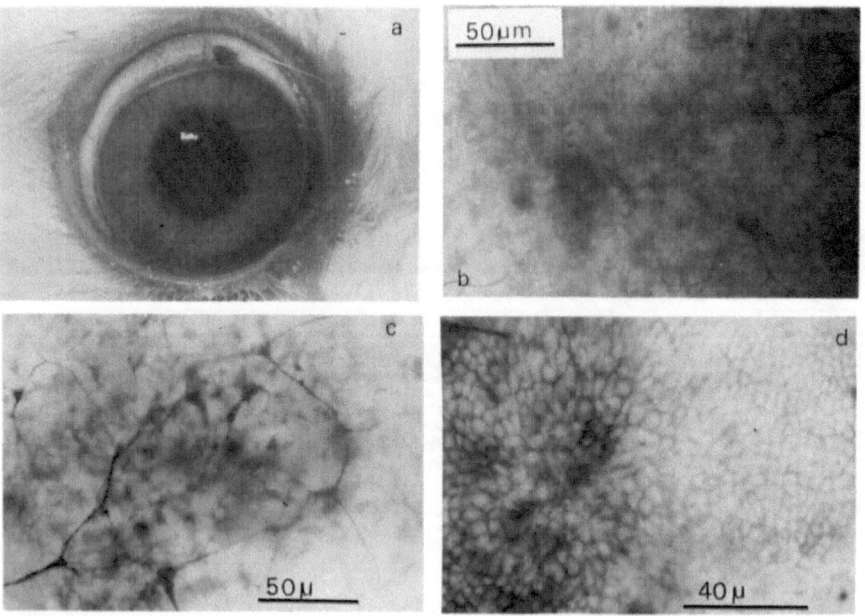

Figure 3. Dendritic Keratitis: (a) Clinical picture of dendritic keratitis, day 3 post-innoculation. Flat mounts (gold chloride): (b) Degeneration of epithelial terminals; (c) Degeneration of subepithelial plexus; (d) Weak wound response near dendritic ulcer.

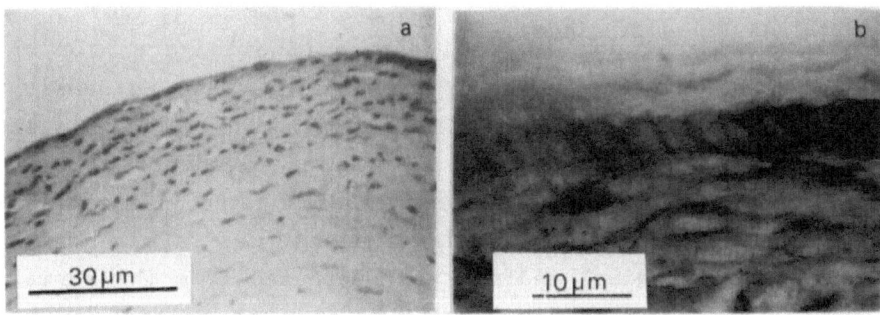

Figure 4. Dendritic keratitis, cross-sections: (a) H & E, showing thin and irregular epithelium, with a moderate mixed cellular inflammatory infiltrate; (b) gold chloride staining, showing sparse terminal endings in the epithelial layer.

4. DISCUSSION

Evaluation of corneal nerve alterations in the rabbit model of herpes simplex type 1 keratitis demonstrated marked peripheral alterations, as evaluated by gold chloride light microscopic evaluation. In dendritic keratitis there was a marked decrease in epithelial nerve endings in the involved cornea, as well as plexus degeneration directly under the ulceration, and deep nerve degeneration. Analysis of the cross-sections occasionally showed abnormalities of the corneal epithelial cells as well as loss of terminal endings in the epithelium. These results were paralleled by decreased corneal sensitivity.

These results suggest that herpes infection in the rabbit cornea leads to direct destruction of the corneal nerves in the involved part of the cornea. Other direct or indirect effects on corneal nerves may also play a role in herpes keratitis and contribute to a change in corneal sensitivity. These studies are in direct contrast to the findings of Metcalf, and may be related to the sampling error, innoculation technique (stromal injection), and/or staining methods.[4] The gold chloride staining clearly demonstrates marked abnormalities in corneal epithelial nerve endings as a result of herpes infection. The corneal nerve alterations noted after dendritic keratitis in the rabbit are in sharp contrast to the changes noted after

54

corneal wound healing.[6] Wounding by epithelial abrasion or superficial keratectomy leads to a marked increase in density of wound oriented terminals by day 3 after injury. Collateral sprouts from the subepithelial plexus were even noted by 24 hours after injury. In contrast, following herpetic infection of the cornea the neural sprouting response was rarely noted. The density of terminal endings was decreased from the normal values. Evaluation on day 3 and day 5 after initiation of keratitis, demonstrated little tendency towards a sprouting response in the herpes model. In addition, degeneration of the epithelial and subepithelial nerves was a notable finding in the herpes model.

Further studies of corneal nerve function in herpes keratitis are needed to evaulate the type of direct damage to the nerve and possible changes in nerve function.

ACKNOWLEDGEMENT: The authors are grateful to Tania Kaminar for her excellent technical assistance.

REFERENCES

1. Walter JR, Shapiro I, Whitehouse F: Pathology of experimental primary herpetic keratitis in rabbits. Am J Opthalmol 41:639-645, 1956.
2. Dawson DR, Togni B, Thygeson P: Herpes simplex virus particles in the nerves of rabbit corneas after epithelial innoculation. Nature 211:316-17, 1966.
3. Tullo AB, Kean P, Blyth WA, Hill TJ, and Easty DL: Corneal sensitivity and substance P in experimental herpes simplex keratitis in mice. Invest Ophthalmol & Vis Sci 24:596, 1983.
4. Metcalf JF: Corneal sensitivity and neuro-histochemical studies of experimental herpetic keratitis in the rabbit. Exp Eye Res 35:231, 1982.
5. Rozsa AJ, Beuerman RW: Density and organization of free nerve findings in the corneal epithelium of the rabbit. Pain 14:105, 1982.
6. Beuerman RW, Kupke K: Neural regeneration following experimental wounds of the cornea in the rabbit. In Hollyfield JG,ed. The Structure of the Eye, 319-330. Amsterdam, Elsevier, 1982.

DISCUSSION :

C.R. Dawson (San Francisco) : Did you examine the long ciliary
  nerves to look for damage at a distance from the cornea ? Is
  it your hypothesis that destruction of the neurons occurs or
  that only the terminal portions of the axons are damaged ?

P.A. Asbell (New York) : Basically, we looked at the cornea itself. We did not look at the nerves, which certainly would
  be of interest. But it appears that there is direct damage to
  peripheral nerves there. How far that damage goes in terms
  of retrograde degeneration, we don't know from this study.

P.C. Maudgal (Leuven) : This is a very interesting study. Could
  you tell us if this nerve damage influences the healing time
  of dendritic and geographic ulcers ?

P.A. Asbell (New York) : One of the current feelings is that the
  epithelial nerves of the cornea are instrumental in maintaining
  a normal epithelium. And if you destroy them, you have less
  normal epithelium and perhaps a longer time in recovery of the
  epithelium. We did not specifically go on to evaluate past day
  20 in this particular study. But we are pursuing that right
  now. I think one of the interesting things just to think about,
  although it is certainly not answered by this study, is whether
  there is a more marked decrease in those patients who have
  more intensive keratitis and those patients who go on to have
  more recurrences. Since we feel that the herpes virus enters
  the eye through the nerves, it presents a bit of a conundrum
  to understand how the virus gets in when in fact there may be
  fewer nerve endings in the eyes that have more clinical recurrent disease. And we have no answer to that. But it is an
  interesting thing to think about and to try to figure out what
  the etiology might be.

ISOLATION OF HERPES SIMPLEX VIRUS FROM CORNEAL DISCS OF PATIENTS WITH
CHRONIC STROMAL KERATITIS

A.B. Tullo, D.L. Easty, C. Shimeld, P.E. Stirling and J.M. Darville,
Departments of Ophthalmology and Microbiology, University of Bristol,
U.K.

1. INTRODUCTION

The dendritic ulcer results from replication of herpes simplex virus
(HSV) in corneal epithelial cells [1,2]. The pathogenesis of herpetic
stromal keratitis (HSK) is however less clear. How much this disease
process is due to viral replication, and how much due to the immune
response to viral antigen [3,4], or other factors such as nerve damage,
is not fully understood.

The removal of corneal discs at keratoplasty provides an opportunity
to attempt identification of the virus in a selected group of patients.
Although it has been possible to demonstrate the presence of virus in
such specimens by electron microscopy, and by immunofluorescence, the
isolation of virus from such specimens has proved difficult.
We have cultured several full thickness corneal discs from patients
with HSK, using a laboratory method normally used to demonstrate
latent infection in neuronal tissue [5].

2. MATERIAL AND METHODS

2.1. Tissue and Culture

Vero cells (African green monkey kidney) were grown continuously in
supplemented medium 199; for detection of virus cell monolayers were
grown in 20 mm square wells in plastic dishes [5].

2.2. Isolation of Virus

After removal corneal discs were placed in sterile balanced saline
solution and kept in a refridgerator at 4°C for up to 48 hours,
excluding the time taken to reach the laboratory, where they were
transferred to 3 mls of GM contining 5% FCS (patient 1) or 20% FCS
(patients 2-9).
The cornea of patient 1 was incubated for 5 days then ground in a

Maudgal, P.C. and Missotten, L., (eds.) Herpetic Eye Diseases.
© 1985, Dr W. Junk Publishers, Dordrecht/Boston/Lancaster. ISBN 978-94-010-8935-7

sterile glass grinder. Supernatant samples were taken at intervals (at least three times per week) from all other specimens until virus was isolated, or for up to 31 days. Several 50 μ samples of the ground specimen (patient 1) or supernatant samples were placed on Vero cell monolayers in multidishes. After incubation in a humidified CO_2 incubator at $35^{\circ}C$ for 48 hours the plates were fixed with ethanol and stained with Giemsa for identification of viral plaques.

2.3. Restriction Endonuclease Analysis
Isolates were analysed by the cleavage of ^{32}P labelled viral DNA with the restriction enzymes; BstI, PvuII and SstI[6].

2.4. Electron Microscopy
Tissues were fixed in 2.5% glutaraldehyde in 0.1 m cacodylate buffer, postfixed in 1% osmium tetroxide.

3. RESULTS

3.1. Virus Isolation
Virus was isolated from six of the nine corneal discs. Six of the patients were female and three were male. All patients except one (patient 2) had a dendritic ulcer at some stage prior to keratoplasty. HSV was cultured from a conjunctival swab of patient 2 taken at the time the patient presented with blepharoconjunctivitis. The period in culture till virus was first isolated ranged from 5 to 11 days.

3.2. Restriction Endonuclease Analysis
All isolates were shown to be HSV type 1, and were all distinguishable from each other.

3.3. Electron Microscopy
1 mm^3 pieces of all corneas which yielded virus were examined by EM. One piece was taken at random from the discs of patients 2 and 4; virus was found in both specimens. Two pieces separated from each other by several mms, were taken from the disc of patients 5 and 6. Virus was found in both specimens of patient 5, and one from patient 6. The number of fibroplastic cells in each specimen was of the order 30-50. Infected cells tended to occur in foci where virus was plentiful in most cells. Few extracellular particles were seen.

Margination of chromatin characteristic of infection with HSV was present. Cytoplasmic changes were also seen in cells which were not infected, however similar changes were observed in the cytoplasm of keratocytes from a normal cornea that was cultured for 5 days. In none of the specimens was the endothelium still present.

5. DISCUSSION

Despite the demonstration of viral antigen by immunofluorescence [4,8], and of virus particles by EM [4, 10, 11, 12], the isolation of virus in stromal keratitis has proved difficult in man [9, 10, 13], and animals [15]. The successful isolation of virus from the discs of 6 out of 9 patients with HSK, which have been previously reported [16], show how such diseased corneas will yield infectious virus when cultured in vitro.

The state and site of the infection with HSV are of considerable interest, and the results of this study permit speculation on three possible origins of the virus. Chronic stromal keratitis is typically preceeded by epithelial disease, as was the case in most of the patients. Once virus has penetrated the stroma, often facilitated by the inappropriate use of topical steroids [17], a chronic low grade infection may be established. The appearance of virus particles on EM has been interpreted as resulting from an abortive form of replication in degenerating keratocytes [8], which may explain the difficulties in isolating HSV. However evidence of active replication has also been reported [9], and on one occasion was found to be present in part of the stroma which had appeared normal on slit-lamp.examination [18]. There is also histological evidence of inflammation inferring an active process, in corneas which were clinically quiescent [13]. In vitro systems have been developed in which persistent infection with HSV can be masked by elevated temperature [19], or by cytosine arabinoside [20], and in which the presence of virus can be demonstrated only after considerably long periods by culture methods similar to that described here. Thus in vitro culture of the cornea may have merely removed the

DETAILS OF PATIENTS AND ISOLATION OF VIRUS

Patient (age in years)	Length of history (years)	Clinical details	Time from removal to culture (hours)	Time of sampling of cultures and isolation of virus (days in culture)
1. Male (46)	6	Dendritic ulcer treated with steroid - chronic ulcerative keratouveitis	48	⑤
2. Female (33)	7	Blepharoconjunctivitis - recurrent disciform keratitis	36	5, ⑥ ⑦
3. Male (56)	7	Dendritic ulcer - chronic stromal keratitis	20	3, 4, 6, 10, 11, 12, 13, 16
4. Female (57)	4	Dendritic ulcer treated with steroid - stromal keratitis - graft (1979) - graft failure - second graft (1982)	48	4, 5, ⑦ ⑧
5. Female (29)	11	Dendritic ulcer - disciform keratitis - vascularisation	20	5, 6, 7, 8, ⑨ ⑩
6. Female (35)	4	Keratouveitis dendritic ulcer - disciform keratitis	30	5, 6, 7, 8, 9, ⑩ ⑬
7. Female (60)	5	Dendritic ulcer treated with steroid - chronic ulcerative keratitis and marked thinning	14	5, 6, 7, 8, 11, 13, 15, 20, 22, 25, 27, 29, 31
8. Female (56)	43	Dendritic ulcer - disciform keratitis - recurrences - vascularised scarred cornea	18	4, 6, 8, 13, 18, 20, 22, 24
9. Male (55)	10	Dendritic ulcer - keratouveitis - scarred quiescent cornea with sectional vascularisation	48	3, 4, 5, 6, 7, 8, 9, ⑪

○ = virus isolated

restrictive influences of the immune system or antiviral drugs which
might mask infection without its eradication.

An alternative to low grade chronic infection,is that of true latent
infection. This is suggested by the delay of up to 11 days in the
isolation of virus. This delay may merely reflect the time taken for
virus particles to pass out through the lamellae of the cornea [9].
Nevertheless the nature of the keratocyte, which does not normally
undergo mitosis is such that viral DNA might become incorporated into
the cell. Lack of access to adequate numbers of specimens has
prohibited the necessary investigation of grinding discs immediately
after removal and placing samples of the resulting suspension onto
indicator cells.

The cornea is not the only site which challenges the apparent
prerogative of sensory neurones as a host cell for latent infection
with HSV. The virus has been isolated from clinically normal skin of
mice latently infected in the dorsal root ganglion supplying the area
[21], and from the footpad of mice [12]. HSV has also been isolated from
the skin of guinea-pigs in which latent infection of the ganglion could
not be demonstrated [23]. Recently the presence of HSV has been reported
in the posterior segment of the mouse eye after lengthy periods in
culture [24, 25].

A third possible source of infection is the influx of virus into the
cornea from the trigeminal ganglion which is generally considered to be
the source of virus resulting in recurrent epithelial disease [26]. Such
latent infection would be expected in patients with HSK, and a 'dribble'
of virus from the trigeminal ganglion into the cornea may explain the
chronic nature of the condition. The demonstration of virus particles
by EM failed corneal grafts [9, 12], and the isolation of virus from the
disc of one of our patients indicates that an extra-corneal source of
virus may be present.

An adequate supply of corneal specimens would allow the method of in
vitro culture to be further developed and compared with other
techniques such as immunofluorescence and DNA hybridisation. An
advantage offered by in vitro culture over other techniques is that
isolates become avialable for further study. It has been suggested
that some strains are more likely to result in stromal disease than
others [17]. It will now be possible to make in vivo and in vitro

62

comparisons of human isolates causing epithelial disease with those recovered from corneal discs.

ACKNOWLEDGEMENTS

The work was supported in part by the Wellcome Trust and South Western Regional Health Authority.

REFERENCES

1. V.R. Coleman, P. Thygeson, C.R. Dawson and E. Javetz. Isolation of virus from herpetic keratitis. Influence of Idoxuridine in isolation. Arch. Ophthalmol. 1969; 8: 22-24.
2. S. Kobayashi, K. Shogi and M. Ishizu. Electron microscopic demonstration of viral partlces in keratitis. Jap. J. Ophthalmol.1972; 16: 247-253.
3. H.E. Kaufman. Herpetic stromal disease. Am. J. Ophthalmol. 1974; 80: 1092-94.
4. T.H. Pettit, R.L. Meyers. Stromal herpes simplex keratitis. Trans. Pac. Coast Otoophthalmol. Soc. 1976; 57: 253-61.
5. T.J. Hill, H.J. Field and W.A. Blyth. Acute and recurrent infection; with herpes simplex virus: model for studying latency and recurrent disease. J. Gen. Virol. 1875; 28: 341-53.
6. J.M. Darville. A miniaturised and simplified technique for typing and subtyping herpes simplex virus. J. Clin. Pathol. 1983; 36: 929-34.
7. T.H. Pettit, S.J. Kimura and H. Peters. Fluorescent anitbody technique in diagnosis of herpes simplex. Arch. Ophthalmol. 1964; 72: 86-98.
8. R.H. Meyers-Elliott, T.H. Pettit and W.A. Maxwell. Viral antigens in the immune ring of herpes simplex stromal keratitis. Arch. Ophthalmol. 1980; 98: 987-904.
9. C.R. Dawson, B. Togni and T.E. Moore. Structural changes in chronic herpetic keratitis. Arch. Ophthalmol. 1968; 79: 740-7.
10. J.F. Metcalf and H.E. Kaufman. Herpetic stromal keratitis - evidence for cell-mediated immune pathogenesis. Am. J. Ophthalmol. 1976; 82: 827-34.
11. B.R. Jones, M.G. Falcon, H.P. Williams and D.J. Coster. Objectives in therapy of herpetic eye disease. Trans. Ophthalmol. Soc. U.K. 1977; 97: 305-13.
13. M.J. Hogan, S.J. Kimura and P. Thygeson. Pathology of hprpes simplex kerato-iritis. Am. J. Ophthalmol. 1964- 57: 551-564.
14. L. Hanna, E. Jawetz and V.R. Coleman. Studies on herpes simplex: VIII. The significance of isolating herpes simplex virus from the eye. Am. J. Ophthalmol. 1957; 43: 125-31.
15. K. Hayashi, and Y. Uchida. Studies on chronic herpetic keratitis - estimation of virus-harbouring ganglion cells. Graefes Archiv. Ophthalmol. 1981; 217: 257-71.
16. A.B. Tullo, D.L. Easty, C. Shimeld, P.E. Stirling and J.M. Darville. Isolation of herpes simplex virus from the corneal dises of patients with chronic stromal keratitis. Trans. Ophthalmol. Soc. U.K. 1984;10: (in press).

17. R. Robbins and M. Galin. A model for steroid effects in herpes keratitis. Arch. Ophthalmol. 1974; 93: 828-90.
18. C.R. Dawson and B. Togni. Herpes simplex eye infections: clinical manifestations, pathogenesis and management. Surv. Ophthalmol. 1976; 21: 121-35.
19. J.J. Kelleher, J. Varani and W.W. Nelson. Establishment of a non-productive herpes simplex infection in rabbit kidney cells. Infect. Immun. 1975; 12: 128-33.
20. F.J. O'Neill, R.J. Goldberg and F. Rapp. Herpes simplex virus latency in cultured human cells following treatment with cytosine arabinoside. J. Gen. Virol. 1972; 14: 189-97.
21. T.J. Hill, D.A. Harbour and W.A. Blyth. Isolation of herpes simplex virus from the skin of clinically normal mice during latent infection. J. Gen. Virol. 1980; 47: 205-7.
22. S.A. Al-Saadi, G.B. Clements and J.H. Subak-Sharpe. Viral genes modify herpes simplex virus latency both in mouse footpad and sensory ganglion. J. Gen. Virol. 1983; 64: 1175-79.
23. M. Scriba. Persistence of herpes simplex virus (HSV) infection in ganglia and peripheral tissues of the guinea-pig. Med. Microbiol. Immunol. 1981; 169: 91-6.
24. H. Openshaw. Latency of herpes simplex virus in ocular tissue of mice. Infect. Immun. 1983; 39: 960-62.

25. C. Shimeld, A.B. Tullo, T.J. Hill, W.A. Blyth and D.L. Easty. Spread of herpes simplex virus and distribution of latent infection after intra-ocular infection.
26. A. Nesburn, M. Cook and J.G. Stevens. Latent herpes simplex infection from trigeminal ganglia of rabbits with recurrent eye infections. Arch. Ophthalmol. 1972; 88: 412-7.
27. A.B. Tullo. Corneal grafting in Bristol 1970-1980. Bristol Medico-Chirurg. J. 1982; 1: 17-20.
28. A.H. Wander, Y.M. Centifanto and H.E. Kaufman. Strain specifity of clinical isolates of herpes simplex virus. Arch. Ophthalmol. 1979; 98: 1458-61.

DISCUSSION :

J.Mc Gill (Southampton) : It is a lovely work. Your rejected grafts had some virus particles in them. Do you think that viral invasion takes place in these grafts ?

A.B. Tullo (Bristol) : Yes; but this is not an original observation. Virus particles have been observed by electron microscopy in failed grafts. One does not always remove all the diseased tissue during keratoplasty, and as I emphasized there is a need for antiviral cover in the postoperative period.

J.McGill (Southampton) : Have you treated any rejected grafts with antivirals and reversed rejection ?

A.B. Tullo (Bristol) : I think if one sees a rejection episode in a patient with a diagnosis of herpetic keratitis, you have to treat it as you would any rejection episode; and obviously you have to be very mindful of the fact that the virus is playing a part. I don't think you have to assume it necessarily, because a lot of these corneas are grossly vascularised anyway. So they are entitled to reject for other reasons.

J.McGill (Southampton) : I have several patients who have shown rejection phenomenon and have kept the steroid levels at the same level, and given them systemic and topical antivirals, in this case acyclovir, and have been able to reverse the rejection signs.

Y. Centifanto (New Orleans) : I like this work very much, and I am very interested in the sequence of events here. First you obtain the corneas and put them into the medium. Then you sample the supernatant. When you see the cytopathic effects in these cultures, then you perform electron microscopy. You mentioned that you recover the virus at eight days, or between five and eleven days. This would be about the time you would expect to begin to see the virus if it were in the latent state. However, you didn't say whether this virus really was latent. Have you done a simple control, such as taking a piece of tissue initially to see if the virus is there or not ?

A.B. Tullo (Bristol) : I think that is the major criticism of the work. The reason why we have not done that is, firstly, that other people have shown that in a small proportion of such cases there is a virus there when it is first removed from the patient. But more importantly, we just haven't had access to a large enough number of specimens to do the study. But I think that is a very fair criticism. Another shortcoming that you pointed out is that it takes 48 hours to observe the indicator cells having cytopathic effects. One then fixes the specimen. So there is further 48 hours before electron microscopy is carried out. So there is delay.

Y. Centifanto (New Orleans) : Do you think the virus is in the latent state ?

A.B. Tullo (Bristol) : One of the differences between the electron microscopy findings in this study and previous ones, and particularly of Kaufman who showed that inflammatory cells tended to aggregate around the keratocytes in which there was a replication going on.

Y. Centifanto (New Orleans) : What did you see ?

A.B. Tullo (Bristol) : We did not see that. We tended to see the isolated cells of which I showed an example with virus particles in it. And no apparent inflammatory response around it. One interpretation of the appearance of replicating virus is that it is an event which occurs after the tissues have been removed from the patient.

Y. Centifanto (New Orleans) : I think this is very good work, and I also think that finding the answer to this problem is fundamental to understanding stromal disease from the virologist's point of view.

L. Missotten (Leuven) : You have shown us a slide with an infected keratocyte. Have you seen virus particles in the other layers of the cornea too ?

A.B. Tullo (Bristol) : No, I have been waiting to answer the question on endothelium. There is a lot of interest in this. I am sure it is very important. None of the specimens, at the time they were fixed for electron microscopy, had endothelium present. I would like to ask anybody else if you remove the disc at keratoplasty and fixed it for routine light microscopy, would you expect to see the endothelium there in such specimens ?

C.R. Dawson (San Francisco) : Certainly.

A.B. Tullo (Bristol) : You would ! So we lost it somewhere !

P.A. Asbell (New York) : Then you did not have the opportunity to look at any EM samples of the cornea just after material removal from the patient.

A.B. Tullo (Bristol) : No. I said if we had done that we would not have got the size of the patient group, which is still small. I think it is obviously a very important thing to do, and in a center where you have access to a large number of specimens, I think it should be done.

P.A. Asbell (New York) : Yes, but it seems a bit surprising since you have 5 samples labeled disciform edema and 4 of the 5 had positive cultures. In general, many feel that disciform edema may be related to an immunological mechanism, rather than to direct viral replication. I have analyzed EM samples of patients with disciform edema, where we did a very superficial corneal biopsy, and we noted no virus in the keratocytes.

A.B. Tullo (Bristol) : Is this during the active stage ?

P.A. Asbell (New York) : Yes. During the acute disease, most of these patients with disciform edema, in my experience, do not come to penetrating keratoplasty. So, I was wondering whether your samples are really typical of disciform edema.

A.B. Tullo (Bristol) : I think this is a very highly selected group of patients, isn't it ? I mean these patients are not a simple disciform keratitis because this is a condition that responds well to treatment, as you say. There are patients who have repeated episodes of disciform keratitis and they have vascularised corneas. So they select themselves. So, I think, we may be talking about slightly different group. But it is a very attractive hypothesis that relatively normal clear cornea can suddenly become opaque and edematous, as if by magic, where an exacerbation of disciform keratitis represents reactivation of the virus from the latent site in the cornea. But it is not yet proven.

C.R. Dawson (San Francisco) : Do you feel that you can tell whether or not there is virus in the stroma by the clinical appaerance of these corneas ?

A.B. Tullo (Bristol) : Well, I am beginning to get a bit of a feeling as to whether we are going to isolate something or not.

C.R. Dawson (San Francisco) : Could you tell us what clinical findings suggest viral infection of the stroma ?

A.B. Tullo (Bristol) : I think it is important to emphasize this selection, the autoselection of these patients, I mean, they should have a strong definitive clinical history; and we have looked at patients without the diagnosis and failed to get the virus out.

GENETIC INFLUENCE FROM CHROMOSOME 12 ON MURINE SUSCEPTIBILITY TO HERPES
SIMPLEX KERATITIS

C. STEPHEN FOSTER, M.D., RICHARD WETZIG, M.D., DAVID KNIPE, PH.D.,
AND MARK I. GREENE, M.D.

From the Hilles Immunology Laboratory, Massachusetts Eye and Ear
Infirmary (Drs. Foster, and Wetzig); the Deaprtments of Opthalmology
(Dr. Foster), Pathology (Dr. Greene); and Microbiology (Dr. Knipe).
Harvard Medical School.

ABSTRACT
    We studied, in a murine model of herpes simplex keratitis, the
influence of certain genes for controlling immunological responses on development of keratopathy after HSV corneal inoculation. We found, using
congenic strains of mice, that the Igh-1 gene locus exerts a powerful
influence on the clinical expression of HSV infection. Mice with Igh-1e
or Igh-1d phenotype routinely developed severe keratopathy after HSV
corneal inoculation, while those congenic strains with Igh-1a or Igh-1b
phenotype were less susceptible to such keratopathy development.
These results are discussed in the context of genetic influence on the
response to herpes simplex infection.

    Herpes simplex keratitis (HSK) is a major cause of corneal blindness
in the world today, in spite of the development, over the past two decades,
of very effective antiviral agents for treatment of an active episode
of dendritic keratitis. The incidence of recurrent HSK and of corneal
scarring secondary to such recurrent episodes has not diminished in the
past 20 years, and, indeed is apparently increasing. The available
evidence suggests that both viral factors and recipient immune host
factors, influence the clinical expression of herpes simplex virus (HSV)
infection. Clarification of the details of the role of the immune system
in the initial response to herpes simplex virus encounter, in the
establishment of ganglionic latency, and in the reactivation process
from latency to active viral replication has been extremely difficult.

    We have chosen to concentrate on an animal model of herpes simples
keratitis in an effort to define certain immunologic responses to HSV.
A variety of genetic events including immune response gene defects has
been implicated in reactivity to several viruses (1). Genetic analyses
of natural killer cell (NK) activity revealed the influence of non-H-2

background seen in murine eradication of HSV-infected targets (2).
The purpose of this report is to describe a genetic association with
the development of clinical lesions after HSV corneal inoculation.

MATERIALS AND METHODS

Mice. Inbred congenic murine strains were employed in these
studies. The background genetics and the H-2, Igh-1 and Igk phenotype
of each of these congenic strains are shown in Table I. Female mice,
6-8 weeks of age, from each of the strains studied, were randomized
into an incomplete block design for corneal inoculation of herpes
simplex virus or placebo control. Six mice from each strain were
employed for each experiment, and at least three replicates of each
experiment were performed.

Table I.   Congenic Murine Strain Genetics

Mouse Strain	Chromosome 17 H-2 Haplotype	Chromosome 12 Igh-1-allotype	Chromosome 6 Lyt 2 Genotype (Igh-V)
Balb/c	d	a	b
CAL-20	d	d	b
C58-AL20	d	d	a
A/J	a	e	b
ABY	b	e	b
AKR	k	d	a
B10	b	d	b
B10.A	a	b	b
B10.D2	d	b	b
C57BL6	b	b	b

Virus. Herpes simplex virus type-1, KOS strain, was grown on
Vero cell layers. An inoculum of 10^7 plaque forming units (PFU) was
employed for these studies.

Inoculation and Clinical Observations. The right cornea of each
mouse was scratched eight times, 4 vertical and 4 horizontal scratch
marks, with a 25 gauge needle under binocular microscopy observation.
Fifty microliters of a suspension of KOS herpes simplex virus type-1
at a concentration of 10^7 PFU/ml was inoculated into the cul-de-sac,
and the lids were compressed over the cornea for five seconds. Daily
masked biomicroscopic observations were performed, and clinical
parameters scored. HSV lid lesions, conjuctival inflammation, epithelial keratitis, stromal keratitis, and anterior chamber cellular
reaction were each graded on a scale of 0-4+. Representative members
of each study sample were randomly killed at various time points;

blood was harvested for herpes simplex antibody determinations and for mononuclear cell isolation, and eyes were harvested for histopathology and were fixed in Karnovsky's fixative, embedded in JB4 plastic, sectioned at 1 μm, and stained with alkali Giemsa or with hematoxylin and eosin. Tissue for immunologic studies was snap-frozen immediately after being obtained, embedded in Tissue Tek II OCT embedding compound (Lab Tex Products, Inc. Naperville, IL), and sectioned at 4 μm. Direct immuno-fluorescence staining was performed with fluorescein-conjugated rabbit antisera to mouse IgG, IgA, IgM, third component of mouse complement and antiserum directed against herpes simplex virus.

Antiherpes Antibody Determination. Serum was isolated from blood collected from the tail veins of mice at various time intervals. A modified, direct enzyme-linked immunosorbent assay was used to measure anti-HSV antibody titres.

In Vitro Lymphocyte Proliferation. In vitro proliferation in res-ponse to HSV was performed as described elsewhere (3). Briefly, 2 x 10^5 mononuclear cells prepared in single cell suspension from draining lymph nodes and suspended in 1.0 ml of RPMI-1640 tissue culture medium were placed in triplicate into wells of micro-culture tissue-culture plates. An additional 0.1 ml of medium, containing appropriate concen-trations of stimulatory mitogens or herpes simplex antigen was added to the appropriate wells. The plates were incubated in a humidified atmosphere of 5% CO_2 in water-jacketed incubator, and blastogenic transformation in response to mitogens and antigens was measured by examining the uptake by proliferating cells of tritiated thymidine 3H-TdR, 0.5 μCi/well, at 3 days for mitogens, and at 7 days for herpes antigen.

Delayed-Type Hypersensitivity (DTH) Responses. DTH responses to HSV-1 foot pad challenge was performed five days after priming. Foot-pad challenge was achieved by injection of 10^7 PFU HSV-1 into the left footpad. Twenty-four hours after challenge, footpad swelling was meas-ured with a Fowler micrometer (Schlesinger Tool, Broklyn, NY). The uninjected right footpad was also measured, and the difference in size was used as an index of DTH. All measurements were done in masked fashion with respect to experimental groups.

Statistical Analysis. Group means, standard errors, and standard errors of the means were calculated in the usual way, and statistical

70

Significance of differences between the means was assessed with Student's
t-test as the statistical instrument. The reported results for each
experiment represent reproducible findings from multuiple repeated experiments (at least 3 replicates of each experiment) employing at least 4
mice in each experimental group during each experimental run.

RESULTS

Lack of Influence of the Major histocompatibility locus on HSV.
Figure I shows the major differences in clinical disease pattern
development between the various murine strains studied, C57 black mice
(H-2b, Igh-1b), both with the B10 background and with the B6 background,
were relatively protected from development of severe keratitis after
HSV corneal inoculation. A/J mice (H-2a, Igh-1e), on the other hand,
routinely developed severe
keratopathy after similar
inoculation. Balb/c mice
(H-2d, Igh-1a) regularly
exhibited a pattern of
initial resolution of
keratitis with subsequent
relapse and development of
keratopathy. ABY (H-2b, Igh-
1e), and AKR (H-2k, Igh-1d)

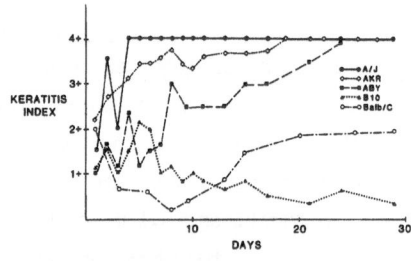

(Figure 1)

mice developed rapid onset and persistance of severe keatopathy. It is
apparent that the major histocompariibility phenotype does not discern-
ably influence susceptibility to HSV-induced keratopathy. C57 B10, and
C57B6 mice are resistant, Balb/C mice are relatively resistant, and A/J,
ABY and AKR mice are susceptible to severe HSV-induced keropathy. To
further evaluate the influence of the H-2 histocompatibility locus on
development of keratopathy, we compared B10 congenics differing only at
H-2 (Figure 2.) There was no
apparent disease difference
among B10 (H-2b), B10.A (H-2a
or B10.D2 (H-2d) congenics.

(Figure 2)

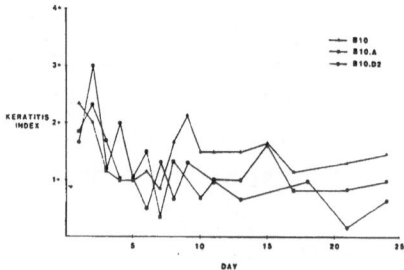

Influence of Igh-1-linked Genes on HSV Keratopathy. In contrast to the above results, the use of Igh-1 allotype congenics showed distinct clinical disease pattern differences. CAL-20 (Igh-1d) had similar disease to A/J (Igh-1e) but dissimilar to Balb/c (Igh-1a) (Figure 3). Further, the availability of new inbred congenic murine strains which have the kappa gene of C58 mice on the C.AL-20 background enabled us to determine that the Igk locus has no apparent significant influence on disease suseptibility. CAL-20 and C58-AL-20 mice are genetically different at the Igk locus, but develop similar degrees of ocular destruction after HSV inoculation into the cornea

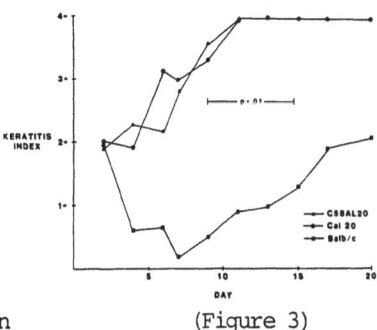

(Figure 3)

Figures 4a & b are representative clinical lesions in resistant (Balb/c Figure,4a)and in susceptible (C.AL-20, Figure 4b)mice. The extensive destruction of the eye (4+ keratopathy)in the C.AL-20 mice is in sharp contrast to the minimal damage in the Balb/c cornea.

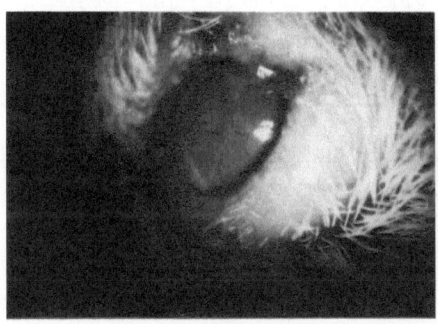
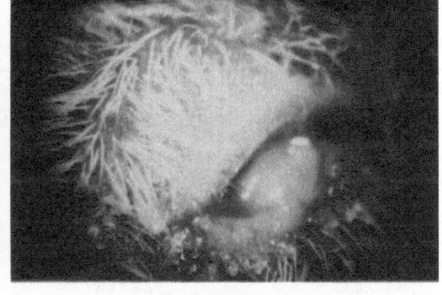

(Figure 4a)   (Figure 4b)

Antibody Responses to HSV. Antiherpes serum antibody levels after HSV corneal inoculation are not significantly different between murine strains, irrespective of H-2 and Igh-1 types regardless of the corneal pathology that develops (Table II). Total HSV-specific immunoglobulin responses after corneal inoculation with HSV are similar in all strains.

Table II.   Anti-herpes Antibody Titers 5 Weeks after Corneal
Inoculation with HSV

Murine Strain	Inoculation Route	Antibody Titer
A/J	Intraperitoneal +	1:128
A/J	Corneal *	1: 64
AB.y	Intraperitoneal	1:256
AB.y	Corneal	1: 64
B10	Intraperitoneal	1:256
B10	Corneal	1: 64
B10.D2	Intraperitoneal	1:256
B10.D2	Corneal	1:256
Balb/c	Intraperitoneal	1:256
Balb/c	Corneal	1:128
Cal 20	Intraperitoneal	1: 64
Cal 20	Corneal	1: 32

Specific anti-HSV antibody titers in serum of mice inoculated
introcorneally (5 x 10^4 PFU) * or intraperitoneally (10^7PFU) +.
Although the CAL20 mice did not develop as good an antibody response
as the Balb/c mice, the data overlap makes the differences statistically insignificant. Antibody determinations prior to 4 weeks post
inoculation were unreliable due to the nearly undetectable amounts
present in serum at this early time.

T Cell Responses to HSV. HSV-specific lymphocyte proliferation
studies indicated that there is a more vigorous, and more rapid development of a T cell dependent response in the murine strains that
resist severe keratopathy after HSV corneal innoculation (Table III).

Table III.   In Vitro Lymphocyte Proliferation Responses to HSV
5 Days After Corneal Priming with HSV.

Murine Strain	CPM	S.I. *
A/J	12933	24
B10	29002	266
Balb/c	24314	121
CAL20	12748	38

$$*S.I.:\ \text{Stimulation Index} = \frac{\text{CPM (counts per minute) with HSV antigen}}{\text{CPM Control}}$$

Control CPM varied from 109 to 537.

Delayed type hypersensitivity in vivo (DTH) responses to HSV corneal
inoculation (Figure 5) were impaired in mice with the Igh-le or
Igh-ld genotype as compared to other congenics.

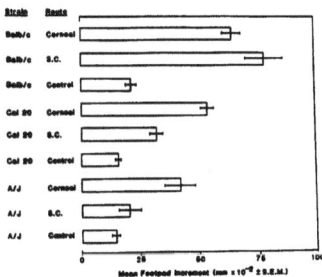

(Figure 5)

Immunofluroescence and Histopathology. The Immunofluorescence and histopathology patterns which develop in corneas from the various murine strains are dramatically different between "susceptible" and "resistent" strains. The initial (up to 2 days after HSV corneal inoculation) response in all strains is characterized by complement deposition (C3) in the superficial corneal stroma and by a neutrophil and lymphocyte peripheral corneal stromal infiltrate; A/J mice, however, subsequently fail to develop a prominent mononuclear response in the cornea. Instead, neutrophils continue to constitute the major cell type migrating into A/J corneas. Immunofluorescence studies show that, compared to the patterns in B10 mice, excessive IgG, IgM, IgA, and C3 commonly accumulate in the corneal stroma of A/J mice and herpes persistence in the epithelium past day 16 after inoculation is common. B10 mice, on the other hand, rapidly develop a prominent mononuclear cell response in the HSV inoculated cornea, with few neutrophils seen by day 5 after inoculation. Macrophages and lymphocytes are the predominent cells. By immunofluorescence and by HSV culture we find B10 mice to harbor few HSV particles after day 7 post inoculation; this is in distinct contrast to A/J mice which frequently continue to have HSV in the cornea 16 - 20 days after inoculation. Balb/c mice, which tend to exhibit clinical keratitis severity intermediate to that of A/J and B10 mice, usually develop a mixed mononuclear cell/neutrophil corneal response; these animals usually show no virus in the cornea past day 7. Exceptions to the typical responses are occasionally seen, in that rarely a B10 mouse will develop clinically severe keratitis. Histopathology of these corneas always shows intense neutrophil infiltration of the corneal stroma, and immunofluorescence always demonstrates extreme amounts of IgG, IgM, and C3 in these corneas. HSV persistence is also occasionally demonstrable.

DISCUSSION

These studies indicate a dominant genetic influence on the clinical response to HSV infection. This genetic effect is imported by Igh-1 linked genes on chromosome 12 of the mouse. These Igh-1 associated clinical responses are mediated by as yet incompletely defined immune responses to limit HSV mediated keratitis. We have no evidence to indicate antibody mediated effects on HSV as explaining these data. We have considered that HSV-induced T cell dependent processes may be contributary.

The work of Lopez et al. has shown that there are major differences in murine susceptibility to the lethal effect of intraperitoneally inoculated herpes simplex Type 1-1 (2). This genetically governed "natural" resistance seems to be mediated by a bone-marrow-dependent cell (apparently a natural killer (NK) or NK-like cell) which rapidly clears the virus, thereby preventing viral dissemination (4). The natural immunity governing such resistance or susceptibility appears to be controlled by two major, independently segregating, non-H2 genetic loci (5). Kirschner et al. (6) have shown that this early "natural" murine resistance or susceptibility to HSV is correlated with the capacity of the specific murine strain's spleen cells to produce interferon, with spleen cells from resistant strains (e.g., B10 or B6) producing much greater amounts of interferon than those from susceptible strains (e.g., A/J or AKR). We believe that the work from our laboratory, reported above, further suggests that, in addition to these differences in natural immunity, major differences exist in the development of an acquired immune response to HSV inoculation.

REFERENCES

1. Lefvin NL, Kauffman RF, and Finberg R. T lymphocyte immunity to reovirus: cellular requirments for generation and role in clearance of primary infections. J Immunol. 127:2334, 1981.
2. Lopez C. Genetics of natural resistance to herpes virus infections in mice. Nature. 258:152, 1975.
3. Rosenberg GL, Farber PA, Notkins AL. In vitro stimulation of sensitized lymphocytes by herpes simplex virus and vaccinia virus.
4. Lopez C, Ryshke R, Bennett M. Marrow dependent cells depleted by 89Sr mediate genetic resistance to herpes simplex virus type-1 infections in mice. Infec and Immun. 28:1028, 1980.
5. Lopez C. Resistance to HSV-1 in the mouse is governed by two major, independently segregating, non-H-2 loci. Immunogenics. 11:87, 1980.

6. Kirschner H, Engler H, Zawatzky R, Schroder CH. Studies of resistance of mice against herpes simplex virus. In: Genetic Control of Natural Resistance to Infection and Malignancy (Eds. Skamene, E, et al.). Academic Press, New York, p. 267, 1980.

DISCUSSION :

H.J. Field (Cambridge) : Is it not the case that the C57-black mouse is resistant to virus infections by many other routes of inoculation ? That is to say this phenomenon may not be specific to the eye.

C.S. Foster (Boston) : It is not a virus specific to the eye. Others, including most notably Carlos Lopez, have looked at the so called natural immune phenomenon, particularly with respect to the natural killer cell activity, and have summarily shown that the black strains of mice resist death from encephalitis after intraperitoneal inoculation compared, for example, to AJ mice. I think that is an important question you ask. An important distinction between their work and ours is that they have shown, and others have confirmed, that there is a pronounced difference in K activity and immediate resistance to the virus. We think that our work suggests that there is also a difference in the acquired immune system.

P.A. Asbell (New York) : It would help elucidate the difference between the role of host genetics and viral genetics. Have you looked at other viral strains, keeping the host genetics the same ?

C.S. Foster (Boston) : Herb and Ysolina sent us a variety of virus isolates which we are very grateful for, and have now a huge stock of viral isolates stored away. The first thing we did when we started this work was to look into mouse system, at keratopathy that resulted from corneal inoculation with a panel of seven different viruses. And in essence, we confirm their observations of striking differences depending on the isolate. We have not gone to the point yet, where we will try to dissect out establishment of latency, reactivation and the role that the relationship between the host reponses and the virus isolate plays. It is ten years worth of work.

D.L. Easty (Bristol) : Have you done any work on the permissiveness of corneal cells in these mice. Are there strain differences ?

C.S. Foster (Boston) : We haven't. But as I mentioned in this
morning session, Doyale Stulting and his colleagues at Emory
have done that, and reported their results at the ARVO meeting
at Sarasota two weeks ago. They showed differences in permissivity in keratocytes from different inbread congenic mouse
strains. It was interesting work. I asked the question about
the AJ mice, for example, which classically develops very severe ocular pathology. And they haven't looked at AJ keratocytes.

SYSTEMIC IMMUNE RESPONSES AFTER OCULAR ANTIGENIC ENCOUNTER

C. STEPHEN FOSTER

Harvard Medical School and the Hilles Immunology Laboratory of
The Massachusetts Eye and Ear Infirmary

INTRODUCTION

The eye has been considered an immunologically "privileged" site
for over three decades. Corneal and anterior chamber (AC) immunologic
privilege concepts are particularly well entrenched in traditional
teaching, since the pioneering work of Medawar (1) and of Woodruff
(2) demonstrated prolonged survival of allogenic transplants in
these sites. In order to explain this relative unresponsiveness to
antigen in these ocular sites, the notion of afferent arc blockade
developed, and many scientists accepted this concept of antigen
"invisibility" from the recipient immune system. Indeed, this concept
has been employed as the explanation for the relatively low incidence
of corneal allograft rejections.

Clinical experience with human ocular disease and with corneal
transplantation quickly calls into question this idea of afferent arc
blockade in the cornea and in the AC. Corneal allograft rejection
reactions occur in approximately 30% of human keratoplasties, even in
the very best prognosis cases with completely avascular corneas and no
inflammation prior to grafting and in the period after postoperative
inflammation resolution. More important, treatment of such rejection
reactions with topical corticosteroids results in successful resolutions
of the allograft rejection episode in 80-90% of these cases. Furthermore, patients who have experienced such a corneal allograft reaction
with successful reversal typically enjoy graft tolerance without
further episodes of rejection indefinitely, even in the absence of
steroid or other drug therapy. Recent evidence has shown, in fact, that
corneal transplant recipients exhibit systemic immunoreactivity against
the transplanted tissue very soon after corneal grafting, even in the
absence of any subsequent clinically evident graft rejection. (3,4).

The importance of understanding the cellular and molecular events
responsible for immunoregulation in the eye seems obvious; yet this is
an area of study which has been relatively neglected over the past

Maudgal, P.C. and Missotten, L., (eds.) Herpetic Eye Diseases.
© *1985, Dr W. Junk Publishers, Dordrecht/Boston/Lancaster. ISBN 978-94-010-8935-7*

three decades. We recently developed a model to study ocular immune responses and to study systemic immune responses to ocular antigenic encounters in the murine system. We took advantage of the previously accumulated information on the immune response of A/J strain mice to the hapten azobenzenearsonate (ABA) (5-7), and studied the response to ABA encounter in the ocular AC and in the vitreous body. We find that initial encounter with ABA coupled to spleen cells in the AC results in suppression of subsequent delayed-type hypersensitivity (DTH) reactions to challenge with ABA. This suppression is hapten-specific and is adoptively transferable to syngeneic naive recipients by T lymphocytes which lack idiotypic surface determinants. These suppressor T lympho-cytes are capable of suppressing both afferent and efferent arcs of the DTH response. Splenectomy prior to ABA priming in the AC prevents the development of tolerance. Vitreous body priming with particulate antigen (ABA-SC) does not result in the generation of these suppressor cells, although vitreous priming with anti-ABA idiotypic antibody, a soluble "mimic" of ABA, does stimulate the development of tolerance.

MATERIALS AND METHODS

Mice. A/J (H-2a, Igh-1e) female mice, 8-10 weeks old, were obtained from Jackson Laboratories, Bar Harbor, ME. Each experimental group consisted of 4 or 5 mice.

Antigen. The diazonium salt of arsanilic acid (Eastman Organic Chemicals Division, Eastman Kodak Co., Rochester, N.Y.) was prepared to give a 10 mM concentration of activated ABA used to derivatize erythrocyte-free A/J splenocytes, as described previously (6). The ABA-derivatized syngeneic splenocytes were washed in Hanks' balanced salt solution to form trinitrophenol conjugates of syngeneic, erythro-cyte-free splenocytes (TNP-SC), as described below.

Immunization and Challenge. A dose 3 x 10^7 derivatized cells in 0.2 ml of Hanks' balanced salt solution was injected in bilateral dorsal sites for immunization 5 days later; challenge consisted in injecting either 25 µl. of activated ABA at 10 mM or 25 µl of TNP-SC totalling 1 x 10^7 cells into the left footpad. Twenty-four hours after challenge, footpad swelling was measured with a Fowler micrometer (Schlesinger's Tool Brooklyn, N.Y.). The uninjected right footpad was also measured, and the difference in size was used as an index for DTH. All measure-ments were done blindly with respect to experimental groups.

Intravenous Induction of Tolerance. Mice in some groups received intravenous tail injections of varying doses of ABA-SC in 0.5 ml of Hanks' balanced salt solution just before subcutaneous immunization.

Intraocular Priming. Capillary tubes were heated and pulled to produce glass needles of 10 μm tip diameter. The needles were attached to a Narishige pipette hub (Labron Scientific Corp. Farmingdale, N.Y.) and thus coupled to a 50 μl Hamilton luer lock syringe. Under 40 X magnification, precise volumes of 10 μl of derivatized cells at 4 x 10^8 cells/ml suspension in Hanks' balanced salt solution were injected into each AC of each mouse. The cornea was entered tangentially so that the oblique needle tract would act as a valve to prevent the egress of injected cells. Subconjunctival priming was similarly performed with volumes of 10 μl. During ocular priming, mice were topically anesthetized with proparacaine hydrochloride. Vitreous priming with ABA-SC or with anti-idiotypic antiserum (anti-ABA) crossreactive idiotype, (a-CRI) was done through a tangential posterior sclerotomy entry site, under microscopic control to ensure avoidance of the crystalline lens and to visually assure delivery of the desired volume of priming material in the vitreous body.

Splenectomies. Splenectomies were performed 3 weeks prior to the experiments of spleen requirement for tolerance induction. Sham splenectomies were done on mice destined to serve as controls in these experiments. Skin and peritoneal wounds were closed with surgical adhesive.

Anti-idiotypic Antiserum (a-CRI). The a-CRI used in some of the vitreous body experiments was the generous gift of Dr. Alfred Nisonoff, Brandeis University, Waltham, Mass. Its preparation, purification, and characterization have been previously described (9).

Splenocyte Transfer. Donor mice received either 6 X 10^6 ABA-SC in the AC or 5 X 10^7 ABA-SC intravenously and were killed 7 days later. Their splenocytes were suspended and washed in Hanks' balanced salt solution. A total of 5 X 10^7 donor lymphocytes were injected intravenously into syngeneic naive recipients. Within 1-2 hours, the recipients were immunized subcutaneously with ABA-SC or TNP-SC.

Anti-Thy 1.2 and Complement Treatment. Mouse monoclonal IgM anti-Thy 1.2 was the generous gift of Phil Lake, George Washington University, Washington, D.C. Its characteristics are described elsewhere (10). Low tox rabbit complement for mice was purchased from Cedar Lane Laboratories, Hornby, Ont., Canada. Splenocytes were treated with anti-Thy 1.2 plus complement or with complement alone, as described previously (7). After treatment and washing in Hanks balanced salt solution, 5×10^7 viable cells were transferred through intravenous tail injection.

Statistical Analyses. Group means, standard errors, and standard errors of the means were calculated in the usual way, and statistical significance of differences between the means was assessed with Student's test as the statistical instrument. The reported results for each experiment represent reproducible findings from multiple repeated experiments (at lease 3 replicates of each experiment) employing at least 4 mice in each experimental group during each experimental run.

RESULTS

The results of subcutaneous sensitization with ABA-SC and footpad challenge with ABA 5 days later is seen in Table I.

Table I. Responses after ocular or intravenous administration of ABA-SC.

Group	Day 1 Priming Site	Day 1 Subcutaneous Immunization	Day 6 Footpad Increment (mm x 10^{-2} + SEM)	% Tolerance	P
I	--	ABA	30 + 5	--	--
II	--	ABA	27 + 3	—	NS
III	AC	ABA	16 + 2	73%	0.0033
IV	IV	ABA	15 + 2	77%	0.0045
V	--	--	10 + 1	--	0.0003

The footpad swelling response is typical of DTH, with response peaking 24-48 hours after challenge and a typical mononuclear cell infiltration, as seen on histopathology. The response is dose dependent, with minimal but consistent sensitization responses to 6×10^6 cells and maximal response to 6×10^7 cells for subcutaneous immunization (Table II).

Table II. Dose-Response Characteristics after ocular or Intravenous
administration of ABA-SC

Dose of hapten-coupled cells	Response to priming, % of positive control		
	after AC	intravenous	subconjunctival
6×10^5	--	91	--
3×10^6	54	--	--
6×10^6	36 (P < 0.01)	47 (P < 0.01)	75
2×10^7	--	42 (P < 0.01)	120
5×10^7	--	39 (P < 0.01)	--

AC Priming Produces Systemic Tolerance. A state of relative
immunologic tolerance results from AC priming. Systemic DTH was markedly
inhibited in mice that received either AC or intravenous injections of
ABA-SC, whereas subconjunctival priming had no such effect (Table I).
In fact, footpad swelling was enhanced if the number of ABA-SC injected
subconjunctivally was increased. Tolerance was also achieved with lower
doses of ABA-SC and with monocular injection, but the magnitude of the
tolerance was smaller. As shown in table III, tolerance also decreases
with decreasing numbers of cells injected intravenously. Intravenous
injection of 5×10^7 ABA-SC led to about the same level of tolerance as
injection of 6×10^6 ABA-SC into the AC.

Table III. Hapten Specificity

Group	Day I Cell Trans. from AC Primed mice	Day 1 Subcut. Immun.	Day 5 Challenge	Day 6 Footpad Increment (mm x 10^{-2} + SEM)	% Suppression	P
I	--	ABA	ABA	30 + 6	--	--
II	5×10^7 SC	ABA	ABA	19 + 4	55%	0.007
III	--	--	ABA	10 + 3	--	0.0009
IV	--	TNP	TNP	25 + 3	--	--
V	5×10^7 SC	TNP	TNP	22 + 8	--	NS
VI	--	--	TNP	6 + 3	--	0.007

Tolerance following AC Priming is Mediated by Hapten-Specific
Suppressor T-Cells. The results in Table III show that the systemic
unresponsiveness to ABA after AC priming with ABA-SC is hapten specific.

The suppressor phenomenon is specific for ABA in that lymphocytes from ABA-primed mice do not inhibit the ability to sensitize to the unrelated hapten trinitrophenol. The lymphocytes suppressing the response to ABA were elimated by treatment with anti-Thy 1.2 plus complement alone (Table IV).

Table IV. Adoptive Transferability is T-Cell Dependent.

Group	Day 1 SC Trans. from AC Primed Mice	Day 1 SC Treatment	Day 5 Subcut. Immun.	Day6 Footpad Increment (mm x 10^{-2} + SEM)	% Suppression	P
I	--	ABA	ABA	38 + 12	--	--
II	5×10^7 normal SC	--	ABA	26 + 10	--	NS
III	5×10^7	--	ABA	14 + 4	75%	0.0034
IV	5×10^7	anti-Thy 1.2 +C	ABA	32 + 6	--	NS
V	5×10^7	C alone	ABA	12 + 4	80%	0.0032
VI	--	--	--	7 + 3	--	0.0005

Therefore, the suppressor cells are thymus-derived and are suppressor T lymphocytes (Ts). These results indicate that a population of hapten-specific suppressor T lymphocytes (Ts) is activated following AC inoculation with ABA-SC.

AC Priming Induces Ts That Block the Efferent Immune Responses. Transfer of AC-induced Ts suppressed the immune response in mice previously sensitized (i.e. sensitized via subcutaneous ABA-SC priming prior to rather than simultaneous with adoptive transfer of donor splenocytes) to ABA-SC. Transfer of Ts from mice primed with 5×10^6 ABA-SC injected intravenously did not suppress the DTH challenge response in previously sensitized mice. Both the AC and the intravenously induced Ts used in this experiment were able to prevent sensitization for DTH in naive mice when given in the afferent mode (i.e. when transferred simultaneously with subcutaneous sensitization priming with ABA-SC). Thus, AC-induced Ts differ from intravenously induced Ts in their ability to block the efferent arm of the immune response (Table V).

Table V. AC-induced Ts are second order-like

Group	Day 1 SC Trans.	Day 1 Subcut. Immun.	Day 4 SC Trans.	Day 5 Footpad Increment (mm x 10^{-2} $\pm$ SEM)	% Suppression	P
I	--	ABA	--	24 $\pm$ 4	--	--
II	--	ABA	AC induced	5 $\pm$ 1	100	0.01
III	--	ABA	IV induced	24 $\pm$ 6	--	NS
IV	--	--	--	8 $\pm$ 3	--	0.03
V	AC induced ABA	--		6 $\pm$ 2	89	0.001
VI	IC induced ABA	--		15 $\pm$ 2	53	0.005

AC Primed Ts Do Not Bear CRI Surface Determinants. It is now well established that Ts induced by intravenous injection of ABA-SC bear CRI surface determinants (11). Treatment of intravenously induced Ts with anti-CRI plus complement prior to transfer prevents transfer of suppression; similar treatment of AC-induced Ts does not abolish transfer of suppression (Table VI). Therefore, AC-induced Ts differ from intravenously induced Ts in that they lack CRI surface determinants.

Table VI. AC-induced Ts do not express cross-ractive idiotype.

Group	Day 1 SC Trans. from AC-Primed Mice	Day 1 SC Treatment	Day 1 Subcutan. sensiti- zation	Day 6 Footpad Increment (mm x 10^{-2} $\pm$ SEM)	% Suppression	P
I	--	--	ABA	38 $\pm$ 2	--	--
II	5×10^7	--	ABA	22 $\pm$ 2	49	0.005
III	5×10^7	aCRI + C	ABA	7 $\pm$ 1	100	0.0001
IV	5×10^7	C alone	ABA	23 $\pm$ 2	44	0.01
V	--	--	--	9 $\pm$ 1	--	0.0001

Splenectomy Prevents the Development of Tolerance following AC Priming. Splenectomy 3 weeks prior to AC priming with ABA-SC prevents the development of tolerance to subsequent encounter with ABA. Simultaneous ABA priming after splenectomy results in sensitization to ABA with DTH responses to·footpad challenge comparable to sham-splenectomized mice (or to unaltered controls) not receiving AC priming with ABA-SC. This contrasts sharply with the suppression of DTH to ABA in non-splenectomized mice primed in the AC with ABA-SC (Table VII).

Table VII. Splenectomy presents induction of tolerance

Group	Splenectomy	Day 1 AC Prime	Day 1 SC Prime	Day 6 Footpad Increment (mm x 10^{-2} + SEM)	% Tolerance	P
I	+	+	+	27 + 2	--	--
II	+	--	+	25 + 5	NS	0.68
III	--	+	+	17 + 3	45%	0.015
IV	--	--	+	20 + 4	NS	0.32
V	--	--	--	6 + 2	--	0.0015

Vitreal Priming with ABA-SC Does Not Produce Systemic Tolerance, but Priming with a-CRI tends to Suppress Subsequent DTH Reactions to ABA. Intravitreal priming with 8 x 10^6 ABA-SC does not result in tolerance but in fact enhances sensitization to ABA. (Table VIII).

Table VIII. Intravitreal priming with ABA-SC does not tolerize.

Group	Day 1 Priming Site	Day 1 Subcutaneous Immunization	Day 6 Footpad Increment (mm x 10^{-2} + SEM)
I	--	ABA	29 + 3
II	Subconj.	ABA	40 + 15
III	Vitreous	ABA	39 + 10
IV	--	--	7 + 7

However, intravitreal priming with 3 mM IBC a-CRI suppressed subsequent DTH reactions to ABA footpad challenge; and the degree of suppression was comparable to that seen after intravenous priming with the same dose of a-CRI (Table IX).

Table IX. Intravitreal Priming with a-CRI Induces Tolerance.

Group	Day 1 Priming Site	Day 1 Subcutaneous Immunization	Day 6 Footpad Increment (mm x 10^{-2} + SEM)	% Tolerance	P
I	--	ABA	17 + 2	--	--
II	Vitreous	ABA	5 + 2	70%	0.05
III	IV	ABA	12 + 2	41%	0.2
IV	--	--	8 + 3	--	0.031

DISCUSSION

We have shown that immune processing indeed occurs after antigen presentation via the AC. Specific systemic tolerance of the antigen, mediated through the activity of antigen-specific suppressor T lymphocytes, occurs after such antigenic presentation.

In our model, the AC injection of ABA-SC was tolerogenic, whereas the subconjunctival route was not. Noting that foreign particles leave the AC through venous channels providing direct access to the spleen, Kaplan and Streilein (12) suggested that suppressor mechanisms that involve enhancing antibodies or suppressor T cells are activated as a result of AC priming. This theory is consistent with the consensus that the route by which antigen is presented determines the nature of an immune response (13,14). Presentation of antigen by antigen-presenting cells activates T cell help for DTH and subsequent events in graft rejection (15). With plentiful numbers of macrophages populating draining lymph nodes, and other antigen-presenting cells in the skin itself, it follows that subcutaneous priming with antigen results in sensitization. In contrast, tolerization should result if antigen bypasses effective encounters with antigen-presenting elements necessary for immunity. AC priming may have this effect in our system. Whereas the active mechanisms that produce tolerance after intravenous priming have been described in detail (11, 17), the cause of tolerance after AC priming has not been elucidated previously.

We have pursued an analogy between intravenous and AC inoculation. Sulzberger (18) originally described specific immune tolerance following intravenous antigen presentation. It is evident that this sort of tolerance is, at least in part, an active form of suppression mediated by thymus-derived lymphocytes (Ts) (19,21). In our model, we know that ABA-SC injected intravenously into A/J mice primes for suppression mediated by a series of cellular interactions involving suppressor T cells and their products (6). The present study demonstrates that AC inoculation also primes for Ts-mediated suppression. The afferent limb of the immune system is clearly intact within the AC. We believe this is the first documentation of a cellular mechanism for the tolerance observed after AC antigen presentation.

The finding the AC priming with antigen differs from intravenous priming in terms of T suppressor cells induced was unexpected.

In this system, AC priming and intravenous priming appear to engender different regulatory responses or different kinetics of the same suppressor pathway. It is possible that sustained release of antigen from the AC, a depot of sorts, produced more efficient suppression. Also, the timing of the antigen release may influence which Ts clone in the succession Ts1, Ts2, Ts3 predominates at any given time. It might also be speculated that the drainage apparatus of the AC, the trabecular meshwork, is not simply a sink emptying into the venous system, but rather a matrix which incorporates special antigen-processing elements of its own. Indeed, one intriguing possibility is that antigen presenting cells special to the suppressor pathway may be present in the trabecular meshwork. Work in progress may resolve this issue.

We believe that our demonstration of second order suppressor cells resulting from AC priming implicates the activation of immune regulation. Through better insight into such inhibitory mechanisms, the problems of corneal graft rejection, ocular infection, and auto-immune uveitis might some day be better managed. In particular, the responses to herpes simplex virus after ocular compartment encounter may be especially provocative.

REFERENCES

1. Medawar, P.B.: Immunity to homologous grafted skin. III. The fate of skin homografts transplanted to the brain, to subcutaneous tissue, and to the anterior chamber of the eye. Br. J. exp. Path. 29: (1948).
2. Woodruff, M.F.A.; Woodruff, H.G.: The transplantation of normal tissue. With special reference to auto- and homotransplantation of thyroid and spleen in the anterior chamber of the eye and sub-cutaneously in the guinea pigs. Phil. Trans. R. Soc. 234:559 (1950.
3. Szabo, G.; Balaza, C.; Leovey, A.; Alberth, B.: Immunological investigations of patients with transplanted cornea. Graefes Arch. klin. exp. Ophthal. 196:169 (1975).
4. Grunnet, N,; Kristensen, T.; Kissmeyer-Nielsen, F.; et al.: Occurence of lymphocytotoxic lymphocytes and antibodies after corneal trans-plantation. Acta ophthal. 54:156 (1976).
5. Nisonoff, A.: Ju, S.T.; Owen, F.L.: Studies of structure and immunosuppression of cross-reactive idiotype in strain A mice. Immunol Rev. 34: 89 (1977).
6. Bach, B.A.; Sherman, L: Benacerraf, B; Greene, M.I.: Mechanisms of regulation of cell-mediated immunity. II. Induction and suppression of delayed-type hypersensitivity to azobenzenearsonate-coupled sysngeneic cells. J. Immun. 121: (1460).
7. Sy.M.S.; Nisonoff, A.; Germin, R.N.; et al.: Antigen and receptor driven regulatory mechanisms. VIII. Supression of idiotypic-negative ABA specific T-cells results from the interaction of an anti-idiotypic Ts2 with a CRI+ primed T-cell target. J. exp. Med. (in press).

8. Greene, M.I.; Sugimoto, M.; Benecerraf, B.: Mechanisms or regulation of cell-mediated immune responses. I. Effect of the route of immunization with TNP-coupled syngeneic cells on the induction and suppression of contact sensitivity to picryl chloride. J. Immun. 120: 1604 (1978).
9. Kuettner, M.G.; Wang, A.L.; Nisonoff, A.: Quantitative investigations of idotypic specificity as a potential genetic marker for the variable regions of mouse immunoglobulin polypeptide chains. J. exp. Med. 135:579 (1972).
10. Lake, P.; Clark, E.A.; Khorshidi, M.; et al.: Production and characterization of cytotoxic Thy-1 antibody-secreting hybrid cell lines. Detection of T-cell subsetts. Eur. J. Immunol. 9:875 (1979).
11. Dietz, M.H.; Sy. M.S.; Greene, M.I.; Nisonoff, A.; benacerraf, B.; Germain, R.N.: Antigen and receptor-driven regulatory mechanisms. VI. Demonstration of cross-reactive idiotypic determinants on azobenzearsonate-specific antigen-binding suppressor T cells producing soluble suppressor factors (s). J. Immun. 125:2374 (1980).
12. Kaplan, J.J.; Streilein, J.W.: Immune response to immunization via the anterior chamber of the eye. II. An analyses of F1 lymphocyte-induced immune derivation. J. Immun. 120:689 (1978).
13. Greene, M.I.; Back, B.A.: Hypothesis. The physiological regulation of immunity. Differential regulatory contributions of peripheral and central lymphon compartments. Cell. Immunol. 45:446 (1979).
14. Claman, H.N.: Hypothesis: T-cell tolerance - one signal ? Cell Immunol. 48:201 (1979).
15. Frei, P.C.; Benecerraf, B.; Thorbecke, G.J.: Phagocytosis of the antigen, a crucial step in the induction of the primary response. Proc natn. Acad Sci USA 53:30 (1965).
16. Weigle, W.O.: Immunological unresponsiveness. Adv. Immunol. 16:61 (1973).
17. Katz, D.H.; Benacerraf, B.: Immunological tolerance, Academic Press, New York (1974).
18. Sulberger, M.D.: Hypersensitivities to arsphenamine in guinea pigs; experiments in prevention and desensitization. Archs Derm. Syph. 20:669 (1929).
19. Zembala, M.; Asherson, GL.: Depression of the T-cell unresponsive mice. Nature, Lond. 244:227 (1973).
20. Claman, H.N.; Miller, S.D.: Requirements for induction of T-cell tolerance to DNFB. Efficiency of membrane-associated DNFB. J. Immunol. 117:480 (1976).
21. Miller, S.D.; Wetzig, R.P.; Claman, H.N.: The induction of cell-mediated immunity and tolerance with protein antigens coupled to syngeneic lymphoid cells. J. exp. Med. 149:758 (1978).

DISCUSSION :

A.B. Tullo (Bristol) : Have you looked at the effect of priming intracamerally; also how can you be sure that the inoculation will be into the cornea only and that you are not doing something to penetrate the anterior chamber ?

C.S. Foster (Boston) : There is no virus in these eyes in the experiments that I have just described. All our work is done using microglass needles. We have developed techniques that allow us to inject, quite precisely if we wish, 1 µL of material into the mouse corneal stroma, without perforating the anterior chamber. The results of the experiments described in the abstract book in fact relate to microtechniques that involve draining aqueous and placing specific amounts of material into the anterior chamber, replacing the aqueous, and doing in such a way that there is no leak, although material is placed in it. The vitreal work is done in that way too. Others have looked at intracameral inoculation of live HSV, and the clinical response is dramatically different from how we are reporting here. What one sees with anterior chamber injection of herpes is almost total destruction of the anterior segment on the site injected, with interesting sparing of ipsilateral retina and a subsequent total destruction of this contralateral retina. We don't see that in this corneal scarification model.

D.L. Easty (Bristol) : In your experiments did you adjust the dosage ? Was virus concentration the same in the two groups of animals ? I wonder whether increasing the dosage of virus inoculum might suppress T cell response.

C.S. Foster (Boston) : We have done both ways. It has been suggested to us that, in fact, the way we set our model system up, we are too stringent. It has been suggested that we don't initially immunise subcutaneously, but in fact try to induce suppressor cells by ocular encounter with antigen first, then come back and immunise, and show a so called defective response. But we have done the experiments in exactly the way that we have done the azobenzene arsenate experiments and it does show, I think, something about the power of the system of generating suppression.

G. Smolin (San Francisco) : Stephen, I was wondering if you have looked at the draining lymph nodes in these animals histopathologically. What type of cells are increased and so on ?

C.S. Foster (Boston) : We have, I am not ready to talk about that yet. We just harvested the regional lymphnodes and spleens, and that relates to your comment, and looking at mononuclear cell subsets using monoclonal antibody and fluorocytometry after cell dispersion, and by immunoperoxidase technique and cryostat sections. But, at this stage the story is far from complete.

THE ROLE OF VIRUS-INFECTED MONONUCLEAR LEUKOCYTES IN THE
PATHOGENESIS OF HERPETIC CHORIORETINITIS OF NEWBORN RABBITS

YUICHI OHASHI, JANG O. OH, KER-HWA TUNG-OU
Francis I. Proctor Foundation, University of California,
San Francisco, California, U.S.A.

With the increase of genital herpes, neonatal herpetic
infection has become an increasingly important problem. In
most clinical cases, herpetic chorioretinitis, which is one
of the ocular manifestations of newborn herpetic infection,
occurs after the skin infection, and, interestingly, HSV-2
has so far been the only isolate (1). In a previous report,
we presented a newborn rabbit model of herpetic chorioretinitis which develops after skin infection by HSV-2 (2). Infectious HSV-2 could be isolated both from mononuclear leukocytes (MNLs) and from the plasma of infected animals.
This result strongly suggested the hematogeneous spread of
the virus to the eye, and it seemed that the virus was, for
the most part, associated with MNLs. The present study was
undertaken to determine the relative importance of virus-
infected MNLs, as opposed to free HSV-2, in the pathogenesis of chorioretinitis in newborn rabbits.

In this study, we used the Curtis strain of HSV-2, and
2-7 day old newborns of New Zealand White rabbits. We used
in vitro-infected MNLs because they can easily be obtained
in large amounts using this method. MNLs were isolated
from normal newborn rabbit blood by dextran treatment and
Ficoll-Paque gradient centrifugation, and infected with
HSV-2 for 18 hours at MOI of 10. After washing to eliminate unabsorbed virus, we used these cells as infected MNLs.
These in vitro-infected MNLs were injected into normal newborn rabbits via the right common carotid artery. For comparison, we also injected various doses of free HSV-2 into
the other newborn litters via the same route. Three days

Maudgal, P.C. and Missotten, L., (eds.) Herpetic Eye Diseases.
© *1985, Dr W. Junk Publishers, Dordrecht/Boston/Lancaster. ISBN 978-94-010-8935-7*

after the injection, the animals were killed for histological examination of the eye. The result of injecting virus-
infected MNLs or free virus into the common carotid artery
indicated that virus-infected MNLs are far more efficient
in producing the chorioretinitis than free virus; free virus required 10 fold more than HSV-infected MNLs to produce
the lesions in 50% of the eyes.

Why were MNLs so efficient in producing the chorioreti-
nal lesions? It has been shown that the nature of the cell
surface changes after infection by HSV. Because of this
change, we postulated that infected MNLs may localize more
readily in the eye than uninfected MNLs. To examine this
possibility, we injected radiolabeled, virus-infected MNLs
into the newborn rabbits and measured the radioactivity retained in the eye. We isolated normal MNLs and divided
them into two fractions. One was incubated with HSV-2 and
the other was incubated without virus. The next day, both
cell fractions were labeled with ^{111}In and were injected
into the newborn rabbits via the right common carotid artery. The radioactivity retained in the eyes was counted
three hours after the injection. The result indicated that
more infected than uninfected MNLs stayed in the right eye.

One possible explanation for this difference may be
that infected MNLs were more securely attached to the vascular endothelium of the eye than uninfected MNLs. We
therefore compared in vitro attachment of virus-infected
MNLs to the cultured vascular endothelial cells with that
of uninfected MNLs. ^{111}In-labeled, infected or uninfected
MNLs were obtained, and these labeled MNLs were then incubated with monolayer culture of vascular endothelial cells
for two hours. After the incubation, unattached MNLs were
washed off, and the residual radioactivity was counted. In
the three repeated experiments, the attachment of infected
MNLs to the endothelial cells was consistently better than
that of uninfected MNLs. This difference was statistically
significant.

In summary, (a) <u>Virus</u>-infected MNLs, rather than free
HSV-2, play an important role in the pathogenesis of chorioretinitis of newborn rabbits, and (b) HSV-2 infected MNLs
attach more securely to the vascular endothelium and are
retained better in the eye than uninfected MNLs.

REFERENCES

1. Oh JO, Minasi P. 1981. Herpetic Chorioretinitis in
    Newborn infants. An experimental study. <u>In</u> Herpetic
    Eye Diseases. R. Sundmacher, editor, JF Bergmann Ver-
    lag. Munich. pp. 191-199.
2. Brick DC, Oh JO, Sicher, SE, 1981. Ocular lesions asso-
    ciated with dissemination of type 2 herpes simplex vi-
    rus from skin infection in newborn rabbits. Invest.
    Ophthalmol. Vis. Sci. 21:681.

94

DISCUSSION :

H.J. Field (Cambridge) : How long after the inoculation did virus appear in retina ?

J.O. Oh (San Francisco) : Three days.

H.J. Field (Cambridge) : Is it absolutely certain that the virus is not invading the central nervous system, and invading retina by the normal neuronal pathways of the optic nerve ?

J.O. Oh (San Francisco) : Are you talking of the in vitro infected cells injected into the carotid artery or a skin infection ?

H.J. Field (Cambridge) : I am talking about the intravenous route.

J.O. Oh (San Francisco) : Intravenous route, yes. We checked the central nervous system sequentially on day 1, 2 and 3; and appearance of virus in the eye as well as brain is about the same. So I don't think that there is any neuronal spread from the brain to the eye.

H.J. Field (Cambridge) : But what about in the optic nerve, were there signs of infection there ?

J.O. Oh (San Francisco) : That we have not checked.

G.O. Waring (Atlanta) : Have you done similar experiments with type 1 herpes ? Does it behave in the same way, the leuko-cytes ?

J.O. Oh (San Francisco) : In our previous study in this particu-lar model of newborn rabbits, the skin infection with type 1, virus did not spread to various organs, including eye, and it did not produce chorioretinitis. Only type 2 strains produ-ced skin lesions and disseminated to various organs including eye and produced chorioretinitis in about 40 % of the infected rabbits.

G.O. Waring (Atlanta) : Have you looked specifically whether or not type 1 gets into leukocytes like this ?

J.O. Oh (San Francisco) : As far as the leukocytes are concerned, virus grows very well, whether HSV type 1 or type 2. There is no difference whatsoever.

The influence of prednisolone on external eye disease, virus proliferation and latent infection in an animal model of herpes simplex keratitis.

D.L. Easty[1], A.B. Tullo[1*], C. Shimeld[1], T.J. Hill[2] and W.A. Blyth[2]
Department of Ophthalmology[1] and Microbiology[2], University of Bristol, UK
* present address; Manchester Royal Eye Hospital

INTRODUCTION

It is well known from clinical experience in man that corticosteroids worsen recurrent ulcerative herpetic keratitis. Therefore, a model of herpes simplex keratitis in immune mice (1) has been used to assess the effect of topical treatment with prednisolone (0.5%) on signs of disease in the external eye. The presence of virus in eye washings and establishment of latent infection were also studied.

METHODS

Inoculation of Mice

Groups of 4 week old male NIH inbred mice were made immune by inoculation with 5×10^5 pfu HSV1 (SC16 strain) intradermally in the right ear (2).Four weeks later the left cornea was scarified through a suspension of 5μl of the same virus containing 3.7×10^6 pfu.

Treatment

Animals were anaesthetised for inoculation, treatment, and examination by slit lamp microscopy. Immediately after inoculation, the eye was treated topically with prednisolone drops or saline twice daily at about 9.00 a.m.and 9.00 p.m. for 10 days (experiment 1) or for 5 days (experiment 2).

Eye Washings

At daily intervals during the acute disease 20 μl of medium 199 was irrigated and aspirated upon the left eye, and the washings were placed on to Vero cell monolayers for virus isolation.

Latent infection

Latent infection was assessed six weeks later in the left trigeminal ganglion subdivided into its three parts (3), and the left superior cervical ganglion by culturing the ganglia in growth medium for 5 days prior to grinding and placing on Vero cells.

Maudgal, P.C. and Missotten, L., (eds.) Herpetic Eye Diseases.
© *1985, Dr W. Junk Publishers, Dordrecht/Boston/Lancaster. ISBN 978-94-010-8935-7*

Table Effect of treatment with Prednisolone during ocular infection on establishment of latent infection in the three parts of the trigeminal ganglion and the superior cervical ganglion (S.C.G.)

TRIGEMINAL GANGLION

	Treatment	I	II	III	SCG
Experiment 1	Steroid	12/16 (75)*	7/16 (44)	2/16 (12.5)	0/16
	Saline	12/16 (75)	2/16 (12.5)	1/16 (6.3)	1/16 (6.3)
Experiment 2	Steroid	19/25 (76)	2/25 (8)	0/25	0/25
	Saline	10/25 (40)	2/25 (8)	0/25	0/25

$$* \frac{\text{number positive}}{\text{number tested}} \ (\%)$$

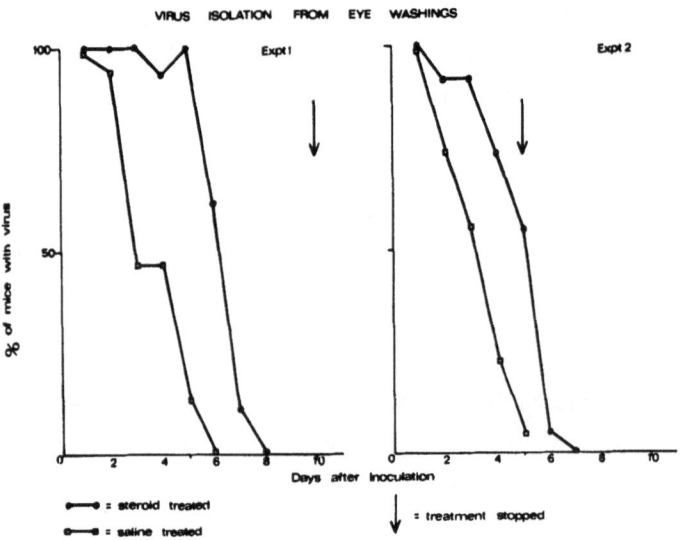

VIRUS ISOLATION FROM EYE WASHINGS

Expt I

Expt 2

% of mice with virus

Days after Inoculation

●—● = steroid treated
○—○ = saline treated

↓ = treatment stopped

Fig. Effect of topical treatment with Prednisolone on shedding of virus in eye washings. Treatment of the inoculated eye began immediately after inoculation of HSV.

RESULTS

External eye disease

All the signs of the inflammatory response of the eye were less marked in steroid-treated animals compared to controls, except the involvement of the lids which became more severe than controls four days after inoculation.

Virus in tears

Treatment with steroid prolonged the period during which virus was isolated from eye washings (Figure).

Latent infection

In experiment 1 latent infection occurred in 9/16 steroid-treated mice at non-ophthalmic sites in the trigeminal ganglion, compared with 3/16 controls ($p < 0.05$). (Table). In experiment 2, steroid treatment increased the incidence of latent infection in the ophthalmic part of the trigeminal ganglion ($p < 0.025$), but the incidence in non-ophthalmic sites was similar in the treated and control group.

CONCLUSIONS

Topical treatment of herpes simplex keratitis in immune mice with prednisolone produced the following effects:

1) decreased severity in the clinical signs of external disease

2) isolation of virus from the eye washings from a larger proportion of mice for a longer period

3) increased incidence of latent infection in non-ophthalmic parts of the trigeminal ganglion (experiment 1), or increased incidence of latent infection in the ophthalmic part of the ganglion (experiment 2).

Keratitis in immune mice provides a suitable model for testing the effect of drugs in herpetic infections. Only by examining virus proliferation and latency as well as assessing clinical disease can the full effect of a drug be assessed.

REFERENCES

1. Tullo, A.B., Shimeld, C., Blyth, W.A., Hill, T.J. and Easty, D.L. (1983) Ocular infection with herpes simplx virus in non-immune and immune mice. Arch. Ophthalmol. 101 961-964.

2. Hill, T.J., Field, H.J. and Blyth, W.A. (1975) Acute and recurrent infection with herpes simplex virus in the mouse: a model for studying latency and recurrent disease. J. gen. Virol. 28 341-353

3. Tullo, A.B., Shimeld, C., Blyth, W.A., Hill, T.J. and Easty, D.L. (1982) Spread of virus and distribution of latent infection following ocular herpes simplex in the non-immune and immune mice. J. gen. Virol. 63 95-101

DISCUSSION :

C.S. Foster (Boston) : Let me just ask if you have information that relates to the influence of topical steroids on reactivation from latency. That is a question that has come up for the last three decades and conflicting views are held by many. Some believe that topical steroids do not enhance the likelihood of reactivation from latency, but certainly can make the disease much worse once spontaneous reactivation occurs.

C. Shimeld (Bristol) : Well, in the few experiments we have done, we never achieved any reactivation. That is all I can say.

SUPPRESSIVE EFFECT OF CYCLOSPORINE ON THE INDUCTION OF SECONDARY HERPES SIMPLEX UVEITIS

JANG O. OH, PETROS MINASI, GUNTHER GRABNER, YUICHI OHASI, Francis I. Proctor Foundation, University of California, San Francisco, California, U.S.A.

When live herpes simplex virus (HSV) was injected intravitreally into the normal rabbit eye, primary uveitis developed, resolving within one month. If such a healed eye was challenged with HSV antigen, secondary uveitis developed within six hours after the challenge. We have shown previously that this secondary uveitis is mediated by an immune reaction that involves HSV antigen, sensitized T lymphocytes, and anti-HSV antibody (1,2). This paper presents our experimental data which indicate that pretreatment of the animal with a T cell suppressor, Cyclosporine (CyA), successfully prevented the induction of secondary uveitis.

Primary uveitis was produced by intravitreal injection of 10^3 PFU of type 1 HSV (Shealey strain) into both eyes of New Zealand white male rabbits and the eyes were allowed to recover from primary uveitis. Blood was collected from these rabbits to obtain neutralizing antibody titers prior to CyA treatment. Then rabbits were divided into two groups; a test group and a control group. Rabbits in the test group received intramuscular CyA, 25 mg/kg body weight, daily for 7 days, while the control rabbits received intramuscular oil daily for 7 days. The oil was used as a solvent for CyA. To investigate whether daily CyA-treatment induces shedding of HSV to tear, eye cultures for HSV were also made daily. Upon completion of daily CyA or oil injections, blood was again collected for anti-HSV antibody titration, and all the eyes of both test and control groups were challenged intravitreally with HSV antigen. The HSV antigen was UV-inactivated, purified HSV-1. Eyes were checked

Maudgal, P.C. and Missotten, L., (eds.) Herpetic Eye Diseases.
© *1985, Dr W. Junk Publishers, Dordrecht/Boston/Lancaster. ISBN 978-94-010-8935-7*

daily for 3 days with a slit lamp for flare and cells in the anterior chamber. The degree of the anterior chamber reaction was graded from 0 to 3+ according to the method of Kimura, Hogan and Thygeson (3). On the third day, animals were killed, and the eyes, trigemial, and superior cervical ganglia were dissected out for virus isolation. Cervical lymph nodes were also obtained for lymphocyte transformation assay.

In control animals, flare appeared in all eyes within 24 hours after the challenge and persisted throughout the experimental period. The mean value of the flare in the control animals was 1.6 on day 1 through day 3. On the other hand, flare in the CyA-treated rabbits was markedly mild, and on day 3, no flare was observed in 9 out of 15 eyes. The mean value of flare in the CyA-treated rabbits was 0.8 on day 1 and 0.6 on day 2 and day 3. The mean value of CyA-treated group was significantly less than that of the control group. The P value was less than 0.01. All the eyes of the control group showed cells in the anterior chambers on day 2 and day 3, whereas cells were present in only 4 out of 15 eyes of the CyA group. The degree of cell infiltration into the anterior chamber was very much milder in the eyes of CyA-treated rabbits than in the control rabbits; the mean value was only 0.3, 0.3 and 0.5 in the test group. It was 1.4, 1.8 and 1.9 in the controls. The P value was less than 0.01.

In these control rabbits, a high degree of lymphocyte transformation was observed following stimulation with phytoheamagglutinin as well as HSV antigen, and no significant changes in antibody titers were noted. On the other hand, the CyA treatment resulted in a marked depression of lymphocyte transformation by both phytohemagglutinin and HSV antigen. However, CyA treatment had no effect on antibody titers. These results appear to indicate that CyA treatment mainly affects T lymphocyte activities.

The daily CyA administration did not induce reactivation
of latent HSV infection. Although trigeminal and superior
cervical ganglia were latently infected with HSV, as indicated by positive HSV isolation in the co-cultivation of
ganglia, no reactivation of latent HSV was detected. This
was evidenced by negative virus isolation from cultures of
conjunctival swabs, eye tissue homogenate, or homogenates
of ganglia.

In summary, a series of intramuscular injections of CyA
significantly suppressed the induction of secondary uveitis
in rabbits. The suppression of secondary uveitis was associated with depressed activites of T lymphocytes. CyA
treatment did not reactivate latent HSV in trigeminal and
superior cervical ganglia.

REFERENCES

1. Oh, JO, 1976. Primary and secondary herpes simplex
    uveitis in rabbits. Surv. Ophthalmol. 21:176.
2. Oh, JO, Minasi, P and Kopal, M, 1982. Immunological
    mechanisms for recurrent herpes simplex uveitis. Invest.
    Ophthalmol. Vis. Sci. 22 Suppl:98.
3. Hogan, M., Kimura, SJ, Thygeson, P, 1959. Signs and
    symptoms of uveitis. Am. J. Ophthalmol. 47 (Part II)
    :155.

DISCUSSION :

P.A. Asbell (New York) : There has been a lot of interest on the possible topical use of cyclosporin, particularly in graft rejection. I wonder if you had any opportunity to look at its topical use in this model.

J.O. Oh (San Francisco) : No, we have not. The main reason was that I didn't know much about the penetration rate of this drug. Now we know that it penetrates very well. So I certainly would like to try.

H.J.M. Völker-Dieben (Leiden) : Perhaps I did not catch it correctly, but if you have a combined treatment, does it mean that you give a two times higher dose in combination for intravitreal and intramuscular, compared to those who had only intravitreal or only intramuscular. So you have an enforced effect, I suppose.

J.O. Oh (San Francisco) : That is true. There may be some larger dosage effect. But in our separate experiments we gave as high as 50 mg of cyclosporin-A, just intramuscular, and it didn't produce as good effect as the combination treatment. I don't know what is the mechanism involved in this case. It is very difficult to explain in view of the mechanisms of the suppressive effects. We know that we have to apply this drug during the reaction period. It is a pretreatment, like cytoxin. Yet we get good results. We are not the only one showing this. As a matter of fact Borel also showed that he could suppress the hypersensitivity reaction only by pretreatment, instead of postchallange treatment. I don't know the underlying mechanism of this effect.

T-CELL SUBSETS IN HERPES ZOSTER CYCLITIS

T.M.RADDA[1],J.FUNDER[1],U.M.KLEMEN[1],U.KÖLLER[2]

1st Department of Ophthalmology[1] and the Institute
of Immunology[2] of the University of Vienna, Austria

INTRODUCTION:

For the pathogenesis of virus-induced uveitis, direct cytotoxic
effects of the virus are considered to be of less importance
than subsequent immunological processes. From experimental
work with animals we know that for these immunological processes T-cell mediated cellular immune reactions are particulary responsible[1]. It was also shown that T-lymphocytopenia
is present during the acute stage of anterior uveitis.[2]
Recently it has been demonstrated that the T-cell modulating
agent Cyclosporin A is effective in therapy of uveitis.[3]
Immunemechanisms including T-cell reactions are under the control of regulatory T-cells. Functional defects of these cells
e.g. imbalance of the helper/suppressor T-cell ratio may thus
also play a role in the pathogenesis of virus induced uveitis.
Lymphocyte stimulation response to mitogens and to various
antigens as well as studies of T-lymphocyte subpopulations
have therefore attracted attention in examining various clinical forms of uveitis[4-11].
The pathogenic heterogenity of the various forms of uveitis
constitutes an obvious difficulty when the results of such
investigation are to be evaluated. We attempted to circumvent
this problem by limiting our studies to one defined form of
uveitis, that is, to cyclitis due to herpes zoster of the
first trigeminal branch.
Recently it has become possible to characterize T-lymphocyte
subsets with the use of monoclonal antibodies. We determined
T-lymphocyte subpopulations in patients with herpes zoster
of the first trigeminal branch using monoclonal antibodies

Maudgal, P.C. and Missotten, L., (eds.) Herpetic Eye Diseases.
© *1985, Dr W. Junk Publishers, Dordrecht/Boston/Lancaster. ISBN 978-94-010-8935-7*

against those antigens which are restricted to the T-helper/
inducer subset (Leu 3 a), to the T-suppressor/cytotoxic subset (Leu 2 a) as well as to a common T-cell antigen (Leu 4a)
Our investigations were carried out on herpes zoster patients
with cyclitis and without uveitis.

MATERIAL AND METHODS:

A total of 23 patients, aged from 38 to 88 years (average
age 62,8) male and female, with herpes zoster of the first
trigeminal branch were divided into two groups: group I were
patients with cyclitis (n = 11), group II patients without
cyclitis (n = 12). In 9 patients, the clinical features of
uveitis were diffuse, in 2 patients additional focal lesions
were found. In 6 patients uveitis was combined with keratitis.
Before therapy was initiated, at the latest on the fourth
day following the appearance of exanthema, blood samples were
drawn by venipuncture from each patient during the active
phase of the disease. Seven patients of each group were available for follow-up investigation and blood samples were taken
during the remission phase (3-6 months after onset of infection).
A group of 20 healthy subjects, matched as to sex and age,
served as controls.

Peripheral blood mononuclear cells were isolated from peripheral
blood by Ficoll Paque (Pharmacia, Uppsala, Sweden) density
centrifugation. T-lymphoytes were characterized with monoclonal
antibodies (MAb) to antigens restricted to the T-helper/
inducer subsets (Leu 3 a) and T-suppressor/cytotoxic subset
(Leu 2 a) as well as to a common T-cell antigen (Leu 4);
(all byBecton-Dickinson)[12].

Six times 10^5 mononuclear cells suspended in 50µl PBS (phos-
phate-buffered saline) supplemented with 1% bovine serum
albumine and 1% sodium azide were added to 50µl of the monoclonal antibody dilution and incubated for 30min at 4°C. Then
the cells were washed twice and stained with fluoresceine con-
jugated $F(ab')_2$ antibody fragments from goat specific for
mouse immunoglobulins. After two final washings the cells
were resuspended in 500 µl of filtered PBS and analyzed.

Cytofluorograhic analyses of T-cell subpopulations were performed on a fluorescence-activated cell sorter FACS 440
(Becton-Dickinson) equipped with a 2-watt Argon Ion Laser.
Light scatter gating was employed in order to limit analysis
to viable lymphocytes.
Frequency and fluorescence profile of cells were determined
using logarithmic signal amplifiers, results were stored in
an ND 624 floppy-disc system (Nuclear Data, Inc.) The results
were expressed as the ratio Leu 3a/Leu 2a. The statistical
significance of the results was calculated with the
Student's t-test.

RESULTS:

In patients with zoster infection and cyclitis the helper
suppressor cell ratio was significantly higher than in normal
controls (p   0,025; Fig.1) In patients with herpes zoster
of the first trigeminal branch with no ocular complications
the helper/suppressor cell ratio was statistically proven to
be lower than in the control group (p   0,005).This difference was mainly due to the high percentage of suppressor cells
in patients with herpes zoster without cyclitis and to the
low percentage in patients with herpes zoster complicated by
cyclitis.

Fig 1

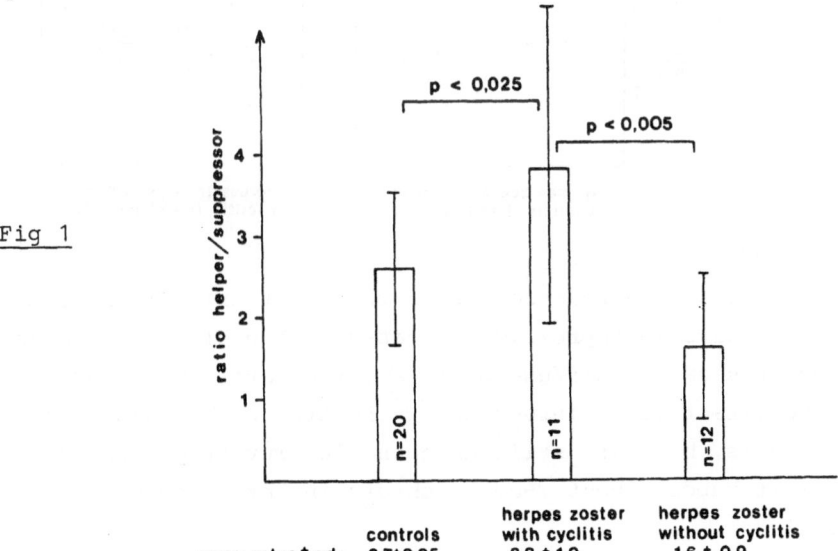

In remission the helper/suppressor cell ratio had the tendency
to decrease in herpes zoster patients with cyclitis whereas
it tended to increase in patients without uveitis (Fig.2)
The relatively high Leu 3 a/Leu 2 a ratio of the control
group has probably two reasons. First the high average age
a fact which was observed to shift the ratio significantly[13];
secondly the percentage used for calculations represents the
peak value of the FACS fluorescence profile, that are the
strongly and uniformly stained cells and not dull reactive
cells.

Fig. 2

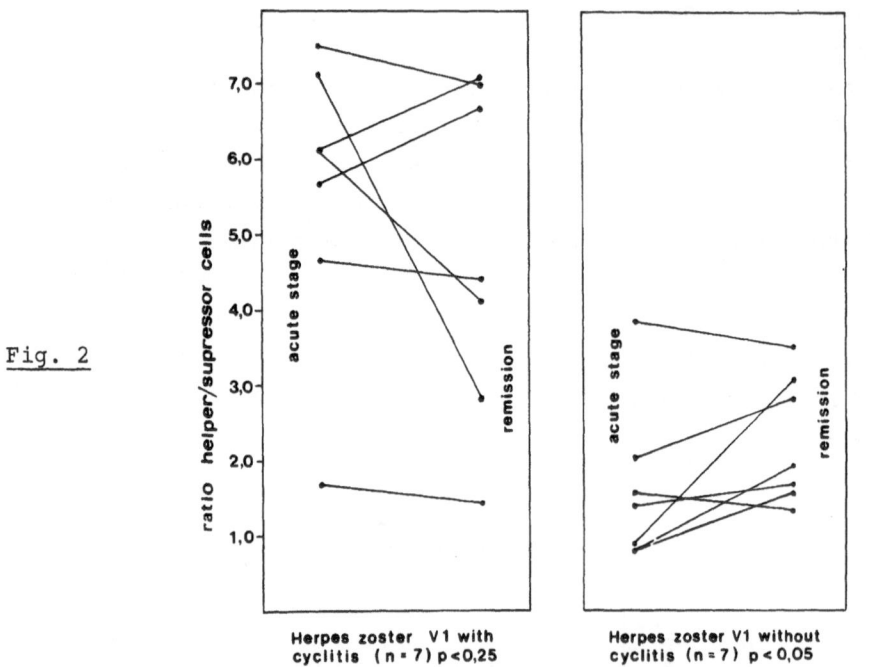

Herpes zoster V1 with
cyclitis (n = 7) p < 0,25

Herpes zoster V1 without
cyclitis (n = 7) p < 0,05

DISCUSSION:

In patients with herpes zoster of the first trigeminal branch,
uveitis occurs in approx. 40% of cases[14]. The clinical picture
of cyclitis can be diffuse or focal, the latter being probably
due to direct viral infection[15]. The true pathogenesis of
cyclitis is, however, still unknown. Our investigation is
the first report about T-cell subsets in herpes zoster
cyclitis.
We found in herpes zoster patients without cyclitis a
distinctly low ratio of Leu 3 a/Leu 2 a due to the presence

of a high percentage of suppressor cells. These results
correlate with studies by Arneborn and Biberfeld (16) and
Reinherz et al (17) who were able to demonstrate that virus
infections of the herpes group lead to an increase of the
number and percentage of Leu 2 a positive cells in the acute
phase. Viral infections are often associated with immunodeficiency states which might be due to both, activation and
increase of suppressor T-cells. Viral infections can activate
a specific T-cell subset and suppress the overall human
immune response.

In our investigation we found that the Leu 3 a/Leu 2 a ratio
was significantly higher in herpes zoster patients with
cyclitis involvement than in a control group. The high ratio
was the result of a considerable decrease in the percentage
of suppressor cells.

Low percentage of suppressor cells and low suppressor cell
activity have been found e.g. in SLE[18], in severe bovel
disease[19] and in multiple sclerosis[20]. This defective T-cell
immune suppression of B-cell activity has been related to
the activity level of disease and this phenomenon was considered to be a condition favouring autoimmune or hypersen-
sitive reaction. As our investigation has shown, a increase
of helper/suppressor T-cell ratio goes hand in hand with
the development of uveitis in the course of varicella/zoster
infection of the first trigeminal branch.

R E F E R E N C E S

1. Ticho, U., Silverstein, A.M., Cole,G.A.:
   Immunopathogenesis of LMC virus-induced uveitis: The
   role of T lymphocytes.
   Invest.Ophthalmol. 13 (1974) 229-231

2. Byrom, N.A., Hobbs, J.R., Timlin,D.M. Combell,M.A.,
   Dean,A.J., Webbley,M., Brewerton,D.A.:
   T and B lymphocytes in patients with acute anterior
   uveitis and ankylosing spondylitis and in their household
   contacts.
   Lancet II (1979) 609 - 613

3. Nussenblatt, R.B., Palestine,A.G., Rook, A.H., Seher, I.,
   Wacher,W.B., Igal, G.:
   Treatment of intraocular inflammatory disease with
   Cyclosporin A
   Lancet 2 (1983) 235 - 238

4. Belfort,R., Moma, N.C., Mendes, N.F.:
   T and B lymphocytes in the aqueous humor of patients with
   uveitis.
   Arch.Ophthalm. 100 (1982) 465 - 467

5. Boone, W.B., Gupta, S., Hansen, J., Good, R.A.:
   Lymphocyte subpopulations in patients with sympathetic
   ophthalmitis and non-granulomatous uveitis.
   Invest.Ophthalmol. 15 (1976) 957 - 960

6. Grabner, G., Berger, R., Knapp, W.:
   Concavalin-A-induced suppressor cell activity in inflamma-
   tory uveal disease
   VIth Congress of The European Soc. of Ophthalmology,
   London, Academic Press, Inc. Ltd. 487 - 491

7. Kaplan, H.J., Aarberg, T.M., Keller, R.H.:
   Etiology of recurrent clinical uveitis. Cell surface
   markers in vitreous lymphocytes. Ber.Dtsch.Ophthalm.Ges.
   78 (1981) 159 - 164

8. Kaplan, H.J.,Aarberg, T.W., Keller, R.H.: Lymphocyte
   sets in clinical uveitis. Invest. Ophthalm. 9 (Suppl.)
   (1980) 33

9. Murray, P.I., Rahi, A.M.S., Dinning, W.J. T-lymphocyte

subpopulations in acute anterior uveitis. Lancet (1983)
1167

10. Nussenblatt, R.B., Salinas-Carmona,M.,Leake,W.,Scher,I.
    T-lymphocyte subsets in uveitis.Am.J.Ophthalm.95 (1983)
    614 - 621

11. Secchi, A.G., Tremolada, F., Antona, C., Malacarne,
    Angi, H.R.
    Lymphocyte subpopulations in uveitis. Ber.Dtsch.Ophthalm.
    Ges. 78 (1981) 165 - 168

12. Ledbetter, J.A., Frankel, A.E., Herzenberg, L.A.:
    Human Leu T-cell differentiation antigens: Quantitative
    expression on normal lymphoid cells and cell lines.
    In: Hämmelling Eds.: Monoclonal Antibodies and T-cell
    Hybridomas. North Holland, Elsevier, 1981

13. Schroff, R.W., Gale, R.P., Fabey, J.F.: Lymphoid
    immaturity and T-subpopulation in balances in human
    disease. B and T cell tumors. Academic Press. Inc. 1982,
    285 - 291

14. Womack, L.W., Liesegang, T.L.: Complications of herpes
    zoster ophthalmicus. Arch.Ophthalmol. 101 (1983) 42-45

15. Sundmacher, R.: Die fokale Iritis durch Herpes simplex
    und Varizellen-Zoster-Virus.
    Ber.Dtsch.Ophthalm.Ges. 78 (1981) 73-76

16. Arneborn, P., and Biberfeld, G.: T-lymphocyte subpopu-
    lations in relation to immunosuppression in measles and
    varicella.Infection and Immunity 39 (1983) 29 . 37

17. Reinherz, E.L., O'Brien, C., Rosenthal, P., Schlossmann,
    S.F.: The cellular basis for viral-induced immunodeficien-
    cy: Analysis by monocloral antibodies.Journal of
    Immunology 125 (980) 1269 - 1274

18. Morimoto, C., Reinherz, E.L., Schlossman, S., Schur,P.H.
    Mills,J.A.,Steinberg,A.D.: Alterations in immunoregula-
    tory T cell subsets in active systemic Lupus erythemato-
    sus.J.Clin.Invest.66 (1980) 1171

19. Elson,C.O., Graeff,A.S., James,S.P.,Stober,W.Reactive
    suppressor T cells in Cohn's disease.Clin.Res.28 (1980)
    275

110

20. Reinherz, E.L., Weiner,H.L. et al.:
    Loss of suppressor T cells in active multiple sclerosis:
    analysis with monoclonal antibodies.
    N.Eng.J.Med. 303 (1980) 125 - 129

Author's adress:
Dr. T.M. Radda et al.
Spitalgasse 2, 1097 Wien, 1. Universitäts-Augenklinik
Austria

DISCUSSION :

G. Smolin (San Francisco) : I am not sure if I understand it exactly, whether or not the patients who had no cyclitits were late
in the disease process and originally had cyclitis and you
are now looking at them after the cyclitis has diminished.
In other words was your examination sequential ?

J. Funder (Vienna) : They are the same patients, after about four
months. But not all of them, I think only six of these 23.

L. Palmisano (Rome) : Did you check immunoglobuline levels and
show any correlation with the effect on suppressor cells ?

J. Funder (Vienna) : No, we didn't.

R. Sundmacher (Freiburg) : In this group were there all types
of iridocyclitis or these were only severe cases with protracted
course ? I am unable to see how the course of a minor, quick
healing iridocyclitis may be reflected by general immune responses.

J. Funder (Vienna) : No, in these patients clinical uveitis disappeared after about three weeks.

EXPERIMENTAL AND CLINICAL PRELIMINARY STUDY OF IMMUNO-
MODULATORS IN THE TREATMENT OF OCULAR HERPES.

J. DENIS, T. HOANG-XUAN, J.F. BONISSENT, K. DOGBE, C. CLAY
(Service d'Ophtalmologie, Hôtel-Dieu, Paris),
D. VIZA, F. ROSENFELD, J. PHILLIPS (Laboratoire d'Immunobio-
logie, Faculté de Médecine Broussais - Hôtel-Dieu, Paris),
and J.M. VICH (Research Group L. Grifols and L.F. Echevarne,
Barcelona).

1. INTRODUCTION

During an ocular herpes infection, the cell-mediated immune
response is the principal mean of resistance of the host, but
it can also be responsible for serious stromal and uveal
lesions. Immunomodulators should be handled with paticular
caution. The efficacy of diverses substances, such as isoprinosine (1), and transfer factor (TF) (4, 6, 7), is still uncertain. However the use of an antiherpes specific transfer
factor (TFd) (8) has decreased the intensity and the frequency
of recurrences both for genital and labial infections (5). In
this report, TFd is compared to isoprinosine during ocular
herpes.

2. TFd AND ISOPRINOSINE

2.1. TFd is a biological moiety which passively transfers cellular immunity. TFd specific for HSV1 was obtained by immuni-
zing a calf with 1 ml HSV1 antigen (Microbiological Associates)
mixed with 10 ml of Freunds complete adjuvant. 25 days later,
the lymphocytes were extracted from the spleen, the lymphatic
lymph nodes and the blood, disrupted by sonication and the
dialysate obtained by filtration through an amicon membrane.
1 unit of TFd is obtained from 10^8 cells.

2.2. Isoprinosine is a complex of inosine and N.N. dimethyl-
amino-2 propanol p-acetaminobenzoic acid in a 1:3 molar ratio
(Delalande Lab.). Isoprinosine stimulates the helper and
suppressor factors of the immune mechanism.

Maudgal, P.C. and Missotten, L., (eds.) Herpetic Eye Diseases.
© *1985, Dr W. Junk Publishers, Dordrecht/Boston/Lancaster. ISBN 978-94-010-8935-7*

3. HERPETIC KERATITIS OF THE RABBIT

3.1. Material and methods

3.1.1. Animal model

- 60 Fauve de Bourgogne rabbits, from 2 to 2.5 kg.
- The HSV1 strain was isolated from the throat of a child ; the viral suspension, prepared in KB cells, had a titer of 10^{-5} CPE 50 %.
- Day 0 : instillation in the right eye of each rabbit of 0.1 ml of viral suspension, followed by closing of the eyelids for 10 to 20 seconds.
- Day 3 : beginning of treatment after examination with a slit lamp. 2 drops of neomycin applied 4 times per day until day 14 to prevent secondary infection.
- Surveillance every 2 to 3 days with a slit lamp. The corneal surfaces, opaque or ulcerated, were graded as follows :

1 : minimal   4 : nearly 3/4
2 : nearly 1/4 of the surface   5 : the total surface
3 : nearly 1/2

The corneal neovessels were graded as follows :

Invasion of the limbus		Progression towards the center of the cornea
1 : minimal		1 : limb invaded
2 : nearly 1/4	+	2 : 1/4 of the corneal radius
3 : nearly 1/2		3 : 1/2
4 : nearly 3/4		4 : 3/4
5 : total		5 : corneal radius

3.1.2. Treatment with TFd, isoprinosine and controls.

On day 3, the 60 rabbits were randomized into 6 groups of 10 rabbits each. The right eye was treated and observed during 2 weeks for groups 1, 2, 3, 4 and a further two weeks for groups 5 and 6.

Group 1 : vaseline oil 4 times / day.

Group 2 : every 2 days (3 times / week), subconjunctival injection of 3 units of TFd, diluted in 0.5 ml of physiological saline.

Group 3 : Antiviral ointment, 1 % 5 iodo 2' deoxycytidine (IDC) 4 times / day.

Group 4 : TFd subconjunctivally + IDC.

Group 5 : 125 mg of isoprinosine (1.25 mg) intramuscularly days 3, 4, 5, 6 and 7, then 17, 18, 19, 20 and 21.

Group 6 : 1.25 ml of sterile saline solution by the same route on the same days.

3.2. Results

3.2.1. TFd administrated subconjunctivally did not modify the evolution of the corneal ulcers (Fig.1). However, cicatrization was favorised by IDC. On the other hand, TFd significantly reduced the formation of stromal opacities and neovessels (Table 1). The association TFd-IDC seems to be synergistic, and almost completely prevents the appearance of stromal lesions (Fig. 1.d).

Table 1. Comparison of lesions in TFd-treated and control rabbits : means of clinical score (standard deviation).

	Group 1 Control n = 10	Group 2 TFd n = 10	Student T test	Group 3 IDC n = 10	Group 4 IDC+TFd n = 10	Student T test
Day 3 ulcers (before tt)	1.94 (0.88)	1.50 (0.85)	NS	1.95 (0.90)	1.70 (0.95)	NS
Days 10-12 opacities (maximum)	2.67 (1)	1.40 (0.84)	$p < 0.02$ S+	0.90 (1.20)	0.10 (0.03)	$p < 0.05$ S+
Day 14 Neovessels	6.11 (3.79)	0.80 (1.32)	$2p < 0.001$ S+++	1.30 (2.16)	0.01 (0.03)	NS (limit)

3.2.2. Isoprinosine administrated intramuscularly did not modify the evolution of the keratitis (Fig. 2).

4. CLINICAL TRIAL ON RECURRENT OCULAR HERPES INFECTIONS
4.1. Patients and methods

- 17 patients having had at least 3 ocular herpes infections were randomly treated, 9 with isoprinosine and 8 with TFd. The treatment was always begun when the patient was in remission.

114

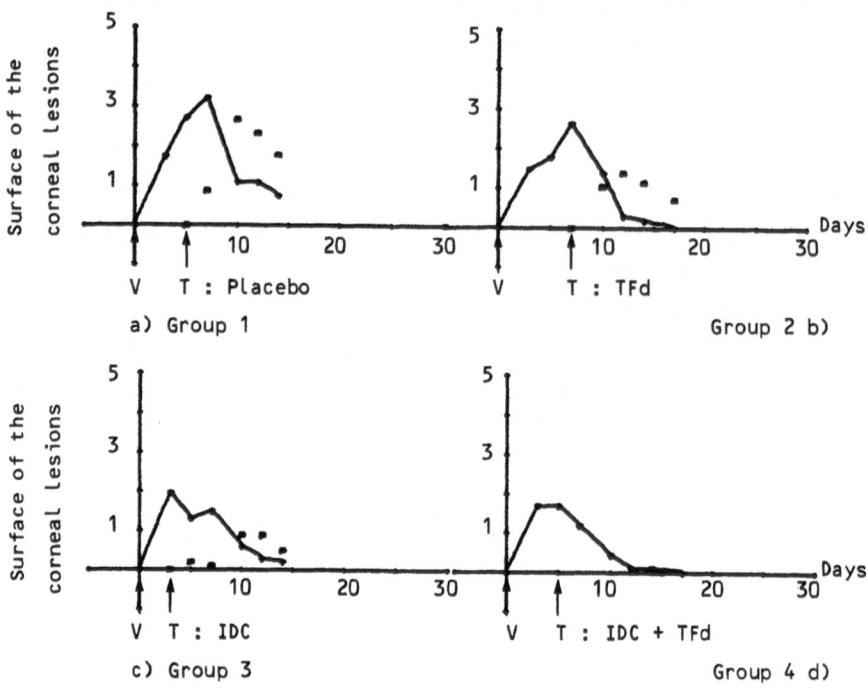

Fig. 1. Treatments with TFd subconjunctivally and controls.

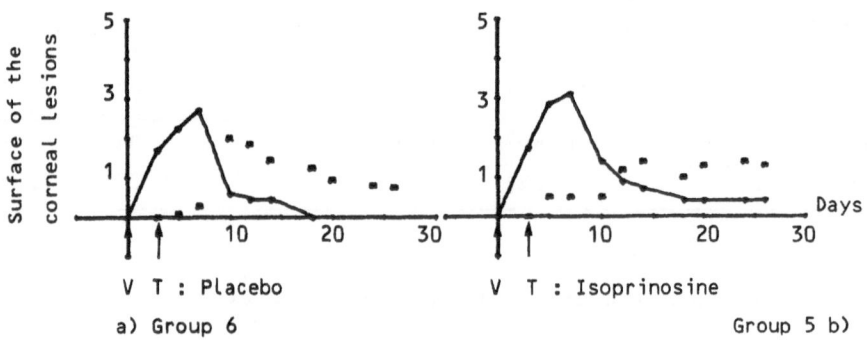

Fig. 2. Treatment with isoprinosine intra muscularly and control.
Evolution of corneal ulcers ——————
and stromal opacities ×××××

V : Virus inoculation.   T : Beginning of the treatment.

- Indications for treatment : increase in the frequency of relapses, the clinical severity, the resistance to the usual treatment with often corticoîds.
- Isoprinosine group : stimulation dose 25 to 50 mg/kg orally for 2 to 5 days every 2 weeks. The duration and the number of courses of treatment is a function of clinical improvement.
- TFd group (TFd specific for HSV1 or HSV1 and HSV2 in severe cases) : average weekly oral dose of 5 units, the dose being attained progressively over 2 months. The treatment lasted 7 to 52 weeks. The cellular immune response was evaluated by the Leukocyte Migration Inhibition Test (LMIT).

4.2. Results

4.2.1. The frequency of relapses seems to be lower with both treatments, with a slight advantage for TFd (Table 2, Fig. 3).

Table 2. Results. Frequency of recurrences.
T = recurrence period before treatment (in months)
T'= follow-up (in months) from the beginning of treatment

$$Q = \frac{\text{number of attacks}}{T} \times 100 \qquad Q' = \frac{\text{number of attacks}}{T'} \times 100$$

Isoprinosine					TFd				
Patients	T	Q	T'	Q'	Patients	T	Q	T'	Q'
1	27	51	23	0	1	9	33	10	0
2	6	33	12	0	2	28	14	9	0
3	12	25	17	0	3	21	14	27	0
4	12	33	17	6	4	36	8	5	0 insufficient T'
5	5	60	25	13	5	12	42	12	25 failure
6	12	58	27	8	6	4	75	13	0
7	12	33	26	4	7	12	25	4	0 insufficient T'
8	12	25	26	0	8	4	50	12	8
9	12	25	28	7					

4.2.2. The action on the opacities is not conclusive with either treatment (Table 3), and there is no correlation between the clinical state and the values of the LMIT.

116

Table 3. Results. Evolution of stromal opacities.

	Isoprinosine n = 9	TFd n = 8
Improved	3	2
Unchanged	6	4
Uninterpretable	0	2

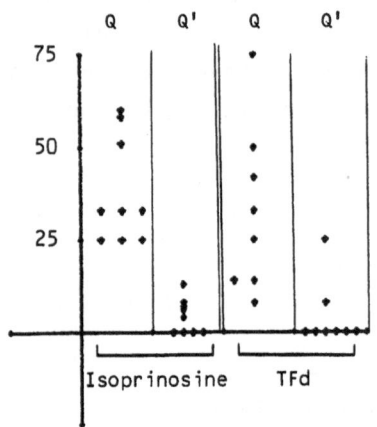

Fig.3. Efficacity on the frequency of recurrences

5. DISCUSSION

5.1. The specificity of the TFd for HSV may explain its therapeutical superiority for ocular herpes over traditional TF (6) and over isoprinosine.

5.2. In the rabbit, TFd administrated according to the protocol described above, has no direct antiviral action on corneal ulcers, but does diminish the stromal inflammatory reaction. It seems TFd causes an inhibition of the migration of lymphocytes and neutrophilic polynuclear cells into the stroma.

5.3. The tolerance to both isoprinosine and TFd in man is good. The repetition of courses of stimulating treatment with isoprinosine results in immunodepression after 3 months. The risk of overdose with TFd seems much lower. Finally, the use of these immunomodulators in association with corticoïds is illogical, and is particularly undesirable for TFd.

5.4. The stimulation can be dangerous for stromal keratitis or uveitis by accentuating the immunopathological phenomena. Preliminary animal experimentation is useful : however, the guinea pig or the mouse are more appropriate than the rabbit for the study of the cellular immune response.

5.5. The antiviral-immunomodulator association is synergis-

tic : IDC-TFd in this study ; TFT-isoprinosine (2) and aci-
clovir-TF (3) in previous reports.

5.6. The action of immunomodulators on the frequency of
relapses is difficult to evaluate because of the large number
of patients needed for a randomised clinical trial and in the
absence of well-defined biological criteria.

5.7. The dialysate, to which we refer in this text as TFd,
contains in fact several molecules : certain transfer a specific cell mediated immunity, others produce a non specific
immune stimulation whereas others inhibit specifically or non
specifically the cellular immune response. The purification of
the immunostimulators should allow an increase in therapeutic
efficacy.

REFERENCES

1. Berkman N, Legoix H, Moubri M, de Saxe E. Action favorable
de l'isoprinosine au cours des affections oculaires virales
et inflammatoires. Nouv. Presse Med. 8, 3829-3830.
2. Colin J, Bonissent JF, Renard G. 1982. Kératite herpétique
superficielle : traitement comparatif par Trifluorothymidine
ou par l'association Isoprinosine-Trifluorothymidine. Bull.
Soc. Ophtalmol. Fr. 82, 779-781.
3. Kohl S. 1983. Additive effect of acyclovir and immune
transfer in neonatal Herpes Simplex Virus Infection in mice.
Inf. Imm. 39, 480-482.
4. Rocha H. 1977. Der Transferfaktor in der Ophtalmologie.
Klin. Mbl. Augenheilk. 171, 63-70.
5. Rosenfeld F, Viza D, Phillips J, Vich JP, Binet O, Aron-
Brunetière R. 1984. Traitement des infections herpétiques
par le facteur de transfert. Presse Med. 13, 537-540.
6. Smolin G, Okumoto H. 1976. Human transfer factor in the
treatment of guinea pig keratitis. Ann. Ophthalmol. 8, 427.
7. Vignat JP, Hainaut J, Bourgeois H. 1978. A propos du
traitement de l'herpès cornéen par les dialysats d'extraits
lymphocytaires. Bull. Soc. Ophtalmol. Fr. 78, 551-554.
8. Viza D, Rosenfeld F, Phillips J, Vich JP, Denis J, Bonissent
JF, Dogbé K. 1983. Specific bovine transfer factor for the
treatment of herpes infections. In : Immunolobiology of
Transfer Factor, Kirkpatrick CH et al. eds, Academic Press,
New York, 245-259.

118

DISCUSSION :

C.S. Foster (Boston) : Seems to work best in patients that are immunosuppressed, and seems to work best in enhancing the cell mediated immune response. We tried in a number of patients and found it to be effective in selective population. We actually could not determine which patients would respond well to systemic Levamisol treatment. But we found that in a number of patients Levamisol did cause amelioration of the course of chronic herpetic disease. I have used isoprenosine in animal model and found the same, as you did. It was ineffective.

T. Huang-Xuan (Paris) : We have no experience of Levamisol treatment.

SUBUNIT VACCINE COMPARED WITH INFECTION AS PROTECTION AGAINST
EXPERIMENTAL HERPES SIMPLEX KERATITIS

B.A. Harney[1], D.L. Easty[1], G.R.B. Skinner[2]
[1] Department of Ophthalmology, University of Bristol, U.K.
[2] Department of Medical Microbiology, University of Birmingham, U.K.

INTRODUCTION

Education about the adverse effects of topical steroid, together
with the development of increasingly effective antiviral agents, has
improved the prognosis of herpes simplex keratitis (HSK). Antivirals,
however, have their limitations, for example; toxicity and the
development of resistance, and an approach aimed at prevention is worth
considering.

There has been some interest in the use of vaccines in the control
of herpes simplex virus (HSV) infections, and in experimental models,
both live (1,2,3) and inactivated (4) preparations have been shown to
protect against corneal infection with HSV. However, live virus carries
the risk of inducing latency, and recurrence at the site of inoculation,
and both live and inactived whole virus vaccines are considered
unsuitable for human use because of their oncogenic potential (5).

We have been investigating a subunit vaccine thought to contain no
biologicaly active DNA (6). We have demonstrated protection against a
primary corneal infection in both the rabbit and the mouse. The vaccine
was effective if used intramuscularly or subconjunctivally in the
rabbit, but not if used topically in the form of drops. The vaccine
elicited humoral and cellular immune responses, and its protective
effect persisted for several months. In the mouse, it reduced the
number of animals found to be latently infected in the trigeminal
ganglion following ocular infection (7,8).

In this experiment, the effects of vaccination on HSV in the rabbit
were compared with those of an ear infection with live HSV.

Maudgal, P.C. and Missotten, L., (eds.) Herpetic Eye Diseases.
© *1985, Dr W. Junk Publishers, Dordrecht/Boston/Lancaster. ISBN 978-94-010-8935-7*

Materials and Methods

Vaccine

The method of preparation for the inactivated subunit antigenoid vaccine Ac NFU (S) MRC was followed (9). For the purpose of this work, the vaccine was prepared in BHK 21 cells. Briefly, cells infected with HSV are disrupted by sonication. Treatment with the detergent Nonidet is thought to strip off important envelope antigens. After formeldehyde treatment, the preparation is ultracentrifuged over a sucrose cushion to pellet down remaining intact virus particles.

Virus

Herpes simplex virus type 1, strain pH, grown in Vero cells was used both for the ear infection and for corneal challenge.

Immunisation schedule

Experimental groups, each consisting of 6 New Zealand white rabbits, were treated as follows:

either 1) injected twice intramuscularly with 1 ml. of vaccine containing the equivalent of 10 infected cells, and aluminium hydroxide adjuvant, with two weeks between injections

or 2) infected in the right pinna by the subcutaneous inoculation of 1.1×10^6 pfu in 0.05 ml. of herpes virus.

A further 6 rabbits acted as controls.

Corneal infection

The corneas of vaccinated, infected and control animals were infected with HSV 6 weeks after the start of the experiment (i.e. 4 weeks after the 2nd vaccination) using the microtitration method of inoculation (1). The virus dose response curve and corneal infectious dose for 50% of inoculations (CID_{50}) were determined for all groups.

Total areas of ulceration as demonstrated by staining with Rose Bengal were measured 4, 7 and 11 days after corneal challenge.

Viral studies

The conjunctival sac was washed using 1.5 mls. of viral maintenance medium and the viral content of the washing was assessed by plaque formation on a Vero cell monolayer.

Immunological Methods

Anti HSV IgG was measured at several stages during the experiment using an ELISA test based on a method described by Bidwell et al. (10).

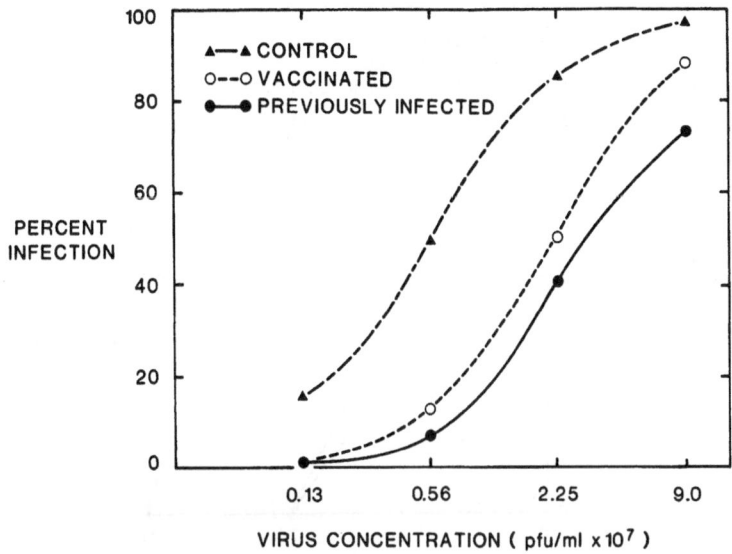

Fig. 1 Virus dose response curves for corneas of control, vaccinated
        and previously infected rabbits two days after corneal challenge

Results
Corneal Infection

Virus dose response curves 2 days after corneal infection showed
significant protection in both experimental groups ($p < 0.05$, method of
Reed and Munsch). CID was 0.6×10^6 for the control, 2.3×10^6 for the
vaccinated, and 3.0×10^6 for the infected group. (Fig.1)

Area of ulceration

In all animals, areas of ulceration reached a maximum at day 7, and
in most cases had cleared by day 11. It was on day 7 that the
differences between groups were most marked, although there was wide
variation between individual animals. By this stage, the previously
infected group showed significantly less ulceration than the controls
($p < 0.001$, t-test) whereas the vaccinated group showed comparable areas
to the controls.

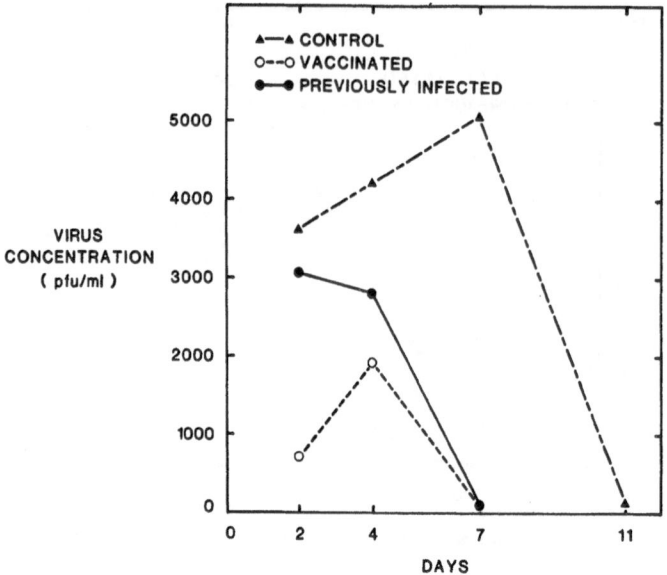

Fig. 2 Virus concentration in conjunctival washings after corneal
infection in control, vaccinated and previously infected
animals.

Viral studies

Average viral content of conjunctival washings was not
significantly different 2 and 4 days after corneal infection, with wide
variation between individuals.   However, by day 7, virus had almost
disappeared from both the immunised groups, but persisted in all the
control animals, in some cases with a high titre (Fig. 2).

Immunological Studies

ELISA Average values for HSV specific IgG antibodies followed a similar
pattern for the two groups, although those for the previously infected
group were consistently higher. Both groups showed a steep rise
following corneal infection, followed by a gradual decrease over the
next few weeks. The one control rabbit which survived till the end of
the experiment, showed levels approaching those of the experimental
group (Fig. 3).

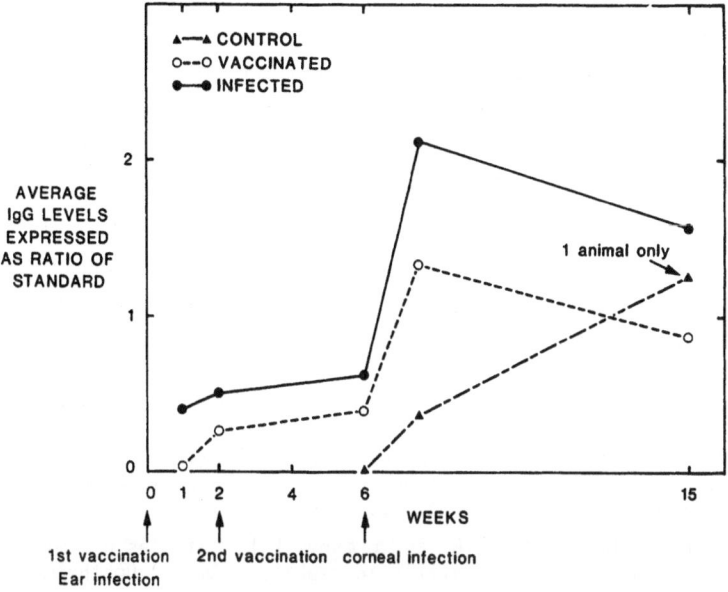

Fig. 3 Average levels of HSV specific IgG antibodies as determined by
ELISA test

Discussion

Replicating virus in this model would be expected to stimulate a
comprehensive systemic immune response comparable to a naturally
occurring situation. The vaccine did well in comparison, especially
when one takes into account that the strain of vaccine used for ear
infection and ocular challenge were the same. At day 2, the results for
the two groups were similar. Very few of the sites at the two lower
concentrations were infected and it seems that there is a level of viral
challenge at which both groups can be expected to show complete
protection.

The advantages of vaccination become less apparent later in the
observation period. In previous experiments, however it has been found
that the degree of residual corneal scarring and neovascularisation
correlates well with the day 2 results (unpublished observation).

There was wide variation in the virus content of conjunctival washings, but in both the immunised groups, virus disappeared earlier than in the controls.

In a previous paper (8), we concluded that as yet there was insufficient evidence to judge whether vaccination might have a role in the modification of recurrent ocular disease. It was argued, however, that this vaccine may well have a role in disease prevention. Although the relatively small proportion of the population suffering from ocular herpes does not in itself justify a large scale immunisation programme, it is probable that a reduction in ocular herpes infection would result if such a programme were to be instituted for the prevention of genital herpes.

REFERENCES

1. Carter, C. and Easty, D.L. Experimental ulcerative herpetic keratitis. I. Systemic immune responses and resistance to corneal infection. Br. J. Ophthalmol. 1981, 65, 77-81

2. Hall, R.L., MacKneson, R.G. and Ormsby, H.L. Studies of immunity in experimental herpetic keratitis in rabbits. Am. J. Ophthalmol. 1955 39, 226-233

3. Okumoto, M., Jawetz, E. and Sonne, M. Studies on herpes simplex virus IX. Corneal responses to repeated inoculation with herpes simplex virus in rabbits. Am. J. Ophthalmol. 1959, 47, 61-66

4. Metcalfe, J.F. Protection from experimental ocular herpetic keratitis by a heat-killed virus vaccine. Arch. Ophthalmol. 1980 98, 893-896

5. Vernon, S.K., Lawrence, W.C., Long, C.A., Cohen, G.H. and Ruben, B.A. Herpesvirus vaccine development: In New Trends and Developments in VAccines. Eds. Voller A. and Friedman, H. MTP Press Ltd., 1978, 179

6. Skinner, G.R.B., Williams, D.R., Buchan, A., Whitney, J., Harding, M and Bodfish, K. Preparation and efficacy of an inactived sub-unit vaccine (NFU BHK) against Type 2 Herpes Simplex Virus infection. Med. Microbiol. Immunol. 1978, 166, 119-132

7. Skinner, G.R.B. Pre-pubertal vaccination against herpes simplex virus infection towards prevention of cervical carcinoma. Blair Bell Memorial Lecture, London, Royal College of Obstetrics & Gynae. 1980

8. Harney, B.A., Easty, D.L. and Skinner, G.R.B. Investigation of a subunit vaccine using an animal model of herpes simplex keratitis. Trans. Ophthalmol. Soc. U.K. 1983, 103, 342-346

9. Carter, C.A., Hartley, C.E., Skinner, G.R.B., Turner, S.P. and Easty, D.L. Experimental ulcerative herpetic keratitis IV. Preliminary observations on the efficacy of a herpes simplex sub unit vaccine. Br. J. Ophthalmol. 1981, 65, 679-682

10. Bidwell, D.E., Bartlett, A. and Voller, A. Enzyme Immunoassays for Viral Disease. J. Infect. Dis. 1977, 136, suppl. 52, 74-78

DISCUSSION :

Y. Centifanto (New Orleans) : I would like to know more about the regimen for applying the vaccine topically. How often do you do this ? I would also like to know if you find antibodies in the tears of both immunized groups, and if you do, are they antibodies of the IgA, IgM, or IgG classes ?

B.A. Harney (Bristol) : In any of my work I have not been able to pick up neutralizing antibodies from tears and I have not managed to develop the ELISA for IgA in tears. So I cannot answer that question.

D. Viza (Paris) : I am not quite certain that I understand your reasoning for using a vaccine to prevent herpes infections. Human herpes is due to a defect in cell mediated immunity (CMI). In our experience, you can not improve this by using a vaccine. The information I have on the Birmingham vaccine and the trial on genital herpes is not very impressive. It was designed to protect healthy volunteers who had been in contact for several years with patients suffering from genital herpes. However, it is well known, and we have several cases among our patients, that some people never develop genital herpes even if they are sexual partners of herpes sufferers for many years. To try to protect, with a vaccine, those who are obviously resistant to herpes infections does not make sense to me.

B.A. Harney (Bristol) : I think in Birmingham study they compared with another group of patients who were not vaccinated. But I think that the Birmingham group themselves made a criticism of their methods and they hope to attempt a placebo controlled trial. These were just the preliminary results. I think they wanted to publish them because the results were so good.

C.S. Foster (Boston) : Dr. Viza, are you suggesting that the tens of millions of patients around the world who have herpes simplex colonization of one ganglion or another somewhere, have that because they have a defect in cell mediated immunity ?

D. Viza (Paris) : Indeed, it is quite probable that all these patients have a cell mediated immunity defect. In fact, in our
hands, the leukocytes of all herpes patients respond very poorly to HSV1 or HSV2 antigens when they are tested in the Migration Inhibition Test. More often than not, they have no antibody levels.

C.S. Foster (Boston) : It is a very well recognized phenomenon
that people who have a viral infection, at the time they show
evidence of clinical disease, they have alterations in their
immunoresponsivity. But to suggest that they are immune deficient, and they were so before they had contact with the virus,
and that immune defect is responsible for establishment of the
viral infeciton is not acurate.

D. Viza (Paris) : There is no evidence that this is correct, on
the contrary. Isn't it ?

C.S. Foster (Boston) : The best available evidence suggests
strongly that in normal population of people, who are well
tested and well characterized immunologically and have totally
intact immune systems, they are still quite capable of being
infected by herpes simplex virus.

D. Viza (Paris) : This depends on the status of the CMI of the
person at the moment he encounters the virus and the amount
of the infecting virus involved. I would like to make two
comments here : We study the CMI of herpes patients during
relapse and during remission. There is no reactivity to viral
antigens neither during relapse nor while the patient is in
remission. The second point concerns the use of a French vaccine (no longer commercially available) or a German vaccine
by some of our patients. These are chronic herpes sufferers
who have tried almost everything without success. The vaccination was also totally ineffective.

C.S. Foster (Boston) : I think the vaccination story, in the development of appropriate vaccine, is a complex story. But I
think the issue of whether or not individuals have a primary
imunodeficiency, that allows them to develop a herpes infection

in the first place, is a terribly important issue. I would like to hear some of the other specialists in the audience, and their remarks about this.

D.L. Easty (Bristol) : Way back we did simple lymphocyte trans- foramtion studies in patients with primary herpes, patients with recurrent disease and patients with stromal disease : only those with stromal disease had any hint of a deficit. Patients with recurrences or primary disease had very good immune responses using this simple technique.

C.S. Foster (Boston) : I think that it is fair to say that there are literally a number of investigators all around the world, who have tried to study populations of humans who have a variety of clinical forms of herpes. They use a variety of in vivo and in vitro assays trying to look at the immune sys- tem, trying to look at the natural killer cells, antibody pro- duction, tear levels of antibody; also in vitro lymphocyte pro- liferation and so on. I think that the human circumstance is so complex, with a variety of viral isolates and variety of genetics in the individuals, and the variety of the clinical patterns of disease, that it is simply not possible in 1984 to be dogmatic and categoric and make broad sweeping statements about the role of immune system in patients with recurrent her- petic disease.

D. Viza (Paris) : I am not certain that I made myself clear. I did not say that herpes patients suffer from a general im- mune deficiency, I said that they have a CMI defect which prevents the recognition of the HSV antigens; this is the only defect so far detectable in these patients. It would be interes- ting to correlate this with HLA phenotypes.

C.S. Foster (Boston) : Yes, I understand. My point is that there are a lot of other investigators who have done similar work and shown no differences between the herpetic patients and normal individuals. That is why I emphasize the complexity in this. Perhaps, there is someone else here who would like to make additional comment.

L. Palmisano (Rome) : We are investigating some patients with serious forms of herpes simplex, labialis and genitalis, and we have noticed a correlation between some aspects of the immune response and the seriousness of the disease. So, I agree with you that you can not identify an immunological profile shared by all those who suffer from relapsing herpes virus infections, but, surely, immunological background in these people is very important, and a selective deficiency, though unknown, must exist. Let us consider what happens with Epstein-Barr virus, which gives infectious mononucleosis in some people, chronic mononucleosis in others, Burkitt's lymphoma in others and, maybe, rheumatoid arthritis in others.

So, even if there is a virus induced immune deficiency, its expression depends upon the background.

C.S. Foster (Boston) : As in the mice.

IMMUNOLOGICAL ASPECTS AND THYMIC HORMONE THERAPY OF HERPETIC KERATITIS

P. PIVETTI-PEZZI[1], P. DE LISO[1], W. CALCATELLI[1], M.C. SIRIANNI[2], M. FIORILLI[2], I. MEZZAROMA[2] and L. PALMISANO[3]

[1]Institute of Ophthalmology II, University of Rome "La Sapienza", Rome, Italy, [2]Department of Clinical Immunology, University of Rome "La Sapienza", Rome, Italy and [3]Istituto di Ricerca Cesare Serono, Rome, Italy.

1. INTRODUCTION

The range of immunological abnormalities which underlie and sustain active infections by herpesviruses is wide (1) and makes the use of immunostimulating agents a promising therapeutic approach to them. Herpetic keratitis represent a quite severe manifestation of herpetic infection, since patients, if not treated, can develop blindness. Some patients with herpetic keratitis have been found to have impaired cell-mediated immunity (CMI) (1,2) and an immunostimulating therapy has also been proposed in the treatment of these patients.

We made a double-blind trial on immunostimulating therapy with the thymic hormone thymostimulin (Tp-1 Serono, Rome, Italy), which is known to potentiate CMI in the immunocompromised host (3) and to reduce the attack rate in people with recurrent herpes labialis (4).

2. MATERIALS AND METHODS

30 patients with herpetic keratitis (HK) were allocated to a double-blind trial with local treatment associated with either Tp-1 therapy or placebo, according to a therapeutic schedule, reported elsewhere (1). One patient of the placebo group missed out-patients checks and he was not considered in this study. 75 % of the patients were suffering from superficial keratitis with or without stromal involvement and the remaining from a deep one. Clinical follow-up ranged from 12 to 24 months. Immunological tests included the evaluation of Sheep Rosette Forming Cells (SRFC) (T lymphocytes) (1) from heparinized peripheral blood, and of the natural killer (NK) activity against the K562 cell line, according to the technique reported in (4).

Statistical analysis was done by CHI_2 test with Yate's correction, Log Rank test and Mann Whitney's "U" test.

Maudgal, P.C. and Missotten, L., (eds.) Herpetic Eye Diseases.
© *1985, Dr W. Junk Publishers, Dordrecht/Boston/Lancaster. ISBN 978-94-010-8935-7*

130

3. RESULTS

The follow-up at 24 months demonstrated a reduction of recurrence rate (p = 0.016) among Tp-1 patients, in comparison with controls (Fig. 1). In addition, SRFC, too, appeared significantly increased among the treated subjects (p < 0.001 at 15th day) (Fig. 2).

DOUBLE-BLIND TRIAL WITH THYMOSTIMULIN IN HERPETIC KERATITIS

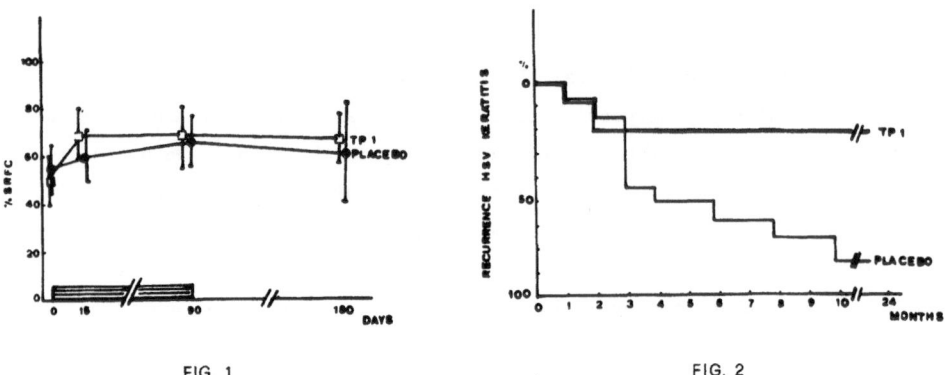

FIG. 1   FIG. 2

4. COMMENT

Our results demonstrate that Tp-1 is able to statistically reduce the relapse rate in patients with HK and is also able to increase the number of E rosettes, in comparison to subjects treated with placebo. The most striking finding is related to the possibility to control long-term and recurrent manifestations, which are responsible of the most severe clinical sequelae of the disease. Other previously used antiviral drugs have been found to effectively control only single attacks of the disease, while they were uneffective on the rate of recurrences. On the other side, Tp-1 has been found to have other different effects on the immune system, among which the ability to enhance interferon production (1) is very important, in view of the management of viral eye infections. In spite of the small number of patients treated by us, the results obtained represent the first example of a double-blind controlled study on thymic hormone therapy of herpesvirus infections of the eye. A study on a larger sample of population will further clarify the potential role of such treatment.

5. REFERENCES

1. Fiorilli M, Pivetti-Pezzi P, Sirianni MC, De Liso P, Testi R, Tamburi S, Russo G, Pontesilli O, Carbonari M, Luzi G. (1984). Thymic hormone therapy of herpetic diseases. In: Proc. of the International Symposium on Thymic Factors Therapy (London, April 25-27, 1983). Academic Press, in press.
2. Businco L, Rossi P, Quinti I, Perlini R. (1980). In: Thymus Thymic Hormones and T Lymphocytes. Aiuti F, Wigzell H (eds.), Academic Press, London, p. 295.
3. Aiuti F, Sirianni MC, Paganelli R, Stella A, Turbessi G, Fiorilli M. (1984). Clin. Immunol. Immunopathol. 30, 11.
4. Sirianni MC, Businco L, Seminara R, Aiuti F (1983). Clin. Immunol. Immunopathol. 28, 361.

PRIMARY OCULAR HSV INFECTIONS IN ADULTS

C.AMEYE, P.C.MAUDGAL AND L.MISSOTTEN

1. Introduction.

A primary herpes simplex virus (HSV) infection usually develops in childhood and remains generally unrecognised as no clinical disease develops in about 50 to 90 % percent cases[1-3]. A subclinical primary infection can only be detected by the appearance of circulating antiherpes antibodies.

Epidemiological data reveal the presence of antiherpes antibodies in 60% of the population under 5 years of age, this incidence increasing to 90% at fifteen years[4].According to other authors[5,6], circulating antiherpes antibodies are found in 40% to 80% of adults. At the age of 60 years, 97% of the population may have developed antiherpes antibodies[6]. The incidence of HSV infection is much higher in the low socio-economic groups living under poor hygienic conditions[4,6-8] and in crowded communities[9].

The incidence of primary infection in the population shows two peaks. The first peak, essentially due to HSV type 1, occurs between 6 months to 5 years of age; and during the second peak, between 16 and 25 years, antibodies to HSV type 2 usually begin to appear[10].

Clinical primary infection is generally mild. Severe generalised and even life-threatening primary infections may occur in the newborn, the atopic patients with immunological disorders or immunosuppressed patients.

Although HSV type 1 has a predilection to cause gingivostomatitis, infections of the upper respiratory tract, ocular and cutaneous infections, and HSV type 2 generally produces anogenital and neonatal infections, both types of the virus may affect any body organ[11].

Inferring from epidemiological data a primary HSV infection in adults, especially a primary ocular infection, would be uncommon. In addition, this condition may not be recognised as ophthalmo-

Maudgal, P.C. and Missotten, L., (eds.) Herpetic Eye Diseases.
© *1985, Dr W. Junk Publishers, Dordrecht/Boston/Lancaster. ISBN 978-94-010-8935-7*

logists are generally unaware of the condition. Moreover, the initial clinical picture of the disease is misleading.

This report presents the clinical features of a primary HSV infection with ocular involvement in six adult patients. All of them had been misdiagnosed by different ophthalmologists.

2. Clinical data.

2.1. Complaints at onset : six female patients, aged between 18 and 37 years, were referred to us with a worsening eye condition which started with an increasing itching and irritation of one eye. In all cases the eye was red. Associated epiphora, sticky yellow mucopurulent discharge and increasing swelling of the eyelids were present.Three patients had a history of eczema, hay fever or allergy.

The referring ophthalmologists had unsuccessfully treated these patients for bacterial conjunctivitis with either topical antibiotics or antibiotic-corticosteroid preparations. In one patient a diagnosis of eyelid cellulitis and allergy had been made. Another patient, who had quickly developed perioral herpes simplex blisters, was advised by her ophthalmologist to instill topical IDU eyedrops every two hours as a prophylaxis.

2.2. General status : All patients complained of marked malaise and fatigue three to four days after the onset of ocular disease. Fever, upto 38,5°C, developed in four patients. Three patients developed sore throat, rhinitis and/or tonsillitis, which had been diagnosed elsewhere as an upper respiratory tract infection with ocular involvement. These patients had also received systemic antibiotics. Another patient had to be hospitalised because of severe headache and malaise as meningitis was suspected. In all patients preauricular lymphnodes were enlarged and tender. Submandibular, cervical, axillary and inguinal lymphadenopathy was present in different patients (Table I).

2.3. Eyelid and skin lesions : All patients had blepharitis with marked swelling of the eyelids. In five patients vesicles and

erosions of the lid margin were observed. Herpetic vesicles
on the periorbital skin, forehead, cheeck, nose, perioral skin
and hand were observed in different patients (Table I).

Table I : Lymphadenopathy and skin lesions in six adult patients
with primary ocular HSV infection.

Regional lymphadenopathy	Number of patients
Preauricular	6
Submandibular	4
Cervical	5
Axillary	3
Inguinal	3
Eyelid and skin lesions	
Blepharitis with marked eyelid swelling	6
Vesicles/erosions on eyelid margin	3
Herpetic vesciles :	
-periorbital	6
-nose	2
-perioral	3
-elsewhere	1

The hospitalised patient, with history of eczema, exhibited eczema-
tous skin changes of the swollen periorbital skin that gradually
extended to the whole face and neck. The herpetic vesicular erup-
tions on the eyelids and on other skin areas generally appeared
from two to six days after the onset of illness.
2.4. Conjunctival and corneal lesions : All patients presented with
red eyes, conjunctival chemosis and follicular conjunctivitis .
The swollen eyelids were stuck together by copious yellow
mucopurulent discharge. Conjunctival pseudomembranes were
present in four patients and subconjunctival hemorrhages in
two patients. In one case there was a conjunctival ulcer on
the lower eyelid.

Corneal lesions developed from two to five days after the onset of ocular symptoms. When we saw the patients, all of them had multiple coarse punctate and stellate corneal lesions. Five patients had one or more dendritic ulcers. In four cases limbal lesions were present. Only one patient had a single large central keratic precipitate.

In all cases follicular conjunctivitis developed in the fellow eye after two to five days. The disease was always mild in the second eye. Keratitis also became bilateral in four patients. Only punctate lesions were observed in the fellow eye.

2.5. Diagnosis : We initially diagnosed HSV infection in these patients on the basis of history and clinical picture. In three patients, who were seen within one week of the onset of disease, antiherpes antibodies were absent in serum. These antibodies had appeared when titers were tested again after one week or 10 days (Table II) interval. HSV was isolated from the eyes of these patients.

Table II : Laboratory data.

Patient	Circulating anti-HSV antibodies			Virus isolation from the eye
	1st titer	Interval	2nd titer	
1	neg.	1 week	1/128	HSV +
2	neg.	1 week	1/64	HSV +
3	neg.	10 days	1/32	HSV +
4	1/4	7 weeks	1/32	–
5	–		–	–
6	–		–	HSV +

The other three patients were seen more than one week after the onset of illness. Serological tests to demonstrate the absence of antiherpes antibodies were not done in two of them, but in one of these patients HSV type 1 was isolated from the eye. The third patient, who was seen 10 days after the onset of disease had an antiherpes antibody titer of 1/4, which is a very low titer. Seven weeks later, this titer was 1/32. Probably the first low titer could have been a beginning stage of antibody production. Although a primary HSV infection has not been demonstrated in the last three patients on the basis of serological tests, their clinical history, and clinical picture is identical to the other three proven cases of primary infection.

3. Management and complications.

All patients were advised bed rest. The eye disease was treated by topical 0,1% BVDU (bromovinyldeoxyuridine) eyedrops to be instilled every hour during the day only.

General symptoms ameliorated in all patients in 7 to 10 days and the ocular disease subsided in four to 21 days. Blepharitis and skin lesions heald in one to three weeks. Stromal infiltration developed in one patient. Lacrimal canaliculitis of the first involved eye developed in two patients during the second week and in a third patient 6 months later. One patient developed recurrent herpes simplex vesicles on the eye lid and lidmargin.

4. Conclusion.

On the basis of these six adult patients, the common features of a primary ocular HSV-infection can be summarised as follows :

1. Unilateral onset of conjunctivitis with severe itching, irritation, redness, epiphora, mucopurulent discharge and eyelid swelling.

2. Systemic symptoms with marked malaise and lymphadenopathy.

3. Vesicles on the eyelidmargins producing ulcerative blepharitis, and skin vesicles on the periorbital skin and other body areas.

4. Involvement of the second eye after two to five days with conjunctivitis or keratoconjunctivitis.

5. Severity of the eye disease and regional lymphadenopathy more pronounced on the side of the first involved eye.

6. Involvement of the cornea after two to five days starting as fine diffuse punctate erosions that develop into coarse punctate keratitis and dendritic ulcers. Presence of limbal lesions.

To conclude, primary ocular herpetic infections may occur in adults, but the initial symptoms are often misleading. Serological evidence of primary infection, and HSV isolation from the eye need time, so that the initial diagnosis has to be based on the clinical examination to commence specific antiherpes therapy.

138

BIBLIOGRAPHY

1. LEOPOLD IH, SERY TW 1963 Epidemiology of herpes simplex keratitis.Invest.Ophthalmol. 2, 298–303.

2. DARRELL RW 1972 Ocular infections caused by the herpes virus group. In Locatcher-Khorazo D, Seegal BC, Microbiology of the eye, St. Louis, CV Mosby, p 302.

3. WHEELER CEJr. 1973 Kaposi's varicelliform eruption. In Denis DJ, Crounse RG, Dobson RL, McGuire J(Eds) : Clinical Dermatology. Vol. 3 Hagerstown, Harper & Row, pp 1–6.

4. BUDDINGH GJ, SCHRUM DI, LANIER JC, GUIDRY DJ 1953 Studies of the natural history of herpes simplex infection. Pediatrics 11 : 595–610.

5. NESBURN AB 1975 Recurrence in ocular herpes simplex infection. Int. Ophthalmol. clin. 15, 101–110.

6. SMITH IW, PEUTHERER JF, MAC CALLUM FO, 1967 The incidence of herpes virus hominis antibody in the population. J. Hyg. 65, 395–408.

7. MAC CALLUM FO, 1959 Generalized herpes simplex in the neonatal period. Acta virol. 3 (suppl.) : 16–21.

8. DUKE-ELDER S, 1965 Diseases of the outer eye. Vol. 8, Part 1, System of Ophthalmology, St. Louis, CV Mosby, p 309.

9. ANDERSON SG, HAMILTON J, 1949 The epidemiology of primary herpes simplex infection. Med.J. Aust. 1, 308.

10.DOWLING RD, HENRY K, 1972 Nonresponsive coeliac disease (clinicopathological Conference) Br.Med.J. 3, 624–631.

11.OSTLER HB, 1976 Herpes-simplex : the primary infection. Surv. Ophthalmol. 21, 91–99.

DISCUSSION :

P. Wright (London) : I think this is a difficult group, as you
   say, in which to make a diagnosis. We have a slightly different piece of evidence derived from looking at patients who
   presented to Moorfields Eye Hospital Casualty Department with
   non-bacterial conjunctivitis with a mixed follicular-papillary
   response in the conjunctival sac. We hoped for useful diagnostic information by doing isolations to herpes, chlamydia and
   adenovirus or from antibody titers. In fact, we got positive
   evidence in only 25 % of cases in this investigation. 75 %
   had no agent that we could determine, which I must say was
   rather a depressing conclusion, but at the same time that
   sets in perspective the rather expensive laboratory investigations that tend to be promoted vigorously by the scientists.

G.O. Waring (Atlanta) : A very naive and simple question. You
   have any idea why people with primary herpes get so many
   dendrites in the cornea, where as in recurrent herpes multiple
   dendrites are not nearly as common ?

C. Ameye (Leuven) : No, I have no explanation. But do you think
   it is so often seen, those dendritic lesions in primary infection?

G.O. Waring (Atlanta) : Certainly when they occur, they are much
   more commonly multiple like that.

C. Ameye (Leuven) : I don't know any explanation for that.

A.A. Tye (Adelaide) : When you say there was involvement of the
   fellow eye, was that with dendrites ?

C. Ameye (Leuven) : Mostly it was punctate keratitis.

R. Sundmacher (Freiburg) : That was a beautiful presentation,
   and I agree with nearly every point you made. Let me just
   bring up one thing with which I disagree : In the course of
   primary herpetic infection you may observe a pronounced follicular reaction. However, I have seen more cases with virtually
   no follicular conjunctivitis. Therefore, this type of reaction
   is by no means pathognomonic for true primary infection. There are other clinical signs which - if they are present - allow
   for the diagnosis of primary herpes. These are (1) confluent
   intermarginal blepharitis, and (2) true limbal dendrites, which

reside more in the conjunctival than in the corneal part of the limbus.

P.C. Maudgal (Leuven) : Your remark about follicular conjunctivitis is correct but it depends at what stage you see the patient. In a beginning conjunctivitis there are no follicles. And in many cases, mostly it was in our cases, they have used topical corticosteroids for red eye. This might suppress the follicular response whereas the disease flourishes further. This danger we intended to point out here.

M.G. Falcon (London) : It is interesting to postulate why this condition should not be common. Figures from London suggested that the incidence of previous exposure to herpes virus has been falling whether it is type 1 or type 2. Seventy five percent used to be quoted; now it is more like 30 %. Why it should be so seldom that we see this primary herpes coming in adults ?

P.C. Maudgal (Leuven) : Serological studies indicate that the incidence of herpes simplex virus infection increases with age. With a rise in the socio-economic standards, and better hygeinic conditions, the incidence of primary infection might decrease, as you have said.

The question as to why primary herpes simplex eye infection is not that common in adults may also be related to the simple fact that the disease, perhaps, is not recognised in the early stages, when the clinical picture is difficult to differentiate from bacterial conjunctivitis. Our patients had been treated with antibiotics and corticosteroids by different ophthalmologists, as they were probably not aware of the condition. Another point is that by the time patient comes to you the typical clinical picture, that we have described here, may have changed. So in these patients one would diagnose herpes simplex eye disease, but not a typical primary infection. This paper emphasizes that we may expect primary ocular herpes infections in adults.

A CASE OF BILATERAL HERPES SIMPLEX EYE DISEASE OF LONG
DURATION

A.A. TYE

1. INTRODUCTION

Herpetic eye disease, of the type causing dendritic ulceration of the
cornea, is well known, and because of its recurrent nature, is one disease in
which long-term treatment of a particular patient is common.   A rather
longer course of treatment may be necessary where bilateral disease exists.
The purpose of this paper is to report such a case.

2.   UNILATERAL DENDRITIC ULCER

To both patient and ophthalmologist it is a fortunate fact that herpes
simplex involvement of the cornea is unilateral, almost exclusively. Despite
years of treatment to one eye, and perhaps with some fears by the patient
that the reverse may be so, involvement of the other eye must be exceedingly rare.   One's own patients provide evidence of this, and I have detailed
relevant information for three of my patients. (Table 1)

PATIENT	AGE (years) FIRST SEEN	DURATION OF ATTEND- ANCE	VISION	
			AFFECTED EYE	NORMAL EYE
C.G.	4	1966- 1984	6/60	6/6
G.P.	24	1961- 1982	6/9	6/6
S.C.	8	1961- 1970	6/36	6/6

Table 1.   Unilateral Dendritic Eye Disease

3.   BILATERAL DENDRITIC ULCER

The case to be described is of a man born in 1922. His general health
was regarded as A1 when he submitted for a medical examination for entry
into the Australian Military Forces in 1941. It was noted then that he did

Maudgal, P.C. and Missotten, L., (eds.) Herpetic Eye Diseases.
© *1985, Dr W. Junk Publishers, Dordrecht/Boston/Lancaster. ISBN 978-94-010-8935-7*

have blepharitis, but vision was quite normal in both eyes. Although he did not enter the army until 1944, he had trouble with his right eye in 1943. Details of this affection are not known, except for the fact that it was a mild one, and the eye healed satisfactorily at home after a week or so.

In 1944 and 1945, whilst in the army, the patient had severe ulcers of his right cornea. Treatment was given in the standard manner of that time, but anti-viral agents were not then available. His army records show that the first attack occurred at a country hospital, and that specialist attention was sought soon afterwards in Sydney. However, the nature of the original attack was not clearly evident from the notes. The diagram below shows the picture of his right cornea shown in one of the attacks, and a linear line of fluoroscein stain is evident. (Diagram 1)

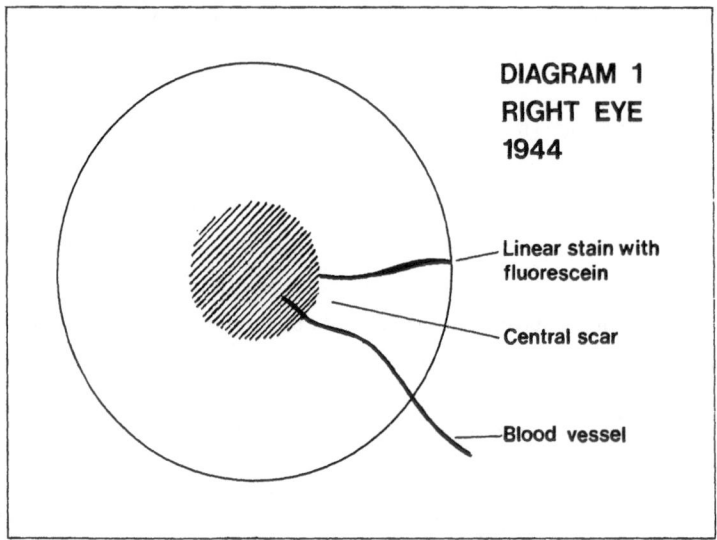

On his discharge from the army in 1945 the eye remained quiet, corneal ulceration recurring in 1962, after an attack of 'flu. The cornea healed slowly. In 1964 a typical herpetic staining pattern recurred. (Diagram 2)

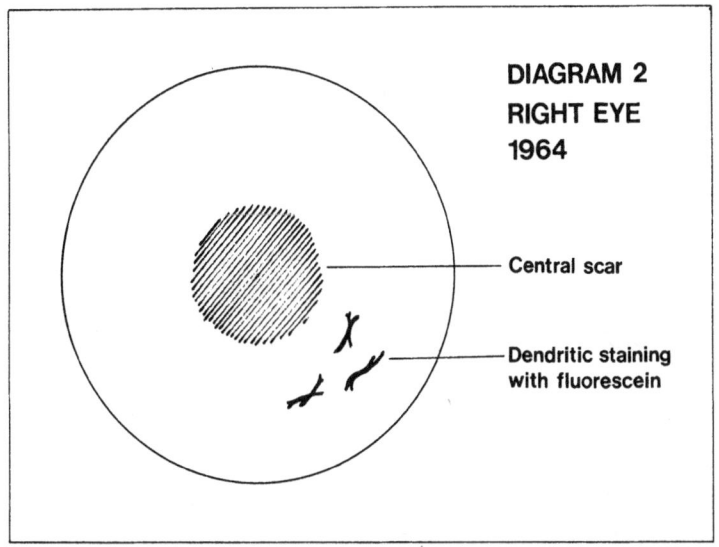

**DIAGRAM 2
RIGHT EYE
1964**

———— Central scar

———— Dendritic staining
with fluorescein

Some 12 years later the right eye was again quiet, but a mature cataract was present. This was removed successfully in 1976, but the corneal scar prevented visual recovery.

In 1980 the left eye showed herpetic ulceration of the cornea for the first time. The dendritic pattern was situated mainly superiorly, and antiviral management (I.D.U. and Vidarabine) was effective in healing. However, disciform keratitis and iritis complicated the picture in 1983. At this time the lower part of the cornea also showed a temporary slight dendritic pattern of ulceration. (Diagram 3)

144

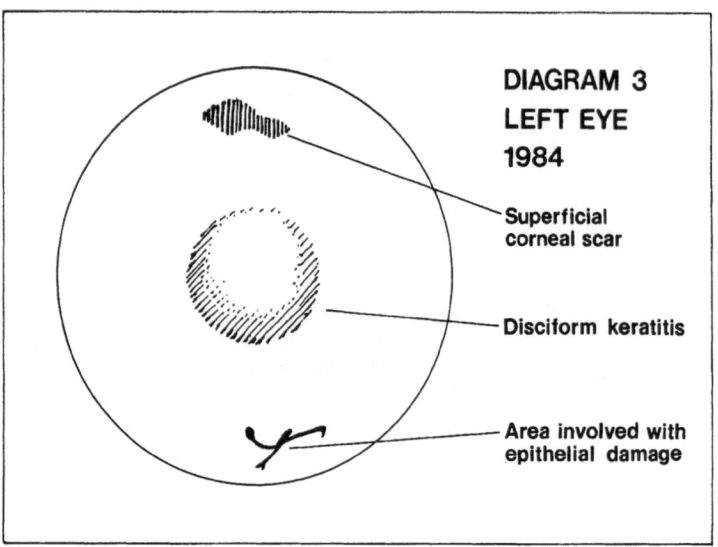

DIAGRAM 3
LEFT EYE
1984

Superficial
corneal scar

Disciform keratitis

Area involved with
epithelial damage

At the time of presenting this report the patient's left vision is good, and a maintenance dose of corticosteroid therapy in local drop form is the only therapy necessary.

4. CONCLUSION

A case of bilateral herpes simplex corneal disease is reported, scanning a 40 year period. It is not possible to say why the condition has affected both eyes. The patient has had mild eczema, but it is unlikely that this has served as a pre-disposing factor.

DISCUSSION :

C.C. Kok-van Alphen (Leiden) : We found about 10 people with
   bilateral herpes in a long period. But why did not you do
   a keratoplasty, because this poor patient will get many recurrences ?

A.A. Tye (Adelaide) : The patient does not particularly want that
   at the moment and I don't want to push too hard.

P.C. Maudgal (Leuven) : I would like to ask Dr. Kok-van Alphen,
   does keratoplasty prevent recurrences ?

C.C. Kok-van Alphen (Leiden) : Of course not. But it will re-establish vision, and recurrences will not be many and in any
   case not painful.

A.A. Tye (Adelaide) : His left vision is good at the moment.
   His exact vision is quite usable.

C.C. Kok-van Alphen (Leiden) : But it is a lot less trouble for
   the patient because you take away quite a lot of the bad tissue.

P.C. Maudgal (Leuven) : Yes, but there are problems of recurrence and possible graft rejection, especially when the vision
   is poor in the fellow eye.

C.C. Kok-van Alphen (Leiden) : Not that bad.

F. Lagoutte (Bordeaux) : We have an interesting case of bilateral
   herpes which occured in a man who has general pemphigus
   with ocular involvement, which is very rare. This is the sixth
   case in the world. He developed superficial corneal herpes
   in both eyes, one three years ago and the other two months
   ago. I think it was induced by corticosteroids, or immuno-sup-
   pressive therapy.

A.A. Tye (Adelaide) : Thanks, that is very interesting.

P. Wright (London) : Yes, I think we all have experience in renal
   transplant patients too, who present to us with severe herpes.
   Atopy and herpes, we all can agree, I think, are patients
   who present with very disagreable very progressive, often
   bilateral herpetic disease. Is that the general feeling ?

Audience : Yes.

J.McGill (Southampton) : You have raised the question how blepharitis possibly can affect herpes. Yes, two ways. One, the blepharitis will upset tear production, you get tear evaporation.
As the cornea dries out, you get erosions. As a chronic herpetic patient is shedding virus intermitantly, these erosions
can be colonized by virus and develop into dendritic ulcers.
And secondly, because you get dry eye from blepharitis, they
get an epithelial disturbance. This is much worse in atopic
patients.

D.L. Easty (Bristol) : We have quite a few patients with atopic
disease and bilateral disease. Sometimes, it is very subtle;
if you go way back in their history they had eczema in childhood when they got their primary infection, which might have
spread bilaterally then. Sometimes it is interesting to look
a bit further into patients; if you evert the tarsal plates,
you can sometimes find evidence of quite major atopic changes
in the tarsal plates. Does this patient have anything like
that ?

A.A. Tye (Adelaide) : Well, we generally do this. We have fairly high incidence of trachoma. Dr. Coster everted the eyelids
at one stage and examined by putting fiber glass under the
top lids. This patient certainly had no chronic changes under
the conjunctiva.

J.McGill (Southampton) : Going back to the problem of lid infections; if they have a chronic lid infection and they are atopic, they have a reduction in tear secretion. They will also
have reduction in local specific and non-specific immunoglobulin, IgA, lactoferrin and lysosome. This will make them more
susceptible to recurrent infection.

From the Department of Ophthalmology

Hamburg—University

(Head: Prof. Dr. J. DRAEGER)

DIFFERENTIAL DIAGNOSIS OF HERPETIC KERATITIS BY MEANS OF A NEW
ELECTRONIC OPTICAL AESTHESIOMETER

J. Draeger, R. Winter, G. Krolzig

Corneal sensitivity triggers one of the most sensitive protection
reflexes of the human body. The threshold in healthy people —
especially in the corneal centre — is exceedingly low. For this reason
pathological changes can be diagnosed particularly early and very
precisely. In particular these measurements allow conclusions about
the general state of the cornea.

In former times the determination of corneal sensitivity was
difficult. In 1895 von FREY introduced the first aesthesiometer:
A "defined" filament was affixed to a wooden handle. With this device
he examined the sensitivity of the normal cornea. Since that time
several workers have tried to improve aesthesiometrie to achieve
better results (SCHIRMER, 1963, LARSON 1970). A semiquantitative
measurement by varying the length of the filament (COCHET and
BONNET, 1961) is possible, but the methodological problem remains:
When using filaments not only does their age matter, but also humidity,
temperature and several other parameters mainly including the skill of
the examiner.

But now by means of a recently developed electronic—optical
instrument a quantitative reproduceable aesthesiometry is achieved
(DRAEGER et al 1976).

Fig. 1:   Electronic—optical aesthesiometer
This apparatus allows the generation and measurement of extremely
small forces. Optical control of the measurement was mandatory to
determine precisely the location of the contact with the corneal
epithelium. By devision of the images in the eye pieces simultaneously
a corneal profile and the lateral location of the contact pin can be
observed. A digital display continously indicates the applied force.
The aesthesiometer fullfills the following criteria:

Maudgal, P.C. and Missotten, L., (eds.) Herpetic Eye Diseases.
© *1985, Dr W. Junk Publishers, Dordrecht/Boston/Lancaster. ISBN 978-94-010-8935-7*

1. High precision, independance from external conditions.
2. Optical control of the contact pin touching the cornea.
3. Continuous alteration of the applied force from 0-1.000 × 10^{-5} N.
4. Dynamically increasing the force whilst on the cornea.
5. Swift and easy handling by one hand only.
6. Exact defined diameter of the contact pin 0,5 mm.

The higher threshold of cornea sensitivity as a main symptome
in herpes simplex was found by KRÜCKMANN in 1895. The reduction of
sensibility was not concerned to the area of the lesion, but was found
throughout the cornea. Only recently SEVERIN (1965) and NORN (1970)
conducted similar studies. They used the aesthesiometer by COCHET
& BONNET, which had still a lof of methodical problems.

We started our examinations with the new aesthesiometer by
DRAEGER to get exact quantitative reproduceable measurements;
looking for the threshold values of the corneal sensitivity we should
get more exact information of the severeness and stageing of herpes
keratitis. Nevertheless the aesthesiometer should bring more reliability
in differential diagnosis.

MATERIAL AND METHODS:
A random sample of patients having attended the University Eye Department of Hamburg for corneal diseases(years: 1976 - 1983). All patients
were examined clinically. Then aesthesiometrie of the cornea was done.
Depending on the course of the disease we repeated the aesthesiometric
measurement. The herpetic keratitises were divided into three groups:
1. Keratitis dendritica - one occurrance, superficial
2. Recurrent keratitis dendritica with superficial and superficial
stromal involvement
3. Severe stromal keratitis.

These groups were compared with patients who suffered from
keratitis caused by bacterial or mycotic infections.

In addition we conducted a study examining patients who suffered
from herpes keratitis in the previous three months to 2 years. Excluded
from this study were patients with other eye disease.

For this study we used the electronic optical aesthesiometer of
DRAEGER. Sensitivity measurements were taken in 5 positions (central

and near the limbus at 3, 6, 9 and 12.00 h). We took measurements from
both eyes of the patients, using the unaffected as control. By this we
were able to determine the individual threshold of every patient.

RESULTS:

Patients suffering from keratitis dendritica the first time showed
no disturbance in their corneal sensitivity. Measurements in the
affected area with the herpetic lesions showed similar results.
Threshold values were about 1×10^{-5} N. This means there was no difference to the contralateral healthy eye.

In recurrent herpetic keratitis we found a distinct disturbance
of sensitivity. While the contralateral eye showed normal sensitivity,
in the affected eye threshold values increased to $10 - 90 \times 10^{-5}$ N with
an average of 52×10^{-5} N. Slitlamp examination showed typical dendritica figures and slight infiltrates in the Bowman and superficial
stroma. In deep stromal keratitis which mostly follows recurrent
herpetic attacks the sensitivity was exceedingly diminished. In many
cases we found values greater than 1.000×10^{-5} N. This was classified as a total loss of sensitivity. Nearly always the sensitivity
of the contralateral eye was normal. In bacterial and mycotic infections we also found a diminished sensitivity. Whereas in these
cases the corneal sensitivity thresholds are raised up to maximal
10×10^{-5} N, which is a diminished sensitivity compared to normal
healthy eyes. In deep stromal keratitis we saw nearly a complete
anaesthesia with a threshold value of 1.000×10^{-5} N. This diminished
value is similar for nearly every place on the cornea.

Fig. 2:　　　　Sensitivity in superficial, recurrent and stromal
keratitis.

These threshold values are not constant in the course of the disease.
So we took measurements to follow-up the inflammatory process. So in
recurrent superficial herpes we found a recovery of the sensitivity
soon after the clinical aspects had normalized. After 4 or 5 months
the sensitivity returned to threshold values of smaller than 8×10^{-5}N,
after 1 year the sensitivity profile had normalized.

Fig. 3:　　　　Course of sensitivity threshold values after
herpes cornea - different recurrencies in epithelial and stromal keratitis.

Even in a deep stromal keratitis we saw first slight and later good improvement of sensibility. The anaesthesia in the beginning of the disease normalized to measurable threshold values of 100×10^{-5} N after 1 year. Two years later there was only a slight disturbance of the sensitivity profile to 10×10^{-5} N. The recurrence rates were different from case to case correlated to the individual stromal alterations.

DISCUSSION:

The loss of sensitivity in herpetic keratitis correlates to severity of the disease. To our surprise a keratitis dendritica with epithelial involvement only showed a normal corneal sensitivity, also in the acute attack. Possibly slight decrease could not be detected, due to mechanical limits of the instrument. The smallest force to touch the cornea is 1×10^{-5} N, that means several times smaller than with the aesthesiometer of COCHET & BONNET, but this is also more than the central threshold value of a normal cornea. So it may be that a value of 1×10^{-5} N indicates a slight disturbance of the sensitivity in comparison to normal corneas.

There is a big difference in threshold values comparing recurrent superficial keratitis with deep stromal keratitis. In deep stromal keratitis the exact threshold value could not be measured as our instrument produces a force of 1.000×10^{-5} N only. This means nearly a complete anaesthesia of the cornea. But really threshold values in this disease can be higher.

SEVERIN (1965) and NORN (1970) also reported comparable results, but they used the older instruments of COCHET & BONNET.

The clinical picture, the aesthesiometric findings and histopathology experiments can be correlated. In the early superficial keratitis dendritica the epithelium is affected only – this means normal sensitivity. In recurrent keratitis dendritica, Bowman's membrane and superficial stromal layers were included in the process. Here the first damage of corneal nerves leads to a slight damaged sensitivity. In deep stromal keratitis the nearly total anaesthesia is a sign of interrupted nerve function.

In the course of the disease, we saw an improvement of the initial diminished sensitivity. The improvement depends on the

severity of the disease. But in the deep stromal recurrent keratitis
an increase of sensitivity is possible, in some cases up to normal.
We correlated these findings with our examinations in healing of
corneal wounds after cataract and keratoplastic surgery (DRAEGER und
MARTIN 1980). A total cutting of the nerves is followed by
complete anaesthesia. Later we saw a slowly increasing corneal sensitivity over several years. Correlating these two phenomen we think that
in herpetic keratitis there may be a loss of functioning corneal
nerves but with healing of the disease a regeneration of nerve fibres
in the cornea may be postulated. This is a very slow process, so it
took over some years for returning to a good sensitivity especially
in the centre. That means, that in superficial keratitis with slight
damaged sensitivity only   the nerve ends should be affected.

A full improvement of the corneal sensitivity is a phenomenon
of periphere nerve fibres. The latency of herpes virus   in the
ganglion does not interfere with the nerve function. The difference
in the sensitivity loss of herpetic eye disease and corneal ulcers
of other ethiology shows us that there must be a specific neurotoxic
factor produced by the virus or the tissue reactions.

REFERENCES:
1. COCHET, P. + BONNET, R.: L'esthesiometrie corneene. Réalisation
    et intere + pratique. Bull Soc. ophth. Fr. 541 (1961).
2. DRAEGER, J., KOUDELKA, A., LUBAHN, E.: Zur Aesthesiometrie der
    Hornhaut. Kl. Mbl. Augenheilk. 169 (1976), 407-421.
3. DRAEGER, J., MARTIN, R.: Renervierung der Hornhaut nach cornealen
    und corneoskleralen Wunden. DOG Symposion, 1980.
4. von FREY, M.: Beiträge zur Physiologie des Sehnerves.
    in: Berichte über die Verhandlungen d. Königl. sächs. Gesell-
    schaft d. Wissenschaften zu Leipzig. Mathem. Class.-Hörsal
    Leipzig 1894, 185-96.
5. KRÜCKMANN, E.: Graefes Arch. Ophthal 1895 Bd. 41, Abs. 45.21.
6. LARSON, M.: Electro-mechanical corneal aesthesiometer. Br. J.
    ophthal. 54 (1970), 342.
7. NORN: Dendritic (herpetic) keratitis. Acta ophthalmologica 48,
    (1970), 383-395.

152

8. SCHIRMER, K.E.: Assessment of corneal sensitivity. Br. J. ophthal. 47 (1963), 488.
9. SEVERIN, M.: Die Hornhautsensibilität bei herpetischer Keratitis. Kl. Mbl. Augenheilk. 146, 683-695 (1965).

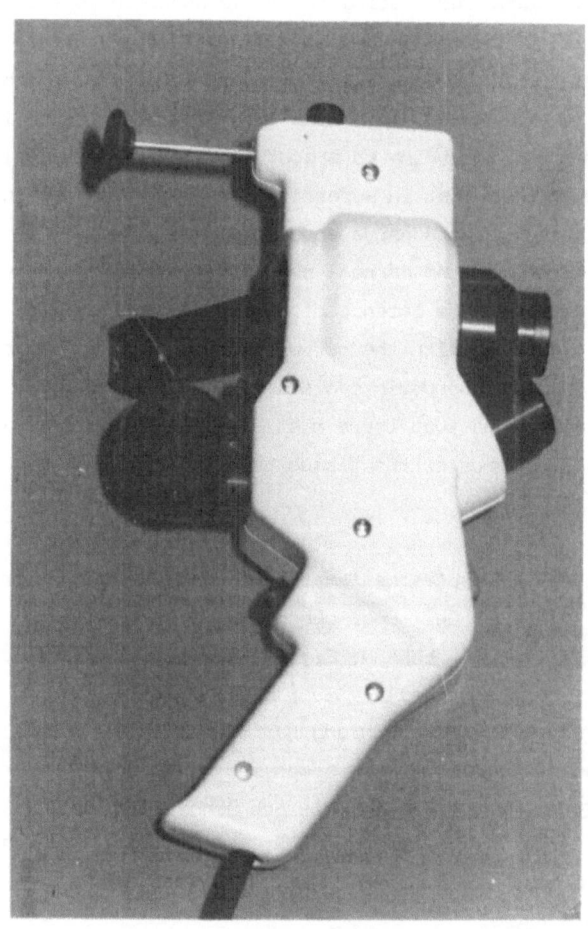

Fig. 1

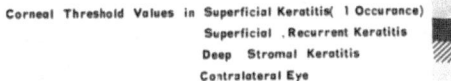

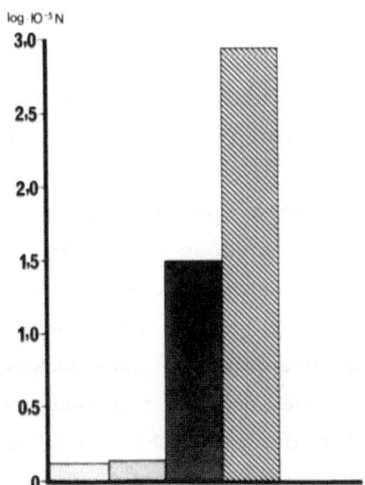

Fig. 2

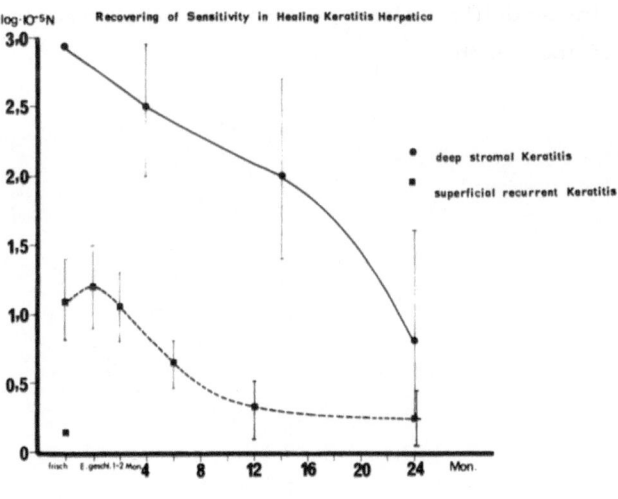

Fig. 3

DISCUSSION :

P.A. Asbell (New York) : It is certainly a very interesting and excellent paper and presentation. I have just one or two
questions. Is the filament you use similar to the Cochet-Bonnet
instrument : a filament that is extended to different lengths to
determine sensitivity?

R. Winter (Hamburg) : There is no filament. That is the difference with other instruments. There is a pin of metal which tou-
ches the cornea with a defined force. You can change the
force by an electromotor.

P.A. Asbell (New York) : It looks very interesting and accurate.
The other question I had is on your results in superficial first-
time or first-noted attacks of herpetic keratitis. Here, you
compared the contralateral normal eye with the infected eye. I
wondered if you can be sure that you were looking at comparable areas. The difference between the two eyes could be related
to the different areas tested, rather than to a real difference
in the two eyes. Work by us and Dr. Beuerman has shown that
corneal sensitivity is not uniform throughout the cornea.

R. Winter (Hamburg) : In general we take measurements at five
points, four in the limbus region and one in the center. You
can control it by the microscope, which is installed in the
machine. In dendritic lesions we also took measurements at
the point of the lesion.

LACRIMAL SECRETION AFTER HERPETIC KERATITIS.

ORSONI, J.G., BONACINI, M., PICCIONI, A.,TOMBA M.C.

Istituto di Oftalmologia dell'Università

IICattedra di Clinica Oculistica

43100 Parma, Italy

INTRODUCTION.

People working in Herpetic Keratitis have often the feeling that a lacrimal secretion impairment follows herpetic infection of the eye.In the first Symposium on herpetic Eye Diseases held in Freiburg in 1980, Shing et al. (4) reported the case histories of 125 patients previously affected by HSV Keratitis and evaluated the Shirmer test in them.The authors concluded that an impairment of lacrimal secretion with high statistical significance could be recorded in these patients.In the same Symposium Kok van Alphen (3) reported graft failure due to hypolacrimation in 25 of 115 cases of keratoplasty after Herpetic Keratitis.The aim of this work was to determine in a continous study the value of lacrimation in its quantitative form in patients who suffered from Herpetic Keratitis.

MATERIAL AND METHODS.

From June 1980 to March 1984 patients affected by Herpes Keratitis examined at the Cornea Service of the Institute of Ophthalmology in the University of Parma were checked both after recovery and in the chronic state .Patients who visit the Cornea Service are partly from the out-patients Service of the Clinic and partly sent for consultation from ophthalmologists in the area.120 patients were examined in this period , but the study was possible only on 74 of them, for a total number of 76 eyes .The patients whom we failed to

Maudgal, P.C. and Missotten, L., (eds.) Herpetic Eye Diseases.
© 1985, Dr W. Junk Publishers, Dordrecht/Boston/Lancaster. ISBN 978-94-010-8935-7

follow-up were lost due to a lack of collaboration or for social reasons.Lacrimal secretion was measured with the Shirmer test I used in the classical way, by leaving the patient with his eyes closed for 5 minutes in a half dark room, utilising Shirmer test paper produced by the Firm Cooper Vision.The patients who healed as well as patients in chronic state were tested every three months .The minimum follow-up was 6 months , the maximum 44 months. The Shirmer test was considered normal up to 15 mm., abnormal under 15 mm. The control group was composed of 90 patients,free from any ophthalmic pathology or/and symptoms.The patients were classified into three categories:1) Epithelial Keratitis which occured only once(EP K)2) Recurring Epithelial Keratitis (EP K RR) 3) Endothelio-stromal Keratitis (END STR K). Age, sex and pathology distribution of patients and of control subjects are summarized in Table 1. As can be seen in Table 2 we have utilized either IDU or TFT or ACV as antiviral drugs both in Epithelial Keratitis and in recurrent Epithelial Keratitis. TFT and ACV were used in association with steroids in endothelio-stromal Keratitis; in only one case were steroids used alone.

RESULTS.

In order to evaluate the incidence of the type of drug used within each group of keratitis with regard to the variable "lacrimation", a one-way analysis of covariance was carried out(2). As seen in Table 4 no statistically significant difference between the different antiviral drugs used has been found.Having therefore excluded any appreciable influence related to the type of treatment used, a covariance analysis (with covariant age) was carried out in order to compare the incidence of the different types of pathology with regard to lacrimation. As can be seen from Table 5 and from the control group (Table 2) the percentage of hypolacrimating patients is higher in the group of patients with recurring epithelial Keratitis.The percentage

TABLE   1

AGE	CONTROLS M	CONTROLS F	EP KERATITIS M	EP KERATITIS F	EP KERATITIS RECURR. M.	EP KERATITIS RECURR. F	END–STR KERATITIS M	END–STR KERATITIS F
20	5	7	2	6	1	0	0	0
21– 40	15	20	4	3	1	2	4	2
41–60	4	18	10	6	5	4	8	1
60	4	17	3	3	5	1	5	1
TOTAL	28	62	19	18	12	7	17	4
	(30%)	(70%)	(51%)	(49%)	(63%)	(37%)	(81%)	(19%)
	90		37		19		21	

AGE, SEX AND PATHOLOGY DISTRIBUTION

TABLE   2

TREATMENT	IDU	TFT	ACV	TOTAL
EP KERATITIS	8	13	16	37
EP KERATITIS RECURRENCE	1	6	12	19
TOTAL	9	19	28	56

TREATMENT	TFT+STER	ACV+STER	STER.	TOTAL.
END–STR KERATITIS	12	8	1	21

DIFFERENT ANTIVIRALS USED IN THE TREATMENT OF
EPITHELIAL AND STROMAL KERATITIS

TABLE   3

AGE	Number of Hypolacrimating subjects	Number of Normolacrimating subjects	Total
20	2	10	12
21-40	9	26	35
41-60	11 (%)	11	22
60	7 (%)	14	21
TOTAL	29 (%)	61	90

LACRIMAL SECRETION IN THE CONTROL GROUP

TABLE   4

AGE	TFT		ACV		IDU		TFT		ACV		IDU		ACV+ STER		TFT+ STER		STER	
	H	N	H	N	H	N	H	N	H	N	H	N	H	N	H	N	H	N
20	0	4	2	2	0	0	0	0	0	0	0	1	0	0	0	0	0	0
21-40	0	3	0	2	1	1	0	0	1	2	0	0	1	1	1	2	0	1
41-60	3	3	3	2	2	3	3	2	3	1	0	0	1	3	2	3	0	0
60	0	0	3	2	1	0	1	0	4	1	0	0	0	2	2	2	0	0
	3	10	8	8	4	4	4	2	8	4			2	6	5	7	0	1
	23%	77%	50%		50%		67%	33%	67%	33%			25%	75%	42%	58%		

EPITHELIAL KERATITIS   EPITHELIAL KERA   END – STR –KERATITIS
                                TITIS RECURRENCE

RELATIONSHIP BETWEEN TREATMENT AND LACRIMAL
SECRETIONS IN DIFFERENT TYPES OF KERATITIS

H = HYPOLACRIMATION
N = NORMAL LACRIMATION

TABLE   5

AGE	EP K H	EP K N	EP K RR H	EP K RR N	END STR H	END STR N
20	2	6	0	1	0	0
21–40	1	6	1	2	2	4
41–60	8	8	6	3	3	6
60	4	2	5	1	2	4
TOTAL	15	22	12	7	7	14
	41%	59%	63%	27%	33%	66%

LACRIMAL SECRETION IN DIFFERENT KERATITIS GROUPS

TABLE   6

	MEAN	STANDARD DEVIATION	ADJ. MEAN
CONTROLS	20.35	8.5	19.98
EP K	18.35	12.45	17.6
EP K RR	13.2	9.98	13.8
END STR K	20.14	9.1	20.6

MEAN VALUE STANDARD DEVIATION AND ADJUSTED MEAN VALUES OF LACRIMAL
SECRETION FOR CONTROLS AND DIFFERENT HERATITIS GROUPS

of these patients (67%) is clearly greater in this group than in the other pathological and control groups.The analysis of covariance indicates that this difference is significant (p=0.05). The comparison of the average amount of tear secretion (mm. of Shirmer test) among the different groups has been carried out by the covariance analysis and further checked with the Dunnet test.The results(Table 6)again point to a decresed lacrimation in the group of patients affected from recurrences.

DISCUSSION.

As already mentioned, observations concerning an impairment of lacrimal secretion after Herpetic Keratitis can be found in the literature (3,4,5). In this study we have focused our attention only on the quantitative alterations of tear production as measured by the Shirmer test. This old test,which is simple to carry out and not expensive, has from time to time been critized, but has not however been replaced by another equally useful one (1).We have divided our patients into three different groups in an effort to differentiate clinical situations which could justify a different behaviour of tear secretion.The results which have been presented allow the following conclusions:

-the various antivirals used have not influenced lacrimal secretion in any significant way;

-the patients who were cured and those who had suffered from an endothelio-stromal Keratitis did not show appreciable reduction of lacrimal secretion in the follow-up period.

A significant reduction of lacrimal secretion was observed only in the group of patients who presented one or more recurrences of the epithelial Keratitis.

Acknowledgements.

The Authors are indebted to statisticians L.Ardia and A.Grignani of

the Biometric Unit of Farmitalia -Carlo Erba ,Milano for the
statistical analysis.

BIBLIOGRAPHY.

1. Clinch, T.E., Benedetto, D.A., Felberg, N.T. and Laibson, P.R.:
Shirmer's test. Arch. ophthalmol. 101, 1383-86, 1983.
2. Gill, J.L.: Design and analysis of experiments in the animal and
medical sciences. The Iowa State University Press, Ames,Iowa USA,1978.
3. Kok van Alphen, C.C. and Volker-Dieben, H.J.M.: Impairment of
tear-production in corneal herpetic diseases. in Sundmacher, R.:
Herpetic Eye Diseases, 211-214, Bergmann, J.F. Verlag, Munchen 1981.
4. Shing D.,Shing, M. and Shinf, R.:Herpetic keratitis causing
lacrimal hyposecretion and xerosis,in:Sundmacher R.:Herpetic Eye
Diseases, J.F.Bergmann Verlag, 211-214, Munchen 1981
5. Wing Chu, Pavan-Langston, D.:Ocular surface manifestations of the
major viruses. I.O.C., 135-167, 19/2, 1979.

DISCUSSION :

O.P. van Bijsterveld (Utrecht) : Dr. Orsoni, I am rather surprised at your Schirmer's test limit between normalcy and disease with regard to dry eyes. If you take a limit of 15 mm, at least in Holland, half of the population would have dry eyes. Moreover, by setting a limit between normalcy and disease, as you did in your study, one is almost forced to analyse the Schirmer data on a nominal scale, which is much less accurate than the interval scale. A second point I want to discuss is that tear function in herpes simplex keratitis is correlated with the number of recurrences and so with the level of the corneal sensitivity. In acute first attacks of dendritic keratitis, the tear function is increased and within 3 months it returns to normal. After repeated attacks, however, the tear function diminishes to levels below normal, and there is a rough positive correlation between the amount of decrease in corneal sensitivity and tear function. Do you have a similar experience ?

J.G. Orsoni (Parma) : We tried to measure the corneal sensitivity, but not in all patients. This is why I did not put the results here. I agree that in the first 3 months you have hyperlacrimation.

O.P. van Bijsterveld (Utrecht) : The reason, why I raise this point is that exactly those cases, who have repeated herpes attacks of the cornea are the ones that are canditates for corneal transplant. Succes in corneal transplantation is in our experience also dependant on tear function and tear function is very often decreased in cases of repeated herpetic attacks.

A COMPUTER-BASED METHOD TO PROVIDE SUBSPECIALIST EXPERTISE
ON THE MANAGEMENT OF HERPES SIMPLEX INFECTIONS OF THE EYE*

Chandler R. Dawson, M.D., Francis I. Proctor Foundation for Research in Ophthalmology, University of California, San Francisco, San Francisco, CA 94143, and John Kastner, Ph.D., Sholom Weiss, Ph.D. and C. Kulikowski, Ph.D., Department of Computer Science, Rutgers University, New Brunswick, NJ 08903, U.S.A.

The treatment of herpes simplex virus (HSV) infections of the eye presents a number of difficult problems. Topical antiviral drugs are effective against viral ulcers of the cornea but may aggravate non-herpetic epithelial defects and do not control herpetic lid vesicles, conjunctivitis, stromal keratitis, or iritis. Corticosteroids suppress stromal keratitis and uveitis but enhance the frequency of viral recurrences. The choice of treatment, then, for individual patients may require considerable expertise.

To provide advice on the management of herpetic eye disease to ophthalmologists, we have developed a computer-based model of the clinical reasoning which provides recommendations on diagnosis and treatment. This model includes of questions to elicit clinical findings, disease categories (diagnosis) and treatments. In a consultation session, the clinical findings of an individual case are obtained by questions directed to the ophthalmologist. The computer program then generates recommendations on diagnosis and management from these data. The model now includes 30 diagnostic categories and 51 therapeutic regimens. It was developed with a generalized program for the construction of consultant systems called EXPERT (1).

---

* Supported in part by NIH grants EY.00427 and RR.643.

Maudgal, P.C. and Missotten, L., (eds.) Herpetic Eye Diseases.
© 1985, Dr W. Junk Publishers, Dordrecht/Boston/Lancaster. ISBN 978-94-010-8935-7

Computer-assisted decision-making is directed at analyzing problems in specific domains of knowledge which ordinarily require human expertise. Such "expert" systems have been widely applied to problems in the diagnosis and treatment of medical problems. Many computer-based models of clinical reasoning utilize production rules to express the causal reasoning of a medical expert; these rules are usually in the form "if a set of conditions, then a set of conclusions".

Like other expert models, this model of herpes eye infections was first developed with production rules which describe the reasoning process in detail. For example, one of the rules is as follows:

IF there is a marginal ulcer of the corneal epithelium and a history of ocular herpetic infections, and corneal anesthesia over the lesion,

THEN it is highly probable that the patient has active herpetic infection of the cornea.

The initial consultation system then consisted of production rules with a control strategy provided by the EXPERT program. The herpes program was tested for validity by comparing its recommendations for 56 patients with advice from specialists at the Francis I. Proctor Foundation.

Precedence tables to select among competing treatments

A specific diagnosis does not necessarily indicate a single treatment but usually a group of competing treatments. During the development of the model of ocular herpes we identified four sets of competing treatments (Table 1). In each set the treatments are mutually exclusive so it is necessary to choose between them.

TABLE 1. SETS OF TREATMENTS FOR OCULAR HERPES SIMPLEX VIRUS INFECTIONS

	INDICATIONS	TREATMENTS
Set A	Antiviral medications	1. Aciclovir
		2. Trifluridine
		3. Vidarabine
		4. Idoxuridine
Set B	Debridement or antivirals	1. Gentle wiping debridement
		2. Prophylactic antiviral
		3. Full antiviral treatment
Set C	Initiating cortico-steroids	1. Do not initiate steroid
		2. Initiate topical steroid
Set D	Patient on treatment with topical cortico-steroid	1. Discontinue steroid
		2. Taper steroid dosage
		3. Increase steroid dosage

To analyze the effect of contraindications on the choice of treatment, competing treatments were initially placed in the order of preference in the absence of any contraindications. This preferred order of treatments is applied if nothing is known about a particular case. For topical antivirals this order has been established by clinical trials (2, 3, 4).

The specific contraindications to the use of a given set of treatments were then listed in order of importance. These contraindications are attributes of individual patients. Their order was determined by common sense judgments and by testing against actual cases.

Each set of treatments and contraindications can be represented as a table, with the treatments listed in preferred order across the top

166

and the contraindications listed at the side in order of importance
(Table 2). Precedence tables summarize a mass of clinical data in a
simple form so that all factors affecting selection of a particular
treatment can be considered.

TABLE 2. PRECEDENCE TABLE TO SELECT AN ANTIVIRAL DRUG TO TREAT
HERPES SIMPLEX EYE INFECTIONS

CONTRA-INDICATIONS	ANTIVIRAL DRUGS (IN ORDER OF PREFERENCE)			
	ACICLOVIR (ACV)	TRIFLURIDINE (TFT)	VIDARABINE (VIRA-A)	IDOXURIDINE (IDU)
1. Drug not available	X	X	X	X
2. Pregnancy (5)				X
3. Antiviral resistance	X	X	X	X
4. Recent corneal surgery (6)		X	X	X
5. Severe drug allergy	X	X	X	X
6. Moderate drug allergy	X	X	X	X
7. Mild drug allergy	X	X	X	X

(X Indicates which contraindictions may apply to individual cases)

For an individual patient, these contraindications are applied
starting with the least important (i.e. the lowest ranked) and proceed-
ing up the list to the most important. If a contraindication to a
particular treatment applies to a specific patient, that treatment is
ranked lowest when the next higher contraindication is applied. Thus
the most important contraindication is evaluated last and has the
greatest effect on the selection of treatment.

Precedence tables have a number of advantages:

- They constitute a formal statement of the knowledge regarding a set of alternative treatments.

- They are a useful means to transmit expert medical knowledge

- They can be modified easily to include new treatments and contraindications

- For computer models of clinical reasoning, they are very efficient and require less computer memory than do production rules (7)

- Their use does not require a computer

Consultation with the EXPERT computer model of HSV eye infection

The herpes model was developed on large computers at Rutgers University, but has been reduced in size to fit onto floppy disks for the IBM-PC or Apple II personal computers. It is available through the Proctor Foundation in San Francisco or the Department of Computer Science at Rutgers University.

References

1. Kulikowski, C.A. and Weiss, S.M.: Representation of Expert Knowledge for consultation: The CASNET and EXPERT projects. pp.21-56, In Artificial Intelligence in Medicine. Szolovits, P., editor. Westview Press, Inc. Boulder, Colorado, 1982.

2. Pavan-Langston, D., et al.: Am. J. Oph. 80:495, 1975.

3. Pavan-Langston, D. and Foster, C.S.: Am. J. Oph. 84:818, 1977.

4. Tormey, P., et al.: Trans. Ophth. Soc. U.K. 101:6-9, 1981.

5. Itoi, M., et al.: Arch. Ophth. 93:46, 1975.

6. Lass, J.H., et al.: Am. J. Oph. 88:102-108, 1979.

7. Kastner, J.K., et al.: Therapy selection in a expert medical consultation system for ocular herpes simplex. Computers in Biol. and Med. (in press).

NEW ANTIVIRAL DRUGS FOR THE TREATMENT OF HERPESVIRUS INFECTIONS

E. DE CLERCQ (Rega Institute for Medical Research, Katholieke Universiteit, Leuven, Belgium).

1. INTRODUCTION

Several antiherpes agents are routinely used for the topical treatment of herpetic eye infections : i.e. idoxuridine (IDU) as 0.1 % eyedrops, trifluridine (TFT) as 1 % eyedrops, vidarabine (AraA) as 3 % eye ointment, acyclovir (ACV) as 3 % eye ointment, and, in some countries (Federal Republic of Germany and France) 0.15 % eyedrops of ethyldeoxyuridine (EDU) and iododeoxycytidine (IDC), respectively.

In recent years, various new antiviral agents have been developed which are highly potent and selective in their activity against herpes simplex virus type 1 (HSV-1) or type 2 (HSV-2) and varicella-zoster virus (VZV). This includes bromovinyldeoxyuridine (BVDU), bromovinylarauracil (BVaraU), fluoroiodoaracytosine (FIAC), fluoromethylarauracil (FMAU), dihydroxypropoxymethylguanine (DHPG) and glycylacyclovir (glycyl-ACV).

The structural formulae of both the old and new generation of antiherpes drugs are presented in Fig. 1. They can all be considered as pyrimidine or purine nucleoside analogues, ACV and DHPG being acyclic nucleosides in which C-2 (DHPG) or C-2 and C-3 (ACV) of the sugar moiety have been deleted, and glycyl-ACV being a prodrug of ACV.

2. ANTIVIRAL POTENCY

As based on the minimum inhibitory concentration required to inhibit virus-induced cytopathogenicity or focus formation in cell culture, BVDU, BVaraU, FIAC and FMAU surpass all other compounds in their potency against HSV-1 and VZV (Table 1). From these data, BVDU, BVaraU, FIAC and FMAU would appear particularly promising for the treatment of HSV-1 and VZV infections, in casu herpes simplex keratouveitis and ophthalmic zoster.

Obviously, the antiviral potency of an antiviral drug in vitro does not necessarily reflect its efficacy in vivo. Due to limited bio-availability (absorption, tissue distribution, half-life), the drug may be less effica-

Maudgal, P.C. and Missotten, L., (eds.) Herpetic Eye Diseases.
© *1985, Dr W. Junk Publishers, Dordrecht/Boston/Lancaster. ISBN 978-94-010-8935-7*

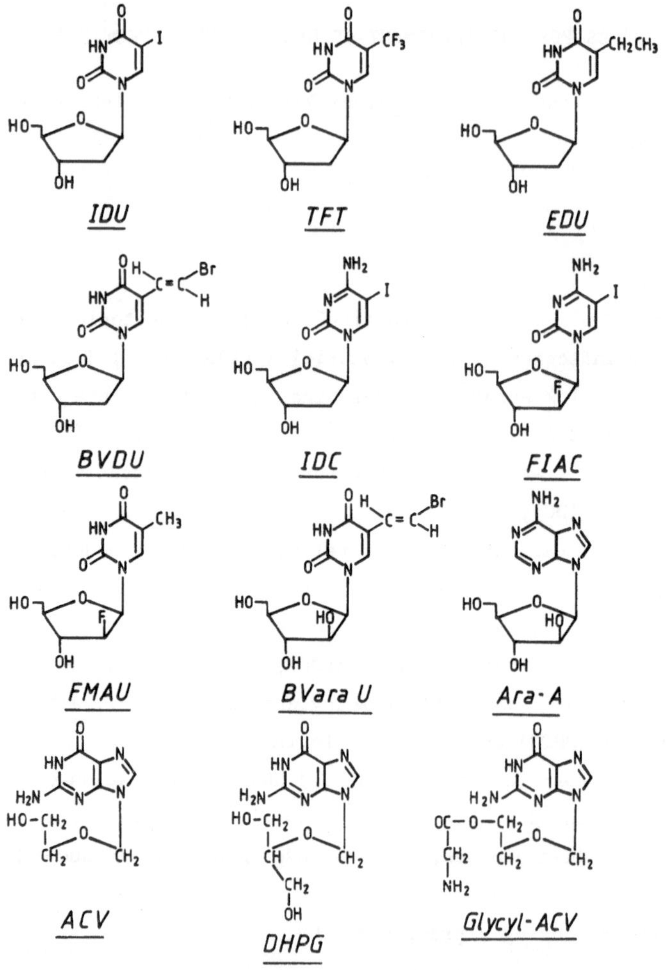

FIGURE 1. Structural formulae and abbreviations of antiherpes drugs.
IDU : idoxuridine, 5-iodo-2'-deoxyuridine.
TFT : trifluridine, 5-trifluoromethyl-2'-deoxyuridine.
EDU : 5-ethyl-2'-deoxyuridine.
BVDU : (E)-5-(2-bromovinyl)-2'-deoxyuridine.
IDC : 5-iodo-2'-deoxycytidine.
FIAC : 1-(2'-fluoro-2'-deoxy-β-D-arabinofuranosyl)-5-iodocytosine.
FMAU : 1-(2'-fluoro-2'-deoxy-β-D-arabinofuranosyl)-5-methyluracil.
BVaraU : 1-β-D-arabinofuranosyl-5-(2-bromovinyl)uracil.
AraA : vidarabine, 9-β-D-arabinofuranosyladenine.
ACV : acyclovir, 9-(2-hydroxyethoxymethyl)guanine.
DHPG : 9-(1,3-dihydroxy-2-propoxymethyl)guanine.
Glycyl-ACV : 9-[(2-glycyloxy)ethoxymethyl]guanine.

Table 1. Comparative efficacy of antiviral drugs against HSV-1 and VZV in cell culture (primary rabbit kidney cells and human diploid fibroblasts, respectively).

Compound	Minimal inhibitory concentration[a] (μg/ml)	
	HSV-1	VZV
IDU	0.1	1.4
TFT	0.7	0.8
EDU	0.5	1.5
BVDU	0.001	0.002
IDC	0.06	1.3
FIAC	0.003	0.003
FMAU	0.003	0.003
BVaraU	0.1	0.001
AraA	7	1.6
ACV	0.03	4.6
DHPG	0.06	1.5
Glycyl-ACV	0.1	...

[a]Required to reduce virus-induced cytopathogenicity (HSV-1) or focus formation (VZV) by 50 % (based on the lowest representative value reported in each case). Data taken from De Clercq (1984), De Clercq et al. (1980), Shigeta et al. (1983) and Colla et al. (1983).

cious in vivo than could be expected from its potency in vitro. In addition, the relative efficacy of the antiviral compounds may vary considerably from one system to another, depending on the pharmacokinetic factors involved, i.e. hindrance in crossing the blood-brain barrier in the treatment of herpetic encephalitis.

Of all in vivo systems, epithelial HSV-1 keratitis most closely mimics the in vitro situation, especially if the compounds are applied topically as eyedrops, since under these conditions they are present in an aqueous medium in direct contact with the virus-infected corneal epithelium, thus very much alike a cell culture system.

3. MECHANISM OF ANTIVIRAL ACTION

All "new generation" antiherpes drugs, i.e. BVDU, BVaraU, FIAC, FMAU, ACV, DHPG and glycyl-ACV (the latter upon release of ACV), share a common mechanism of action, in that they are preferentially phosphorylated by the virus-induced dThd(dCyd) kinase which restricts their further action to the virus-infected cell (Fig. 2). Hence, virus mutant (TK⁻) strains which are deficient in the expression of dThd(dCyd) kinase or virus mutants which express a dThd kinase with altered substrate specificity are not

172

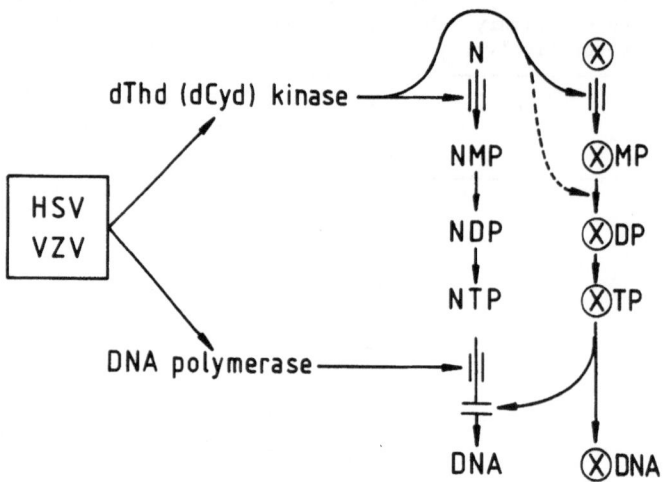

FIGURE 2. Highly simplified scheme for the mechanism of action of selec-
tive antiherpes drugs such as BVDU, FIAC, FMAU, BVaraU, ACV and DHPG.
N : normal nucleoside, i.e. dThd (2'-deoxythymidine) or dCyd (2'-deoxy-
    cytidine).
(X): nucleoside analogue, i.e. BVDU, FIAC, FMAU, BVaraU, ACV or DHPG.
MP, DP and TP correspond to the 5'-monophosphate, 5'-diphosphate or 5'-
triphosphate, respectively.
According to De Clercq (1982b) (modified).

sensitive to the inhibitory effects of these nucleoside analogues. Upon
conversion to their 5'-triphosphate, the nucleoside analogues interfere
with viral DNA synthesis. They may either inhibit viral DNA polymerase by
competing with the natural substrates, i.e. dTTP, dCTP or dGTP, or be incorporated into viral DNA (Fig. 2). While BVDU may be incorporated internally via an internucleotide linkage, ACV is incorporated externally at
the 3'-terminal and thereby shuts off chain elongation. FIAC and FMAU may
be incorporated internally or externally, whereas BVaraU, if incorporated,
would only be incorporated at the 3'-terminal. To what extent DHPG is incorporated into DNA is not clearly established. Anyhow, the antiherpes
drugs are targeted at the viral DNA and their antiviral action may be attributed at least in part to their incorporation into viral DNA. This has
been clearly demonstrated for BVDU which causes a virus yield reduction
that is directly proportional to the amount of BVDU incorporated into viral DNA (Mancini et al., 1983).

4. SPECIFIC ATTRIBUTES

The new antiherpes agents BVDU, BVaraU, FIAC, FMAU, DHPG and glycyl-ACV
possess some attractive advantages over the older antiherpes drugs. With a
minimum inhibitory concentration of 0.001 µg/ml (Table 1), BVDU still
stands out as the most potent inhibitor of HSV-1 in cell culture; however,
BVDU is about 1000 times less active against HSV-2. An additional advantage of BVDU is that it is very well absorbed when given orally. In contrast, ACV is poorly absorbed from the gut. However, higher blood drug levels of ACV may be achieved upon oral administration of its prodrug, deoxyacyclovir; deoxyacyclovir would be converted in the organism to acyclovir
by xanthine oxidase. An advantage of glycyl-ACV over ACV is its 30-fold
greater solubility (Colla et al., 1983) which permits the use of glycyl-
ACV as eyedrops (whereas ACV has to be given as an ointment) in the topical treatment of herpetic keratitis. Glycyl-ACV may also be suitable for
intramuscular administration in the systemic treatment of HSV and VZV infections at drug concentrations, i.e. 3 x 5 mg/kg/day, at which ACV has to
be given intravenously.

With a minimum inhibitory concentration of 0.001 µg/ml (Table 1),
BVaraU is the most potent inhibitor of VZV in cell culture : it is slightly more potent against VZV than BVDU (Machida et al., 1982) but less potent against HSV-1 and HSV-2. Moreover, the antiviral activity of BVaraU
depends to a large extent on the nature of the cell substrate (De Clercq,
1982a). The great promise of DHPG resides in its activity against cytomegalovirus (CMV) (Tocci et al., 1984) and its markedly greater antiviral
efficacy upon oral administration than ACV (Field et al., 1983). The enhanced antiviral activity of DHPG over ACV is presumably related to a more
rapid conversion to its triphosphate. FIAC and FMAU also yield promise as
anti-CMV agents (minimum inhibitory concentration : approximately 0.05 µg/
ml (Colacino and Lopez, 1983; Mar et al., 1984)). Furthermore, FMAU is an
exquisitely effective agent for the systemic treatment of HSV-1 encephalitis (Schinazi et al., 1983).

5. TREATMENT OF EXPERIMENTAL KERATOUVEITIS

Of the newly developed antiviral agents, glycyl-ACV, FMAU, FIAC and in
particular BVDU have emerged as efficacious agents for the topical treatment of HSV-1 keratouveitis : BVDU proved superior to IDU in the topical
treatment of epithelial keratitis (Maudgal et al., 1980), and superior to

TFT in the topical treatment of stromal keratitis (Maudgal et al., 1982a) and iritis (Maudgal et al., 1982b). BVDU was also more effective than glycyl-ACV in suppressing epithelial and stromal HSV-1 keratitis, and iritis therewith associated (Maudgal et al., 1984a). BVDU proved also superior to BVaraU in the topical treatment of epithelial HSV-1 keratitis (P.C. Maudgal : personal communication, 1984). Boisjoly et al. (1983) reported BVDU to be effective in the topical treatment of keratouveitis due to infection with an ACV-resistant HSV-1 mutant, and Trousdale et al. (1983) found the response of herpetic keratitis to treatment with FMAU similar to that obtained with ACV but significantly better than those attained with IDU or AraA. FIAC was also found efficacious in the topical treatment of superficial herpetic keratitis (Trousdale et al., 1981), but in these studies it was not compared to other antiviral drugs.

6. POTENTIALS FOR CLINICAL USE

A number of antiherpes drugs are currently marketed for the topical treatment of herpetic eye infections and several others have proven efficacious for this purpose in animal models (Table 2). Based on its antiviral potency in cell culture (Table 1), BVDU may be considered as a prime candidate for the topical treatment of HSV-1 keratitis. This assumption has been borne out by rabbit experiments in which BVDU was found superior to IDU, TFT, (glycyl)-ACV and BVaraU. The efficacy of BVDU in the topical treatment of herpetic keratitis has also been established in man, i.e. if

Table 2. Potentials of antiviral drugs for the topical treatment of herpetic eye infections.

| Compound | Formulation | | Efficacy demonstrated | | Licensed for clinical use |
	eye drops	eye ointment	experimentally	clinically	
IDU	0.1 %	0.5 %	+	+	+
TFT	1 %	2 %	+	+	+
EDU	0.15 %	0.3 %	Limited data available		+ (FRG)
BVDU	0.1-0.5 %		+	+	
IDC	0.15 %	1 %	Limited data available		+ (France)
FIAC	0.1-1 %		+		
FMAU	0.2 %		+		
BVaraU	0.1-0.5 %		+		
AraA		3 %	+	+	+
ACV		3 %	+	+	+
DHPG					
Glycyl-ACV	1 %		+		

given as 0.1 % eyedrops (Maudgal et al., 1981b). Although BVDU has not been directly compared to other antiviral drugs, it is noteworthy that it has been used successfully in those patients that had become clinically resistant to IDU, TFT or AraA (Maudgal et al., 1984b).

BVDU may also be useful in the systemic treatment of herpetic eye infections, i.e. HSV-1 uveitis or ophthalmic zoster (Maudgal et al., 1981a). Ideally, the management of these conditions should be based upon combined topical and systemic (i.e. oral) BVDU therapy. Oral BVDU administration at 7.5 mg/kg/day for 5 days, seems quite appropriate for the therapy of disseminated or localized herpes zoster (Wildiers and De Clercq, 1984) and when combined with topical 0.1 % BVDU eyedrops, it may achieve optimal benefit in the treatment of HSV-1 and VZV infections of the deeper eye tissues.

REFERENCES

Boisjoly HM, Park N-H, Pavan-Langston D, De Clercq E. 1983. Herpes simplex acyclovir-resistant mutant in experimental keratouveitis. Arch. Ophthalmol. 101, 1782–1786.
Colacino JM, Lopez C. 1983. Efficacy and selectivity of some nucleoside analogs as anti-human cytomegalovirus agents. Antimicrob. Agents Chemother. 24, 505–508.
Colla L, De Clercq E, Busson R, Vanderhaeghe H. 1983. Synthesis and antiviral activity of water-soluble esters of acyclovir (9-[(2-hydroxyethoxy) methyl]guanine). J. Med. Chem. 26, 602–604.
De Clercq E. 1982a. Comparative efficacy of antiherpes drugs in different cell lines. Antimicrob. Agents Chemother. 21, 661–663.
De Clercq E. 1982b. Selective antiherpes agents. Trends in Pharmacol. Sci. 3, 492–495.
De Clercq E. 1984. Biochemical aspects of the selective antiherpes activity of nucleoside analogues. Biochem. Pharmacol., in press.
De Clercq E., Descamps J, Verhelst G, Walker RT, Jones AS, Torrence PF, Shugar D. 1980. Comparative efficacy of antiherpes drugs against different strains of herpes simplex virus. J. Infect. Dis. 141, 563–574.
Field AK, Davies ME, DeWitt C, Perry HC, Liou R, Germershausen J, Karkas JD, Ashton WT, Johnston DBR, Tolman RL. 1983. 9-{[2-Hydroxy-1-(hydroxymethyl)ethoxy]methyl}guanine : a selective inhibitor of herpes group virus replication. Proc. Natl. Acad. Sci. USA 80, 4139–4143.
Machida H, Kuninaka A, Yoshino H. 1982. Inhibitory effects of antiherpesviral thymidine analogs against varicella-zoster virus. Antimicrob. Agents Chemother. 21, 358–361.
Mancini WR, De Clercq E, Prusoff WH. 1983. The relationship between incorporation of E-5-(2-bromovinyl)-2'-deoxyuridine into herpes simplex virus type 1 DNA with virus infectivity and DNA integrity. J. Biol. Chem. 258, 792–795.
Mar E-C, Patel PC, Cheng Y-C, Fox JJ, Watanabe KA, Huang E-S. 1984. Effects of certain nucleoside analogues on human cytomegalovirus replication in vitro. J. Gen. Virol. 65, 47–53.

Maudgal PC, De Clercq E, Descamps J, Missotten L. 1984a. Topical treatment of experimental herpes simplex keratouveitis with 2'-O-glycylacyclovir. A water-soluble ester of acyclovir. Arch. Ophthalmol. 102, 140–142.

Maudgal PC, De Clercq E, Descamps J, Missotten L, De Somer P, Busson R, Vanderhaeghe H, Verhelst G, Walker RT, Jones AS. 1980. (E)-5-(2-Bromovinyl)-2'-deoxyuridine in the treatment of experimental herpes simplex keratitis. Antimicrob. Agents Chemother. 17, 8–12.

Maudgal PC, De Clercq E, Descamps J, Missotten L, Wijnhoven J. 1982a. Experimental stromal herpes simplex keratitis. Influence of treatment with topical bromovinyldeoxyuridine and trifluridine. Arch. Ophthalmol. 100, 653–656.

Maudgal PC, De Clercq E, Missotten L. 1984b. Efficacy of bromovinyldeoxyuridine in the treatment of herpes simplex virus and varicella-zoster virus eye infections. Antiviral Res., in press.

Maudgal PC, Dralands L, Lamberts L, De Clercq E, Descamps J, Missotten L. 1981a. Preliminary results of oral BVDU treatment of herpes zoster ophthalmicus. Bull. Soc. belge Ophtal. 193, 49–56.

Maudgal PC, Missotten L, De Clercq E, Descamps J, De Meuter E. 1981b. Efficacy of (E)-5-(2-bromovinyl)-2'-deoxyuridine in the topical treatment of herpes simplex keratitis. Albrecht von Graefes Arch. Klin. Ophthalmol. 216, 261–268.

Maudgal PC, Uyttebroeck W, De Clercq E, Missotten L. 1982b. Oral and topical treatment of experimental herpes simplex iritis with bromovinyldeoxyuridine. Arch. Ophthalmol. 100, 1337–1340.

Schinazi RF, Peters J, Sokol MK, Nahmias AJ. 1983. Therapeutic activities of 1-(2-fluoro-2-deoxy-β-D-arabinofuranosyl)-5-iodocytosine and -thymine alone and in combination with acyclovir and vidarabine in mice infected intracerebrally with herpes simplex virus. Antimicrob. Agents Chemother. 24, 95–103.

Shigeta S, Yokota T, Iwabuchi T, Baba M, Konno K, Ogata M, De Clercq E. 1983. Comparative efficacy of antiherpes drugs against various strains of varicella-zoster virus. J. Infect. Dis. 147, 576–584.

Tocci MJ, Livelli TJ, Perry HC, Crumpacker CS, Field AK. 1984. Effects of the nucleoside analog 2'-nor-2'-deoxyguanosine on human cytomegalovirus replication. Antimicrob. Agents Chemother. 25, 247–252.

Trousdale MD, Nesburn AB, Su, T-L, Lopez C, Watanabe KA, Fox JJ. 1983. Activity of 1-(2'-fluoro-2'-deoxy-β-D-arabinofuranosyl)thymine against herpes simplex virus in cell cultures and rabbit eyes. Antimicrob. Agents Chemother. 23, 808–813.

Trousdale MD, Nesburn AB, Watanabe KA, Fox JJ. 1981. Evaluation of the antiherpetic activity of 2'-fluoro-5-iodo-ara-C in rabbit eyes and cell cultures. Invest. Ophthalmol. Vis. Sci. 21, 826–832.

Wildiers J, De Clercq E. 1984. Oral (E)-5-(2-bromovinyl)-2'-deoxyuridine treatment of severe herpes zoster in cancer patients. Eur. J. Cancer Clin. Oncol. 20, 471–476.

DISCUSSION :

J. Colin (Brest) : We compared in a double blind study IDC and acyclovir in herpetic superficial keratitis. There was no significant difference between the two drugs.

E. De Clercq (Leuven) : That is very nice. Did you use the 0,15 % IDC eye ointment Cébé-viran or did you use IDC eye-drops ?

J. Collin (Brest) : It was 1 % ointment.

E. De Clercq (Leuven) : O.K. Well, perhaps for those who are interested to know, IDC is readily deaminated in vivo to IDU. So, the activity that you measure is probably due to IDU.

R. Sundmacher (Freiburg) : Just for my information, would you please give me the reference for the controlled BVDU clinical studies. I think I missed them.

E. De Clercq (Leuven) : The clinical studies I referred to were not controlled. Such controlled trials are planned and a direct comparative study of BVDU versus TFT eyedrops is underway.

P.C. Maudgal (Leuven) : I think it will be of interest to the audience if you could little bit elaborate on the toxicity of these compounds on the basis of their mechanism of action or their biochemical activity.

E. De Clercq (Leuven) : I would not go into any details but just make a general comment. This brings me back to the mechanism of action. Because the compounds I described are targeted on specific viral enzymes, they should have reasonable selectivity in their mode of action. Hereby I refer to the newer compounds such as acyclovir, BVDU and also FIAC, FMAU and all related compounds. IDU, TFT, and also Ara-A to certain extent lack this selectivity. They are or not really interacting with any specific viral enzymes; for that reason they do not show much selectivity in their antiviral activity. This is the distinction I wanted to make between the old generation of antiherpes compounds, which affect normal cell metabolism and virus replication indiscriminately, and the new generation of antiherpes compounds, which are targeted at the specific viral enzymes.

OCULAR HERPESVIRUS INFECTIONS AND THE DEVELOPMENT OF VIRUS DRUG-
RESISTANCE

H.J. Field.   Department of Clinical Veterinary Medicine, University
          of Cambridge, UK.

1. Treatment Resistance in Ocular Herpes.   In the two decades during
which nucleoside analogue chemotherapy has been used in the management
of ocular herpes there have been numerous accounts of a marked failure
of the disease to respond to treatment.   These observations may have
been frequent because in eye disease changes in clinical response can
be readily monitored by the physician compared with other manifestations of the infection.   In some cases viruses were isolated from
treatment failures which were subsequently found to be resistant to
particular nucleoside analogues (e.g. Idoxuridine;   IDU) when tested
in vitro (reviewed by McGill, 1977).   In other cases, however,
'treatment-resistance' could not be correlated with decreased
sensitivity when the virus isolates were tested against the therapeutic
drug in tissue-culture (Coleman et al., 1968;   Jawetz et al., 1970).
We are still ignorant as to whether subtle changes had occurred in
these virus populations, which were undetectable, or whether other
mechanisms - host factors - accounted for the failure of treatment.
With the introduction of new more selective and more potent nucleoside
analogues such as acyclovir;   ACV and bromovinyldeoxyuridine;   BVDU
the importance of acquired drug resistance has again been called into
question.

2.   Mechanisms of drug resistance
2.1.   Changes in DNA-polymerase. All the 'useful' nucleoside analogues
used in the chemotherapy of herpes simplex (and ophthalmic zoster)
together with the pyrophosphate analogue, phosphonoformic acid;   PFA
share the common feature that they or their products (i.e.   nucleoside
triphosphates) interact with herpesvirus-induced DNA polymerase (Darby
and Field, 1984).   In all cases mutation(s) in the virus genes coding

Maudgal, P.C. and Missotten, L., (eds.) Herpetic Eye Diseases.
© *1985, Dr W. Junk Publishers, Dordrecht/Boston/Lancaster. ISBN 978-94-010-8935-7*

for DNA-pol can result in a change in the enzyme and this can confer
resistance to particular inhibitors. Such mutants have been selected
from drug-treated tissue cultures and characterized. In some cases
there is found to be a change which confers co-resistance to several
drugs e.g. PFA and ACV (Field et al, 1980) but commonly the resistance
is specific for the drug used for selection and in some cases the
viruses acquire hypersensitivity to certain alternative inhibitors
(Coen et al, 1983). It must be stressed that the DNA-pol has vital
functions in virus replication therefore there are considerable constraints upon the range of mutations which can confer resistance
yet are not lethal to the virus. These constraints are likely to
be considerably greater when the virus is replicating in the hostile
environment of the host for example in the tissues of the eye than
in cell cultures. Thus it would be predicted that many resistant
mutants of this type would have reduced (or altered) pathogenicity.

2.2. Changes in expression of thymidine kinase
In addition to DNA-pol a second locus plays an important rôle in
the acquisition of drug resistance namely the virus-induced thymidine
kinase; TK. The drugs ACV and BVDU largely depend on virus TK for
the initial phosphorylation to their respective nucleotides. This,
of course accounts for their selective toxicity for virus-infected
cells. IDU and particularly trifluorothymidine (TFT) are more readily
phosphorylated by host cellular enzymes although virus TK may still
be important in their activation. On the other hand adenine arabinoside;
Ara-A and PFA both work independently of TK and as a result mutations
in the TK-locus are not important for these two drugs. In tissue
cultures TK-defective variants may be selected readily by means of
any of the TK-mediated drugs; such mutants probably occur spontaneously
with a frequency of at least 0.1% in clinical isolates even when
obtained from patients with no obvious history of exposure to nucleoside analogues. TK-defective viruses may be found to be devoid of
detectable TK-polypeptide yet these strains grow with normal characteristics in actively dividing cell cultures. However, without exception
such strains have a markedly reduced capacity to multiply in the
nervous system and do not produce neurological signs when inoculated into

animals (Field, 1983). **It is** notable that several
TK-defective strains were found to multiply readily in primary ocular
infections in animals, for example the rabbit or guinea-pig
(R.B. Tenser, personal communication) although subsequent latent
infections in the trigeminal ganglia were much more difficult to
detect compared with the wild-type strains. In addition to TK-defective
strains - which may fail completely to synthesize the TK polypeptide
in infected cells, it has been discovered that mutations in the TK
structural gene can lead to a much more subtle change in the enzyme,
causing a narrowing or change in its substrate specificity so it
is no longer able to phosphorylate the nucleoside analogue in question
e.g. ACV (Darby et al, 1981) or BVDU (Field and Neden, 1982; Larder
et al, 1983) while retaining the ability to phosphorylate the natural
substrate, thymidine.

2.3.Alternative loci for the acquisition of resistance

In addition to the mutants described above which have single lesions
many viruses have been described which have alterations in both loci
i.e. TK and DNA-pol. However, to date, no changes have been discovered
in any other locus which accounts for the development of resistance.
In the future modifications in other virus-induced products which
contribute to resistance may be identified although it will be difficult to do this if they make only a minor contribution to the overall resistance. An example of a candidate virus enzyme of this type
would be ribonucleotide reductase where changes could possibly enhance
resistance to BVDU.

3. Development of resistance in vivo

The majority of work on the selection, identification and characterization of resistant mutants has been carried out using viruses selected
for resistance in vitro. It seems that resistance occurs much less
frequently in vivo than might be predicted from these experiments.
No doubt this is because the constraints on mutations in vivo are
much more severe than those which apply to the virus growing in the
relative comfort of a rapidly dividing, permissive, cell culture
system. However, the results of experiments in tissue culture systems

182

designed to resemble more closely the natural situation (e.g. serum-
starved, resting cells) and in animal models and the early clinical
data on virus isolates from acyclovir-treated patients all suggest
that resistance to nucleoside (and pyrophosphate) analogues will
become a significant problem eventually. When HSV is passaged in
mice undergoing sub-optimal ACV therapy (Field, 1982) or when X-
irradiated mice with a persistent skin infection are given continuous
oral ACV (Field and Efstathioce,unpublished observations) resistant
virus may be readily isolated. So far these viruses owe their
resistance to a high proportion of TK-defective virions present in
a mixed population. It is notable that similar mixed isolates containing TK^+ and TK^- virions have also been reported recently, obtained
from immunocompetent human patients (McLaren et al, 1983).

We have shown in our own experimental studies that when such mixed
infections establish latent infections in mice, on reactivation,
the ganglia yield similar resistant mixtures of TK^+ and TK^- virions
(Field and Lay, 1984). This has important implications for chemotherapy
since it suggests that TK^- virus, even if in pure culture it has
reduced disease potential, may confer the property of drug resistance
upon a pathogenic strain and the infection could also become recurrent
by means of classical latency and reactivation.

Secondly viruses which express TK with altered substrate specificity
have now been identified among the human isolates (McLaren et al,
1983). These viruses failed to phosphorylate ACV while retaining
normal (or partial) ability to phosphorylate thymidine. So far no
well-characterized ACV-resistant viruses have been found among the
human isolates that owe their resistance to an altered DNA-pol but
no doubt such viruses will emerge in due course.

4.   The prospects for the future of nucleoside analogue chemotherapy
It seems likely that all the resistance mechanisms discussed above
will have a rôle to play in complicating the treatment of ocular
herpes infections. It is therefore important to monitor clinical
isolates with care. Virus isolation and drug testingprocedures should

be such that relatively small changes in virus sensitivity are not
overlooked. For example the dye-uptake method for establishing ACV-
sensitivity (McLaren et al, 1983) may be convenient for semi-
automation for processing large numbers of isolates but is unable
to detect mixtures containing up to 40% TK⁻ virions which may be
extremely important. Another problem is that resistance may be overlooked because of an inappropriate cell culture system. An extreme
example of this is the observation that TK⁻ viruses are sensitive
to TFT in normal cells; the analogue being readily converted to TFT
triphosphate by cellular kinases. However, if TK-defective cells
are used in the test then virus resistance to TFT is revealed (Field
et al, 1981). It is conceivable that the TK-defective cells used
here resemble more closely some resting cell populations important
in the pathogenesis of the infection? This is an extreme example
but similar principles apply to other inhibitor-cell combinations
and may lead to important resistance being overlooked.

When resistance results from the presence of TK⁻ virions then co-
resistance to all TK-mediated drugs will be apparent. Thus TFT,
being less dependent on activation by virus TK may be useful to
counteract the resistant infection and the drugs AraA and PFA work
independently of TK and from this point of view will be useful alter-
natives. For other kinds of resistance it seems likely that small
and subtle changes will occur in TK and DNA-pol probably causing
reduced sensitivity to particular drugs. Thus there is much scope
for the development of alternating or combinations of drugs (Hall,
1984). Better models need to be designed both in vivo and employing
cell cultures in order to devise and test the development of such
strategies to combat drug resistance in the herpesvirus.

References

Coen, D.M., Furman, P.A., Aschman, D.P. & Schaffer, P.A. (1983)
    Mutations in the herpes simplex virus DNA polymerase gene
    conferring hypersensitivity to aphidicolin. Nucleic Acids
    Res. 11: 5287-5297.

184

Coleman, V.R., Tsu, E., & Jawetz, E. (1968) 'Treatment resistance' to idoxuridine in herpetic keratitis. Proc. Soc. New York Acad. Sci. 129: 761-765.

Darby, G. & Field, H.J. (1984) Latency and acquired resistance - problems in chemotherapy of herpes infections. Pharm. Ther. 23: 217-251.

Darby, G., Field, H.J. & Salisbury, S.A. (1981) Altered substrate specificity of herpes simplex virus thymidine kinase confers acyclovir resistance. Nature 289: 81-83.

Field, H.J. (1982) Development of clinical resistance to acyclovir in herpes simplex virus-infected mice receiving oral therapy. Antimicrob. Ag. Chemother. 21: 744-752.

Field, H.J. (1983) The problem of drug-induced resistance in viruses In The 5th Beecham Colloquia eds. C.H. Stuart-Harris & J.S. Oxford. Academic Press, pp. 71-107.

Field, H.J., Darby, G., & Wildy, P. (1980) Isolation and characterization of acyclovir-resistant mutants of herpes simplex virus. J. Gen Virol. 49: 115-124.

Field, H.J. & Lay, E. (1984) The characterization of latent infections in mice after inoculation with herpes simplex virus which is clinically resistant to acyclovir. Antiviral Research (in press).

Field, H.J., McMillan, A. & Darby, G. (1981) The sensitivity of acyclovir-resistant mutants of herpes simplex virus to other antiviral drugs. J. Inf. Dis. 143: 281-285.

Field, H.J. & Neden, J. (1982) Isolation of bromovinyldeoxyuridine-resistant strains of herpes simplex virus and successful chemotherapy of mice infected with one such strain by using acyclovir. Antiviral Res. 2: 243-254.

Hall, M.J. (1984) Opportunities for the development and use of anti-herpes virus drug combinations. J. Antimicrob. Chemother. (in press).

Jawetz, E., Coleman, V.R., Dawson, C.R. & Thygeson, P. (1970) The dynamics of IUDR action in herpetic keratitis and the emergence of IUDR resistance in vivo. Ann. N.Y. Acad. Sci. 173: 282-291.

Larder, B.A., Cheng, Y-C. & Darby, G. (1983) Characterization of abnormal thymidine kinases induced by drug-resistant strains of herpes simplex type I. J. Gen Virol. 64: 523-532.

McGill, J. (1977) Drug resistance and antiviral agents. J. Antimicrob. Chemother. 3: 284-285.

McLaren, C., Corey, L., Dekker, C. & Barry, D.W. (1983) In vitro
      sensitivity to acyclovir in genital herpes simplex virus from
      acyclovir-treated patients. J. Inf. Dis. 148: 868-875.

McLaren, C., Ellis, M.N. & Hunter, G.A. (1983) A colorimetric assay
      for the measurement of the sensitivity of herpes simplex virus
      to antiviral agents. Antiviral Research 3: 223-234.

DISCUSSION :

C.R. Dawson (San Francisco) : Recurrent herpes simplex eye disease is one of the few conditions in which we treat a single
   patient with an antiviral on multiple occasions. Is it likely
   that the patient will acquire a resistant strain ? What is your
   opinion ?

H.J. Field (Cambridge) : I think, from what we know of latency
   and recurrence, I would imagine that the most important thing
   is that the reservoir of latent virus probably forms some kind
   of "template" for future recurrences. But I am not sure, in
   practice, that this will occur. We may observe that during
   the course of treatments the virus will become increasingly resistant. I think it is too early in the clinical experience to know
   whether this will happen or not. It is apparent from early
   data on the sensitivity of isolates that there are strains that
   are already resistant to acyclovir. Part of the explanation
   for this may be that idoxuridine has been around for a long
   time and sometimes there is cross-resistance between the two
   drugs.

C.R. Dawson (San Francisco) : How do you think that the preva-
   lence of resistance might increase in the population ?

H.J. Field (Cambridge) : I am sure it will be rather an insidious
   process. I doubt that there will be spectacular changes in
   the sensivity of the viruses. But with a drug which is not
   totally effective, that is we are always looking at partially
   effective compounds, it is very difficult to determine that they
   are becoming slightly less effective.

A.B. Tullo (Bristol) : Would you care to speculate on why immunodeficient patients are producing resistant strains ?

H.J. Field (Cambridge) : It may be just that there is more virus
replication, therefore there is more opportunity for selection
to occur. I rather doubt that, because with every yield of
virus from a cell, there is probably a proportion of thymidine
kinase defective virus. The yield of virus from a single cell
is of the order of 1000 virions and the rate is about 0.1%.
The fact that these defective strains can persist is probably
telling us something about the biology of the infection. Actually, they are not that debilitated : they grow normally in
tissue culture. But they certainly have differences in ability
to interact with differentiated cells, especially neural tissue,
I think.

J.McGill (Southampton) : Concerning the question of resistance
we looked at several isolates from different attacks in people
with herpes simplex keratitis and the in vitro sensivity of each
isolate was the same. It did not alter at all.

H.J.Field (Cambridge) : I think there are plenty of similar data
and I am sure this is right. The reason are clear, rapid
emergence of highly resistant virus is not a problem. But I
think you have still got to be very careful when analysing
the data of particular laboratories. I am not exactly sure
how you do your assays, but in some cases, high multiplicity
is used, and this will not reveal mixtures. Indeed, you may
get complementation within particular infected cells. In conclusion, I just had a very quick look through the marketing information of the Burroughs Wellcomme and I find no reference at
all there among the management of eye disease to the development of resistance.

RELEVANCE OF VIRAL THYMIDINE KINASE FOR CLINICAL RESISTANCE TO ANTIVIRAL DRUGS WHEN TREATING HERPES SIMPLEX EYE INFECTIONS.

Karlström A.R., Källander C.F.R., Gronowitz J.S. and P.J. Wistrand[1].
Department of Medical Virology, Box 584, Biomedical Center, S-751 23 Uppsala, and [1]Department of Ophthalmology, The University Hospital, S-751 85 Uppsala, Sweden.

1. INTRODUCTION

Herpes simplex virus (HSV) type 1 normally infects the upper part of the body especially the oral cavity, the lips and sometimes also the eye. After primary infection the virus establishes latency but may then give recurrent localized infections i.e. cold sores and in some individuals infections of the cornea, which may lead to blindness (Dawson & Togni 1976).

The oldest drug for treatment of HSV eye infections is 5-iododeoxyuridine (IUdR), a substance synthetized by Prusoff already in 1959 and found by Kaufman et al. in 1962 to be therapeutically active (cf. Fischer & Prusoff 1984). IUdR is dependent on phosphorylation by thymidine kinase (TK) for its antiviral activity (cf. Fischer & Prusoff 1984).

During recent years the increased knowledge of virus specific enzymes and their differences from the cellular counterparts have led to the synthesis of several other antiviral nucleoside analogues interfering with thymidine (dThd) metabolism, such as E-5-(2-bromovinyl)-2'deoxyuridine, 9-(2-hydroxyethoxymethyl)guanine (Acyclovir), and 9-(3,4-dihydroxybutyl)guanine (cf. Fischer & Prusoff 1984).

With the increased clinical use of antiviral agents, it has been found that the HSV infections can become resistant to therapy. Two different mechanisms for induction of resistance have been discussed; selection of therapy resistant virus already present at the start of treatment; and mutation by therapy followed by selection. Therapy resistant HSV strains have been induced in cell culture systems and characterized in great detail; strains totally devoid of TK inducing capacity and strains inducing low TK levels have been reported. However, different results from strains isolated from patients resistant to IUdR have been reported (Coleman et al 1968, Jawetz et al 1970, Hirano et al 1979). A detailed biochemical characterisation of such strains is also lacking. Moreover, it is important to know whether these strains can establish latency.

Maudgal, P.C. and Missotten, L., (eds.) Herpetic Eye Diseases.
© *1985, Dr W. Junk Publishers, Dordrecht/Boston/Lancaster. ISBN 978-94-010-8935-7*

Studies in animals have shown that TK negative strains cannot establish latency, however, strains with low TK activity can. Moreover, recent results indicate that TK positive virus may complement TK negative ones and thereby could make latency of the TK negative strain possible (Tenser et al 1981).

Earlier reports on in vitro induced therapy resistance indicate that mutations in the TK locus are common, while alterations in the viral DNA polymerase gene are less frequent (Coen et al,1982). Because of this, we decided to analyse and compare in vivo isolates from patients responding well or poorly to antiviral therapy with reference to the TK activity and its characteristics.

Our earliest procedure for typing of HSV isolates was based on the differential IUdR sensitivity of HSV type 1 and type 2. During these studies an eye isolate C915, sampled after IUdR treatment of a keratitis in a 50-year old person, was found to be TK negative (Gronowitz et al 1982).

2. MATERIALS AND METHODS

2.1. Cells and media. Early passages of human embryonic fibroblast (HEF) or green monkey kidney (GMK) cells were grown in 1 ml tubes and used for primary isolations. Propagation of virus isolates and titrations were performed on VERO cells. All cells were cultured with Eagle MEM supplemented with 10% calf serum. Before isolation or virus infection the calf serum was omitted.

2.2. Virus isolation and propagation. Corneal cell scrapings were transferred to tubes containing Eagles MEM and directly transported to the virus diagnostic laboratory, where two tubes with GMK and HEF, respectively, were inoculated. The isolate was typed and passaged once in order to achieve a higher titer. Virus from this second passage was titrated and then used for enzyme preparation.

2.3. Enzyme preparation. TK preparations were done in a manner similar to that described earlier (Gronowitz et al 1982), except for the use of a new buffer system based on HEPES (Gronowitz et al 1984). From one VERO cell culture tube, containing about 3×10^5 cells, 200 µl of enzyme preparation was prepared.

2.4 Enzyme assays. All TK assays were performed with the recently described system (Gronowitz et al 1984). In the assays, the final concentration of ATP and CTP was 4.6 and 2.5 mM respectively, and the final concentration of the substrate IUdR was 1.1×10^{-7} M. Thymidine concentrations in M (Fig.1), giving 50% inhibition of ^{125}I-IUdR phosphorylation were calculated from analyses using three different concentrations. Enzyme activities are given as units per µl undiluted enzyme preparation. One unit is 1.2×10^{-18} katal giving circa 1000 cpm per hour assay when using ^{125}I-IUdR, with a specific activity of 130-160 Ci/mmole (Gronowitz et al 1984).

2.5 Typing of isolates. This was done using serological typing of TK employing isozyme specific antisera (Gronowitz et al 1982, Källander et al 1983)

3. RESULTS

3.1. Isolates and patient data. Sixteen HSV isolates from fifteen unselected patients with eye infection were obtained. Two other isolates C915, and J1 were also included (Table 1). C915 is the TK negative mutant described above. J1, a HSV type 1 strain, was found to possess a TK with altered K_m values for IUdR ($2.3 \pm 0.7 \times 10^{-7}$ M) and dThd ($8.2 \pm 0.1 \times 10^{-7}$ M), similar to those of HSV type 2. Relevant clinical data on all isolates are also given in the table. From this it may be noted, that a poor therapeutic response was found in all six patients with more than one recurrence, while a good response was obtained in 7 out of 10 patients with a primary eye infection having their first recurrence.

Table 1. Clinical data on patients with HSV eye infection, and TK activity induced by their isolates, measured with ATP and CTP respectively as phosphate donors.

Age years	type of eye infection	recurrence number	type of therapy	therapy effect	isolation day in relation to therapy	sample code	TK activity with ATP as phosphate-donor	% activity[3] with CTP as phosphate-donor
83	recurrence	3	IUdR+	poor	3	N010	115	99
			ARA-A		7	N019	90	119
83	recurrence	3	IUdR+ACV	poor	0	X012	52	81
73	recurrence	2	ACV	poor	0	X217	65	109
66	recurrence	18	IUdR	poor	0	N003	50	90
50	recurrence	3	IUdR+ster[1]	poor	0	N034	42	78
47	recurrence	13	IUdR	poor	0	T148	107	99
32	recurrence	1	IUdR	good	0	N011	72	105
19	recurrence	1	IUdR+ACV	good	3	X075	93	106
25	unknown		IUdR	unknown	2	J1[2]	79	112
69	primary		IUdR	good	0	M597[2]	55	84
50	primary		IUdR	poor	70	C915[2]	14	8
44	primary		ACV	poor	0	X093	62	117
43	primary		IUdR	good	14	N082	ND	ND
42	primary		IUdR	poor	0	N035	68	124
29	primary		ACV	good	0	T346	63	109
29	primary		ACV	good	0	X314	109	106
5	primary		ACV	good	0	X309	56	96
						Mock	9	2
						11 clones derived from N003 mean	34 ± 13	105 ± 30

[1] steroids
[2] these eye isolates were sampled earlier but incorporated in the study. C915 was sampled from a kidney transplanted patient, and has been reported (J.Clin.Microb 1982, 15:3 pp 366-371).
[3] % CTP mediated activity was calculated after correction for ATP and CTP activity in mock-infected cells.

190

3.2. <u>TK inducing capacity</u> In order to compare the TK inducing capacity of the different isolates, three cell culture tubes were infected with each isolate. When 80% cytopathic effect was seen, a raw extract of enzyme was prepared by freeze thawing, using three different stabilizing buffer systems. Similar levels of enzyme activity were obtained from all three tubes, infected with the same isolate, indicating that the enzyme was stable during preparation (data not shown). The TK activities induced by the different isolates are given in Table 1. Compared to mock infected cultures, isolates were found which induced more than a 10-fold increase in TK activity, as well as isolates which induced only a slight increase in TK activity. One of the clinically resistant isolates, N003, which was found to induce a fairly low TK activity, was cloned and recloned at an early passage. These clones were found to induce equally low TK levels, showing that the recurring infection in fact was caused by virus particles with a low TK inducing capacity.

3.3. <u>Capacity of viral TKs, to utilize cytidinetriphosphate (CTP) as phosphate donor.</u> The enzyme activity with 2.5 mM CTP as phosphate donor, was compared to that with 4.6 mM ATP. As seen from Table 1, all TKs utilized CTP with similar efficiency, except for the TK prepared from C915. This indicates that the TK in all preparations, except for that of C915 and that of mock infected cells, were of viral origin, and had no modifications in the phosphate donor site as detected by this procedure.

3.4. <u>Thymidine (dThd) inhibition of IUdR phosphory-</u> <u>lation.</u> The results do not exclude the possibility that isolates with low TK inducing capacity, owe this to a decreased affinity for IUdR, at the same time as the enzyme has a high dThd phosphorylating capacity. Therefore the capacity of dThd to block the phosphorylation of IUdR was analysed for all isolate TKs. No difference was found between the isolates from the group of patients responding to therapy and those who did not (Table 1, Fig.1). However, with the exception for TK derived from C915 and mock infected cells (Fig.1), one isolate N003 and its clones required a 2-3 times higher dThd concentration for 50% inhibition of IUdR turnover.

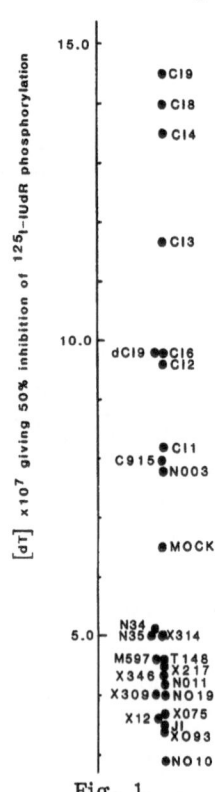

Fig. 1

4. DISCUSSION

A good therapeutic response was recorded in 7 out of the 10 patients with primary eye infection, or having their first recurrence, while a poor therapeutic effect was found in all six patients with two or more recurrencies. In the latter group the recurring virus is probably in some way modified. However, irrespective of resistance, the isolates were found to induce various levels of TK activity, similar with respect to use of phosphate donor. The only deviating isolate with respect to CTP mediated phosporylation of IUdR was C915, the earlier reported TK negative isolate. It should be noted, that C915 was sampled from an immunosuppressed patient after kidney transplantation, and therapy resistance may be easier induced if the duration of the infection is prolonged due to poor immune status. The isolates were also equally sensitive to competition by dThd of IUdR phosphorylation, with the exception of N003. TK induced by this isolate, as well as by its clones, required higher dThd concentrations for inhibition of IUdR phosphorylation. The reason for this is not obvious. Most isolates were sampled before therapy was started. However, three isolates were sampled after 3 to 7 days of therapy, and still the TK:s induced by these isolates were similar to those of the others. Surprisingly small differences with respect to the characteristics of TK were thus found between isolates from resistant and non-resistant patients. If, after all, the observed therapy resistance is related to alteration of viral TK, this could perhaps be determined by further studies of other parameters, such as the cytidine kinase and thymidylate kinase functions of this enzyme. Further, resistant isolates should be analysed for alterations in other possible steps involved in the induction of therapy resistance, e.g DNA polymerase.

However, apart from the above, the difference in therapeutic effects in patients with primary or first recurrence and those with several recurrencies may be due to differences in age and immune status.

REFERENCES
Coen DM, Schaffer PA, Furman PA, Keller PM, St Clair MH. 1982. Biochemical and genetic analysis of acyclovir-resistant mutants of herpes simplex virus type 1. Proc. of a Symposium on Acyclovir, Am.J.Med. 98:351-360.

Coleman VR, Tsu E, Jawetz E. 1968. "Treatment resistance" to Idoxuridine in herpes keratitis. Proc.Soc.Exp.Biol.Med. 129: 761-765.

Dawson, CR. & Togni, B. 1976. Herpes Simplex eye infections: Clinical manifestations, pathogenesis and management. Surv. Ophthalmol. 21:121-135.

Fischer, PH. & Prusoff, WH. 1984. Chemotherapy of ocular viral infections and tumors. In Handbook of Exp.Pharmacol., vol 69, pp 551-583. Ed. ML Sears, Springer-Verlag, Berlin.

Gronowitz JS, Källander CFR, Jeansson S, Wallin J. 1982. Rapid typing of herpes simplex virus based on immunological specificity of viral thymidine kinase and typing according to sensitivity to iododeoxyuridine. J.Clin. Microbiol. 15:366-371.

Gronowitz JS, Källander CFR, Diderholm H, Hagberg H, Pettersson U. 1984. Application of an in vitro assay for serum thymidine kinase: Results on viral disease and malignancies in humans. Int.J.Cancer 33: 5-12.

Hirano A, Yumura K, Kurimura T, Katsumoto T, Moriyama H, Manabe R. 1979. Analysis of herpes simplex virus isolated from patients with recurrent herpes keratitis exhibiting "Treatment resistance" to 5-iodo-2'-deoxyuridine. Acta virol. 23:226-230.

Jawetz E, Coleman VR, Dawson CR, Thygeson P. 1970. The dynamics of IUDR action in herpetic keratitis and the emergence of IUDR resistance in vivo. Ann.N.Y.Acad.Sci. 173: 282-291.

Källander CFR, Gronowitz JS, Olding-Stenkvist E. 1983. Rapid diagnosis of varicella-zoster virus infection by detection of viral deoxytyhmidine kinase in serum and vesicle fluid. J.Clin.Microbiol. 17:280-287.

Tenser RB, Ressel S, Dunstan ME. 1981. Herpes simplex virus thymidine kinase expression in trigeminal ganglion infection: Correlation of enzyme activity with ganglion virus titer and evidence of in vivo complementation. Virology 112:328-341.

DISCUSSION :

H.J.Field (Cambridge) : May I ask a question and make a couple of comments? You did not tell us whether there was any in vitro evidence of resistance- you did not mention the sensitivity of the isolates. The other points I would like to make are that, as I understand it from your methodology, you are using a high multiplicity infection in your isolation and production of the TK extracts. Therefore, you would not be able to measure, say 75% proportion of TK⁻ virus among a TK⁺ background. Two other points: taking IDU, you looked at the idoxuridine phosphorylation but one would imagine from past experience that IDU-resistance is probably more likely to result from resistance in the polymerase locus.Finally, you did not look at acyclovir phosphorylation, which could be very important.

P.J.Wistrand (Uppsala) : You are right, we did not look at these things. The resistance to IDU is being determined presently.

A RAPID MICROMETHOD FOR EVALUATING THE SENSITIVITY OF OCULAR HERPES
SIMPLEX STRAINS TO ANTIVIRAL DRUGS

M. LANGLOIS, J. DENIS, J.Ph. ALLARD, M. AYMARD

1. INTRODUCTION

Treatment for Herpes Simplex virus (HSV) infections was now possible
with the use of different antiviral agents. Recently, Acyclovir (ACV) has
been introduced as a potent and selective anti Herpes agent with low host
cell toxicity. A micromethod for evaluating the drug sensitivity of the
HSV strains in vitro was established. This study reports the preliminary
results observed with ACV.

2. MATERIALS AND METHODS

2.1. Vero monkey kidney cells were grown in medium 199 supplemented with
5 % fetal calf serum.

2.2. The laboratory strains of HSV1 and HSV2 were both obtained from
Dr ROIZMAN (University of Chicago) (F-HSV1 and G-HSV2).

2.3. Clinical specimens. We have studied 37 HSV strains (36 types 1 and
1 type 2) collected from 30 patients suffering from different types of
ocular herpetic infections ; we have also examined 10 HSV2 strains isolated from genital lesions or urine samples. All these strains were typed
by direct immunofluorescence test.

2.4. Selection of ACV resistant mutants in vitro was performed on 2 sensitive HSV1 ocular strains. They were grown in Vero culture in the presence
of ACV.

2.5. Viral inhibition assay. The assay derived from the microtiter ver-
sion of the neutral red dye-uptake method described by Mc LAREN et al (5)
Briefly, dilutions of drug (100 µl/well), Vero cells suspension (60 µl/
well, ≃ 30.000 cells) was successively dispensed into 96- well microti-
tre plates. Tenfold dilutions of virus being tested were prepared and

This work was supported by I.N.S.E.R.M.

Maudgal, P.C. and Missotten, L., (eds.) Herpetic Eye Diseases.
© *1985, Dr W. Junk Publishers, Dordrecht/Boston/Lancaster. ISBN 978-94-010-8935-7*

40µl of each dilution were added. Controls were also included. Plates were allowed to incubate for 2 days at 37°C in 5 % CO2 prior to the addition of neutral red. Unincorporated dye was removed by rinsing with PBS and the neutral red incorporated by viable cells was eluted into citrate-ethanol buffer. The OD were read at 540 nm on a multichannel spectrophotometer and all the data were directly analysed on a micro computer. The relation between CPE and OD was linear (correlation coefficient = 0,98). We determined the dilution containing approximately 30 TCID 50 or the nearest one. Then results were calculated by linear regression analysis which yields the 50 % inhibitory dose of the drug. The sensitivity of virus was expressed as an ID50 value that is the concentration of drug (µg/ml) reducing viral CPE by 50 %).

3. RESULTS

3.1. Sensitivity of HSV strains to ACV. The mean ID50 of ACV for F-HSV1 strain was determined in consecutive assays to be 0,16 µg/ml ($\pm$ 0,04). The ID50 values of ACV for 36 HSV1 ocular strains ranged from 0,11 to 0,88 µg/ml, with a mean ID50 of 0,31 µg/ml ($\pm$ 0,18) and a median value of 0,23 µg/ml. The ID50 values for the 29 strains isolated before any treatment with ACV ranged from 0,11 to 0,77 µg/ml (mean = 0,30 µg/ml $\pm$ 0,16). Some of HSV1 ocular strains were isolated after therapy with ACV occurred 1 to 2 years ago. The ID50 values for these 7 strains ranged from 0,15 to 0,88 µg/ml (mean = 0,35 µg/ml $\pm$ 0,25). Then the results obtained before and after ACV were not significantly different. 18 patients have been treated with ACV : we observed a good correlation between in vitro and clinical results. The mean ID50 of ACV for G-HSV2 strain was 1,41 µg/ml ($\pm$ 0,35). Among the ocular strains only one was typed as HSV2. Its ID50 value was 0,48 µg/ml. We have also examined 10 genital HSV2 strains. ID50 values ranged from 0,70 to 1,29 µg/ml with a mean of 0,93 µg/ml ($\pm$ 0,19) an a median value of 0,88 µg/ml. All these strains were isolated before any treatment with ACV.

3.2. ACV resistant mutant strains. The first sensitive HSV1 ocular virus, C2 strain, was serially passaged through 1 and 100 µg/ml of ACV. The ID50 value of ACV for C2 sensitive strain was 0,11 µg/ ml ($\pm$ 0,05). The ID50 value for the different C2R (ACV-resistant mutants) strains were of 32, 77, 83 then 86 µg/ml (up to about 300 to 800 fold). The second virus, DV1 strain was passaged once through 1 µg/ml of ACV. The ID50 value for

DV1 sensitive strain was 0,39 µg/ml ($\pm$ 0,25). For the DV15, the ID50 value was of 70 µg/ml (up to about 200 fold).

4. DISCUSSION

The virus being tested was titrated in the assay in order to shorten the test and our method of computation allowed us to evaluate the 30TC ID50 required in the reaction. Then we avoided the prior titration of the virus. It was difficult to compare the data obtained in different laboratories because several factors may markedly influenced the values for virus sensitivity (type of assay, nature of cells) (3,4,5). But it was said that the ID50 values as reported (CPE reduction assay) were approximatively 10 fold higher than values obtained by plaque reduction assay (1,5). In our assay, the HSV1 strains appeared to be a little more sensitive than HSV2 strains. This phenomenon was observed in most of the studies (1,2,5). However we have noted that ID50 value of ACV for the HSV2 ocular strain was lower than ID50 values determined for G-HSV2 and the 10 genital isolates. Among the 47 viruses we have tested (HSV1 and HSV2), 44 (93 %) were sensitive to ACV concentrations <1 µg/ml, and 3 HSV2 genital strains were inhibited by ID50 values <1 µg/ml (but >2 µg/ml). On the contrary, ID50 values obtained with ACV resistant mutants were always $\geqslant 30$ µg/ml. Then it could be possible to screen isolates in choosing appropriate concentrations of drugs.

REFERENCES

1. Collins P, Appleyard G, Oliver NM. 1982. Sensitivity of Herpes virus isolates from Acyclovir clinical trials. Am. J. Med., 73, 380-382.
2. Crumpacker CS, Schnipper LE, Zaia JA, Levin MJ. 1979. Growth inhibition by Acycloguanosine of Herpes viruses isolated from human infections. Antimicrob. Agents Chemother., 15, 642-645.
3. De Clercq E. 1982. Comparative efficacy of anti Herpes drugs in different cell lines. Antimicrob. Agents Chemother., 21, 661-663.
4. Field HJ. 1983. A perspective on resistance to Acyclovir in Herpes Simplex virus. J. Antimicrob. Chemother., 12, Suppl.B, 129-135.
5. Mc Laren C, Corey L, Dekker C, Barry DW. 1983. In vitro sensitivity to Acyclovir in genital Herpes Simplex viruses. J. Infect. Dis., 148, 868-875.

A REVIEW OF ACYCLOVIR IN THE MANAGEMENT OF HERPES SIMPLEX
VIRUS INFECTIONS OF THE EYE

P.J. REES (Wellcome Research Laboratories, Beckenham, Kent, England).

1.   INTRODUCTION

Acyclovir (Zovirax[R]) is a potent and highly selective antiviral agent
against herpes simplex types 1 and 2 (Elion et al., 1977; Schaeffer et al., 1978)
and has now been widely used in both systemic and topical application. Its
selectivity derives from the fact that the initial stage in the activation of the
drug requires phosphorylation by a herpes virus-specified thymidine kinase while
normal cellular enzymes do not phosphorylate acyclovir to any significant
extent. Acyclovir monophosphate is subsequently converted to a triphosphate
which is a more potent inhibitor of herpes virus DNA polymerase than of cellular
DNA polymerase (Elion, 1983).

The first demonstration of the antiviral efficacy of acyclovir (ACV) in man
came from a double-blind, placebo-controlled study by Jones et al. (1979). ACV
was shown to completely prevent early recurrences of herpes simplex dendritic
ulceration following minimal wiping debridement in comparison with a 58%
recurrence rate in the corresponding placebo group.

2.   ACYCLOVIR IN THE TREATMENT OF DENDRITIC KERATITIS

Following the initial demonstration of the antiviral efficacy of ACV a
number of double-blind studies were conducted to compare topical ACV with
other topical antiviral agents in the treatment of herpes simplex corneal
epithelial disease. Coster et al. (1980) compared ACV and idoxuridine (IDU) and
found no significant difference in median healing times or in the proportion of
patients cured. The multicentre trial reported by McCulley et al. (1982)
similarly found no significant differences in healing between patients treated
with ACV or IDU though the incidence of superficial punctate keratopathy was
significantly lower in the ACV group. A comparative trial by
Collum et al. (1980) showed ACV to be significantly better than IDU both in
terms of the proportion of patients healed and the mean healing times achieved.

Maudgal, P.C. and Missotten, L., (eds.) Herpetic Eye Diseases.
© *1985, Dr W. Junk Publishers, Dordrecht/Boston/Lancaster. ISBN 978-94-010-8935-7*

Mean healing times were similarly reported to be significantly shorter for patients receiving ACV than for IDU recipients in the study by Colin et al. (1981). Klauber and Ottovay (1982) compared the efficacy of ACV and IDU in a group of patients containing a high proportion with stromal involvement. They found significant differences in favour of ACV in both the overall cure rate and in median healing times.

Comparative studies conducted by Yeakley et al. (1981) and Pavan-Langston et al. (1981) failed to demonstrate any significant differences between ACV and adenine arabinoside (Ara A) in the treatment of herpes simplex epithelial keratitis. A similar result was obtained from the study of McGill et al. (1981) though trends in the rate of healing favoured acyclovir. ACV and Ara A were found to be similarly effective in terms of overall cure rate by Young et al. (1982) but the rate of healing was significantly faster in patients treated with ACV.

A single comparative study of ACV and trifluorothymidine (TFT) showed both drugs to be equally effective in both overall cure rate and mean healing times (La Lau et al., 1982).

These trials of ACV have provided a large body of evidence showing the drug to be well tolerated and effective in the treatment of epithelial herpes simplex keratitis. It is at least as effective as the other antiviral agents used. Given the nature of dendritic ulceration, which tends to resolve rapidly when treated with an antiviral agent, it is perhaps not surprising that overwhelming differences in efficacy have not been reported. There have, however, been suggestions from a number of these studies that ACV may offer greater advantages in the treatment of deeper herpetic eye disease.

3.   DEEP HERPES SIMPLEX EYE INFECTION

Poor drug penetration into the aqueous humour following topical application of IDU or Ara A was reported by Pavan-Langston et al. (1973). In a more recent study, Poirier et al. (1982) compared the intraocular penetration of the more soluble Ara AMP, TFT and ACV in patients with intact corneal epithelium who were about to undergo cataract extraction. No TFT was detected in the aqueous humour and only meagre levels of Ara A were found. Topical ACV, however, penetrated the cornea and produced substantial levels in the aqueous humour with a mean concentration of 7.5 μM, well in excess of the potentially therapeutic concentration of the drug for herpes simplex virus.

A series of 20 patients with presumptive herpetic iridocyclitis, treated with either topical ACV or IDU, was reported by Wilhelmus et al. (1981). The uveitis of all 10 patients receiving ACV resolved within 1 to 8 weeks while 4 of the 10 IDU recipients worsened and required steroid therapy. In an open study by Tormey et al. (1981), 20 patients with an ulcer and associated stromal infiltrate and 7 patients with 8 episodes of disciform keratitis were treated with topical ACV. All those with ulcers and associated infiltrate healed in an average of 12.3 days. Six of the 8 attacks of disciform keratitis healed in a mean time of 17 days; the remaining 2 patients required topical steroids to lead to resolution. Another open study (Van Ganswijk et al., 1983) reported the use of topical ACV and steroids in 25 patients with long standing deep stromal herpetic keratitis which had failed to respond to other antiviral therapy. All patients healed within 2 to 4 weeks.

A double-blind, randomised trial of ACV versus ACV plus steroid in the treatment of herpetic disciform keratitis was conducted by Collum et al. (1983). They found that the combination of ACV and steroid was significantly better than ACV alone, resulting in 100% healing in a median time of 21 days. Eleven of the 19 patients who received ACV alone had to be withdrawn because their condition remained static or worsened. It is, however, interesting to note that the disciform keratitis was controlled in 8 patients (40%) using ACV alone, while previous attempts to control this condition without steroids have failed in a high proportion of cases (Falcon, 1983).

The precise mechanisms leading to the development of stromal involvement and deeper manifestations of herpetic ocular infection remain unclear. Direct viral invasion and replication may play a part and immune, inflammatory responses almost certainly have a significant role. The results of the above studies, although limited, suggest that ACV alone may be able to control deeper herpetic eye involvement in a proportion of patients. In those cases where it may be considered advisable to add steroids to control inflammation, the possibility of continuing virus replication within the cornea and its likely stimulation by steroids requires the continued presence of an effective antiviral cover. The good corneal penetration of ACV to produce potentially therapeutic levels in the aqueous humour may offer significant advantages in these circumstances.

4. THE POTENTIAL FOR SYSTEMIC THERAPY WITH ACYCLOVIR

The low toxicity of ACV renders it suitable for systemic use and both oral and intravenous formulations have been widely used in the treatment of herpes simplex cutaneous infections. Many patients with herpes simplex keratitis may be unable or unwilling to comply with relatively frequent applications of ophthalmic ointment and in these cases systemic administration of ACV may offer a rational alternative therapy. Furthermore, systemic treatment may be a more logical approach in attempting to control deeper herpes simplex eye infections. Anecdotal evidence suggests that both intravenous and oral acyclovir may be effective in controlling herpes simplex ocular infection (Van Der Meer and Versteeg, 1982; Sundmacher, 1983; Grutzmacher et al., 1983). The use of intravenous ACV is limited by the need to hospitalize the patient but oral ACV offers the potential of systemic outpatient therapy.

In a recent study (Hung et al. 1984a) the levels of ACV in the aqueous humour of patients undergoing cataract extraction were determined following oral administration of 400 mg ACV five times daily. The concentration of ACV in the aqueous humour (mean 3.26 μM) was approximately half that found following topical application (Poirier et al., 1982) but was, nonetheless, well in excess of the normal in vitro ED50 range for herpes simplex virus type 1. In a further trial (Hung et al., 1984b) 31 patients with herpes simplex dendritic ulcers were treated with minimal debridement, followed by oral ACV or placebo for 7 days. At the end of treatment there was no significant difference in the proportion of ulcers healed in the two groups but the rate of healing was significantly faster in the patients treated with ACV. No adverse reactions to oral ACV were reported in either of the above studies.

The pharmacokinetic and therapeutic evidence available to date suggest that oral ACV may have a potential role as an alternative to topical therapy. Further controlled clinical trials are currently underway.

5. TOXICITY AND TOLERANCE OF ACYCLOVIR OPHTHALMIC OINTMENT

Adverse reactions reported from clinical trials in which a total of 665 patients have received ACV ophthalmic ointment are summarised in Table 1. The incidence of adverse reactions is remarkably low and compares favourably with the other antiviral agents available. The most commonly reported adverse reactions were superficial punctate keratopathy and burning or stinging following application of the ointment. These reactions are common to many ophthalmic preparations and are believed to be due to the ointment base and not the drug.

No patient treated in any of the clinical trials of ACV has had to be withdrawn from therapy because of adverse effects.

Table 1. Summary of adverse reactions in 665 patients

Adverse reaction	Number of cases	%
Superficial punctate keratopathy	84	12.6
Burning/stinging	34	5.1
Conjunctival hyperaemia	2	0.3
Follicular conjunctivitis	2	0.3
Palpebral allergy	2	0.3
Punctal occlusion	1	0.15
Watering	1	0.15

6.   CONCLUSIONS

There is now a substantial body of controlled clinical trial data demonstrating the efficacy of topical ACV in the treatment of superficial herpetic eye disease. Intraocular penetration of topically applied ACV is far superior to that of the other antiviral agents available and this, combined with its extremely low toxicity, may make ACV particularly appropriate for the treatment of deeper herpetic eye infections where longer periods of therapy may be envisaged. Oral administration of ACV has been shown to produce potentially therapeutic levels in aqueous humour and may offer the possibility of an alternative to topical therapy.

REFERENCES

Colin J, Tournoux A, Chastel C and Renard G (1981) Superficial herpes simplex keratitis. Double-blind comparative trial of acyclovir and idoxuridine. Nouv. Presse Med. 10, 2969-2975.
Collum LMT, Benedict-Smith A and Hillary IB (1980) Randomised double-blind trial of acyclovir and idoxuridine in dendritic corneal ulceration. Br. J. Ophthalmol. 64, 766-769.
Collum LMT, Logan P and Ravenscroft T (1983) Acyclovir (Zovirax) in herpetic disciform keratitis. Br. J. Ophthalmol. 67, 115-118.
Coster DJ, Wilhelmus KR, Michaud R and Jones BR (1980) A comparison of acyclovir and idoxuridine as treatment for ulcerative herpetic keratitis. Br. J. Ophthalmol. 64, 763-765.
Elion GB (1983) The biochemistry and mechanism of action of acyclovir. J. Antimicrob. Chemother. 12 (Suppl. B), 9-17.
Elion GB, Furman PA, Fyfe JA, de Miranda P, Beauchamp L and Schaeffer HJ (1977) Selectivity of action of an antiherpetic agent, 9-(2-hydroxyethoxymethyl)guanine. Proc. Natl. Acad. Sci. USA 74, 5716-5720.

Falcon MG (1983) Herpes simplex virus infections of the eye and their management with acyclovir. J. Antimicrob. Chemother. 12 (Suppl. B), 39-43.

Grutzmacher RD, Henderson D, McDonald PJ and Coster DJ (1983) Herpes simplex chorioretinitis in a healthy adult. Am. J. Ophthalmol. 96, 788-796.

Hung SO, Patterson A and Rees PJ (1984a) Pharmacokinetics of oral acyclovir (Zovirax) in the eye. Br. J. Ophthalmol. 68, 192-195.

Hung SO, Patterson A and Rees PJ (1984b) Oral acyclovir in the management of dendritic herpetic corneal ulceration. Br. J. Ophthalmol. in press.

Jones BR, Coster DJ, Fison PN, Thompson GM, Cobo LM and Falcon MG (1979) Efficacy of acycloguanosine (Wellcome 248U) against herpes simplex corneal ulcers. Lancet i, 243-244.

Klauber A and Ottovay E (1982) Acyclovir and idoxuridine treatment of herpes simplex keratitis - a double blind clinical study. Acta Ophthalmol. 60, 838-844.

La Lau C, Oosterhuis JA, Versteeg J, Van Rij G, Renardel de Lavalette JGC, Craandijk A and Lamers WPMA (1982) Acyclovir and trifluorothymidine in herpetic keratitis: a multicentre trial. Br. J. Ophthalmol. 66, 506-508.

McCulley JP, Binder PS, Kaufman HE, O'Day DM and Poirier RH (1982) A double-blind multicenter clinical trial of acyclovir vs. idoxuridine for treatment of epithelial herpes simplex keratitis. Ophthalmol. 89, 1195-1200.

McGill J, Tormey P and Walker CB (1981) Comparative trial of acyclovir and adenine arabinoside in the treatment of herpes simplex corneal ulcers. Br. J. Ophthalmol. 65, 610-613.

Pavan-Langston D, Dohlman CH, Geary P and Sulzewski D (1973) Intraocular penetration of Ara A and IDU - therapeutic implications in clinical herpetic uveitis. Trans. Am. Acad. Ophthalmol. 77, 455-466.

Pavan-Langston D, Lass J, Hettinger M and Udell I (1981) Acyclovir and vidarabine in the treatment of ulcerative herpes simplex keratitis. Am. J. Ophthalmol. 92, 829-835.

Poirier RH, Kingham JD, de Miranda P and Annel M (1982) Intraocular antiviral penetration. Arch. Ophthalmol. 100, 1964-1967.

Schaeffer HJ, Beauchamp L, de Miranda P, Elion GB, Bauer DJ and Collins P (1978) 9-(2-hydroxyethoxymethyl)guanine activity against viruses of the herpes group. Nature 272, 583-585.

Sundmacher R (1983) Oral acyclovir therapy for virologically proven intraocular herpes simplex virus disease. Klin. Mbl. Augenheilk. 183, 246-250.

Tormey P, McGill J and Walker C (1981) Use of acyclovir in herpes simplex corneal ulcers. Trans. Ophthal. Soc. U.K. 101, 6-8.

Van Der Meer JWM and Versteeg J (1982) Acyclovir in severe herpes virus infections. Am. J. Med. 73 (1A), 271-274.

Van Ganswijk R, Oosterhuis JA, Swart-Van Den Berg M and Versteeg J (1983) Acyclovir treatment in stromal herpetic keratitis. Doc. Ophthalmol. 55, 57-61.

Wilhelmus KR, Falcon MG and Jones BR (1981) Herpetic iridocyclitis. Int. Ophthalmol. 4, 143-150.

Yeakley WR, Laibson PR, Michelson MA and Arentsen JJ (1981) A double-controlled evaluation of acyclovir and vidarabine for the treatment of herpes simplex epithelial keratitis. Trans. Am. Ophthal. Soc. 79, 168-179.

Young BJ, Patterson A and Ravenscroft T (1982) A randomised double-blind clinical trial of acyclovir (Zovirax) and adenine arabinoside in herpes simplex corneal ulceration. Br. J. Ophthalmol. 66, 361-363.

DISCUSSION :

L.M.T. Collum (Dublin) : Could I just make two comments. In
   reference to our study you mentioned that a number of patients
   with stromal disease resolved, and you suggested that it was
   possibly acyclovir that was partly responsible for this. That
   might be the case. But, I'll just point out that a good number
   of these patients will resolve spontaneously. In other words
   stromal herpes is a self-limiting disease. And I think it is
   somewhat dangerous to draw any conclusion. Of course, you
   might be right in saying that stromal disease is influenced by
   acyclovir.
P.J. Rees (Beckenham) : I would not wish to draw firm conclusions
   from the small amount of data available, but I think stromal
   keratitis is an indication which should be investigated further.
L.M.T. Collum (Dublin) : The second point was about Peter Tormey's paper. Concerning the stromal reaction, I think distinction should be drawn between a stromal disease entity like disciform keratitis and the very superficial stromal reaction that
   occurs with dendritic or geographic ulceration. There is
   probably a very definite difference between those two. If the
   superficial stromal reaction cleared up with acyclovir, it does
   not necessarily follow that the pure disciform will respond.
   It may well do, and I am sure people will disagree with me.
   And the sort of iritis that is there, possibly it is not pure
   herpetic iritis, but an irritative uveitis that you get with any
   corneal lesion.
P.J. Rees (Beckenham) : The purpose of my presenting that data
   was to indicate that acyclovir may not necessarily be limited
   to the treatment of purely superficial infections. The study
   reported by Tormey et al. included 8 patiënts with disciform
   keratitis, 6 of whom resolved on acyclovir alone. As I have
   said, whether the deeper manifestations are due to viral replication or to immune responses, if you are going to use steroids
   in these patients then you need an effective antiviral cover.

204

Acyclovir is one of the few compounds currently available that
can give that cover.

P.C. Maudgal (Leuven) : I agree with Dr. Collum. In fact, I
noticed that in the iridocyclitis study IDU was used as a comparative drug. We know it does not penetrate the cornea, and
you have shown that there were six patients in this group who
responded to IDU treatment.

P.J. Rees (Beckenham) : That again brings home the point ·that
we need larger properly controlled clinical studies. I think
the suggestion from that study is that the patients who responded on IDU were, in fact, spontaneously resolving.

P.C. Maudgal (Leuven) : In your data you have shown that acyclovir penetrates into the eye whether you administer it systemically or topically. By both routes you have sufficient antiviral
concentration of the compound in the aqueous humor. I don't
understand why should we treat the whole body when by just
applying the drug to the eye you can achieve sufficient concentration in the aqueous.

P.J. Rees (Beckenham) : This is something that Louis will be covering himself later on this morning. A number of patients are
either unable or unwilling to comply with the treatment regime
which requires regular application of the ointment. Some patients
find it very difficult to apply ointment to the eye. Others find
it inconvenient to have to stop work during the day to apply
the ointment and because it leaves the vision blurred for some
time afterwards. In those cases I think if you give them ointment it is unlikely that they get effective therapy because they
are unlikely to comply. I don't think the oral therapy will
be widely used for the treatment of eye infections but in those
patients where you suspect compliance with the ointment may
be a problem then oral therapy could possibly serve as an
effective alternative.

P.C. Maudgal (Leuven) : Let us go a step further. In stromal
disease or iridocyclitis vision is already affected. Whether
you apply ointment or not, it does not make a great difference.
A final comment I wanted to make concerns the relative inef-

ficacy of acyclovir for the treatment of experimental stromal
herpetic keratitis. Dr. Kaufman and his group have shown
that topical acyclovir was not effective in their stromal keratitis model unless it was combined with vidarabine. Our own
results of experimental study (unpublished) show that acyclovir has a significantly better healing effect on stromal disease than placebo, but at the same time it was significantly
less effective than trifluridine. I fail to understand why acyclovir is not as effective as trifluridine when there is evidence
that it has a good ocular penetration and a better in vitro
antiherpes activity than trifluridine.

P.J. Rees (Beckenham) : I don't think we have any comparative
data in man which is the ultimate test, of course. There is
always a danger in overinterpreting or extrapolating too far
from animal models. All the available data we have in man
would suggest that the intraocular penetration of acyclovir is
superior to that of the other antiviral agents currently available and on that basis would suggest that acyclovir should ultimately become the treatment of choice.

F. Lagoutte (Bordeaux) : I want to ask to Dr. Collum if you drew
any distinction in the duration of stromal keratitis : corticosteroids are neccessary when stromal keratitis is of long duration, when it is associated with a very high inflammatory response. In the beginning, when there is only virus proliferation and less inflammatory response, acyclovir alone could have
good results.

L.M.T. Collum (Dublin) : This is possible. We didn't draw much
distinction, we simply took the patients at random and put
them into the trial. Analysing the data afterwards, we quan-
titated the duration of symptoms before therapy. If my memory
is correct, the two groups were comparable.

J.McGill (Southampton) : Some of your patients in your trial may
have had steroids sometime in the past. And I have found
repeatedly that if they have had steroids at any time, there
is no way that people with stromal disease can be treated just
with antivirals. They have to have steroids, that is for any

subsequent attack for the rest of their lives. And I think this is important. You must not treat with antivirals alone, the stromal disease just gets worse.

L.M.T. Collum (Dublin) : Some of our patients had had steroids in the past, we didn't really draw distinction. Perhaps we should have.

A COMPARISON OF THE ANTIHERPES ACTIVITIES IN VITRO AND IN VIVO OF FOSCARNET AND MONO- AND DIHYDROXYBUTYLGUANINE:

R. Datema, A.-C. Ericson, A. Larsson, K. Stenberg, A. Nyqvist-Mayer*, F.Y. Aoki**, N.-G. Johansson, and B. Öberg. Depts. of Antiviral Chemotherapy and *Pharmacy, Research and Development Laboratories, Astra Läkemedel AB, S-151 85 Södertälje, Sweden, and **Dept. of Clinical Microbiology, The University of Manitoba, Winnipeg, Canada R3E 0W3.

THE ROAD TO NEW GUANOSINE ANALOGS

Herpes viruses induce a new DNA polymerase, which is used as a target for the development of antiherpes drugs. These selective antiherpes drugs can be pyrophosphate analogs or nucleoside analogs. Pyrophosphate analogs such as foscarnet (phosphonoformic acid) inhibit the enzyme directly, and, in contrast to nucleoside analogs, do not need prior metabolisation. Foscarnet was developed as an inhibitor of the Herpes simplex virus DNA polymerase, but all human herpes viruses appeared susceptible to inhibition (see 1 for a review). Foscarnet inhibits the DNA polymerases by interfering with the pyrophosphate exchange reaction, with an uncompetitive inhibition with respect to the four substrates, the deoxyribonucleoside triphosphates. Concentrations giving 50 % inhibition of viral enzymes are 0.3-0.5 μM, whereas for inhibition of cellular enzymes 100 times higher concentrations are needed.

When tested as an inhibitor of herpes virus replication in cell culture, the results appear somewhat disappointing when the ID_{50} for HSV-1 replication in Vero cells (50 μM) is compared, for example, with those of the nucleoside analogs BVDU (0.03 μM) or ACV (0.3 μM). The efficacy in vitro of nucleoside analogs is however strongly cell type-dependent (2), whereas foscarnet, being independent of cellular metabolism to exert antiviral effects, has similar ID_{50}'s for different cell lines. In the infected cells foscarnet selectively inhibits viral DNA synthesis (3), showing that it is a selective antiherpes agent.

The high ID_{50} value of foscarnet might be caused by its poor cellular penetration. To achieve a steady state level of intracellular

Maudgal, P.C. and Missotten, L., (eds.) Herpetic Eye Diseases.
© *1985, Dr W. Junk Publishers, Dordrecht/Boston/Lancaster. ISBN 978-94-010-8935-7*

foscarnet (for concentrations of 1-5 mM) 4-8 hours are required, whereas
nucleoside analogs equilibrate within minutes. After removal of foscarnet,
the drug leaves the cells with the same, slow kinetics as found for its
uptake, suggesting a passive mechanism.

High concentrations of foscarnet (>1 mM) cause inhibition of cellular DNA synthesis, and this could be measured as concentration-dependent
cell-cycle effects (4, 5). These effects were reversed after removal of
foscarnet.

Despite the meagre anti-herpes effects in cell-culture, foscarnet
showed good efficacy in the topical treatment of cutaneous or genital
herpes infections in experimental animals (1). In fact, the effect of
foscarnet in these infections was superior to those of nucleoside analogs
with higher cell-culture efficacies. Yet, in some animal models, notably
herpetic keratitis and encephalitis, and in systemic herpes virus infections in mice, foscarnet was not particularly active. A new synthetic
program that might lead to antivirals complementing the in vivo effects
of foscarnet and making combination therapy possible, resulted in a
series of guanosine analogs that, like ACV, need prior activation by
herpes virus-induced thymidine kinase (TK) to inhibit DNA synthesis in
infected cells.

THE MODE OF ACTION OF HBG AND DHBG

As shown in Table 1 acyclic guanosine analogs with a hydroxybutyl
(HBG) or dihydroxybutyl (DHBG) side chain are good substrates for HSV-1
TK. HBG and DHBG were shown to compete with thymidine in selective

Table 1. Enzyme kinetic parameters of some 9-substituted guanosine -
analogs (from ref. 6, 7, 8)

Nature of acyclic side-chain	K_i (μM)		Relative rate of phosphorylation	
	HSV-1 TK	HSV-2 TK	HSV-1 TK	HSV-2 TK
$-CH_2CH_2OH$	171	-	$\leqslant$5 %	-
$-CH_2CH_2CH_2OH$	41	-	$\leqslant$5 %	-
$-CH_2CH_2CH_2CH_2OH$	2.1	28.9	10 %	65 %
$-CH_2CH_2CH_2CH_2CH_2OH$	15	-	$\leqslant$5 %	-
$-CH_2CH_2CHOHCH_2OH(R)$	1.5	5.7	73 %	165 %
$-CH_2CH_2CHOHCH_2OH(S)$	1.5	3.7	46 %	24 %

phosphorylation by herpes virus TK (6, 7, 8). No activity towards cellular TK was observed. HBG and the two forms of DHBG, the R- and S-form, were investigated further for their antiherpes effects in different cell-lines, with different virus strains, the ability to reverse their antiherpes effect in cell-culture with thymidine (9), their ability to inhibit cellular and viral DNA synthesis in infected and uninfected cells, their effects towards TK⁻-strains of HSV and towards CMV, their penetration rates through skin ex-vivo, and their anticellular properties.

These results are summarized in Table 2. The results imply that to exert their antiviral activity the compounds have to be phosphorylated by HSV-induced TK. The antiviral effect coincides with inhibition of viral and cellular DNA synthesis in infected cells. The amount of DNA synthesized in uninfected cells is not influenced by HBG and DHBG at antiviral concentrations.

Table 2. Comparison of antiviral activities of R-DHBG, S-DHBG and HBG in cell culture (concentrations in μM)

Parameter	R-DHBG	S-DHBG	HBG
HSV-1 infected Vero cells			
ID_{50} plaque red.	2.3	13.1	0.8
ID_{50} plaque red. in presence of 50 μM thymidine	6.3	-	40
ID_{50} viral DNA synthesis*	2.5		0.6
ID_{50} cell. DNA synthesis*	25		3.6
HSV-1 infected cont. cell lines			
ID_{50} plaque red.	0.2-14.5	4.0-33	0.8-16
HSV-1 TK⁻-infected Vero cells			
ID_{50} plaque red.	230	160	180
CMV-infected HEL cells**			
ID_{50}	400	400	400
HSV-2 infected Vero cells			
ID_{50} plaque red.	4.0	20	8.0
Uninfected Vero cells			
ID_{50}, cell. DNA synthesis*	>500		>500
ID_{50}, cell growth	500	1000	250

* Measured only for the racemic R,S-mixture
** Pers. commun. Dr. B. Wahren.

Although similar in vitro (plaque reduction in different cell-lines and with different HSV-strains, inhibition of DNA synthesis) and in affinity towards purified viral TK, the guanosine analogs behaved strikingly different in vivo: When studied in animal models, only R-DHBG emerged as an active antiviral compound.

EFFECTS IN VIVO OF HBG AND DHBG

A 5 %-cream of R-DHBG gave a 36 % reduction in cumulative score in cutaneous HSV-1 infections in guinea pigs. For S-DHBG this value was 9 %, whereas HBG was without effect even when dissolved in DMSO. This latter result was not predicted from the cell-culture data. Therefore, we compared the through-skin penetration rates and lag-phases for penetration of R-DHBG and HBG in infected and uninfected guinea pig skins ex vivo. However, no significant differences were found, suggesting that both drugs become available to the epidermal cells in the skin at the same rate. It is, therefore, possible that the rate of phosphorylation of HBG and R-DHBG by HSV-1 TK, which is lower for HBG (9 % rel. to thymidine) than for R-DHBG (75 % rel. to thymidine), determines whether or not sufficient amounts of HBG can be trapped intracellularly as phosphorylated material.

The difference in phosphorylation rates of HBG and R-DHBG by HSV-2 TK is only 2.5-fold (see Table 1). Nevertheless, HBG was without effect in systemic HSV-2 infections in mice, whereas R-DHBG at 30 mg/kg/day orally decreased the percentage cumulative mortality to ca 30 %. In this particular model pharmacokinetic differences were, however, observed and the lack of efficacy of HBG may in part be due to its more rapid clearance from serum.

In the treatment of herpetic keratitis in rabbits, HBG showed only marginal effects (4), whereas R-DHBG showed promising results (5). DHBG was further evaluated in different pharmaceutical formulations. Eye-drops, suspensions and ointments with concentrations of DHBG ranging from 0.3 to 3.0 % were compared. Eye-drops containing 0.3 % DHBG had a moderate effect. Increasing the concentration to 0.5 % by an increase in pH and addition of a thickening agent gave improvement: it reduced the keratitis score with 75 % after 24 h and healing was complete after five days of treatment. The best effect was obtained with a 3 % DHBG ointment (Fig. 1) giving a rapid decline in keratitis score and an almost complete healing after three days of treatment.

211

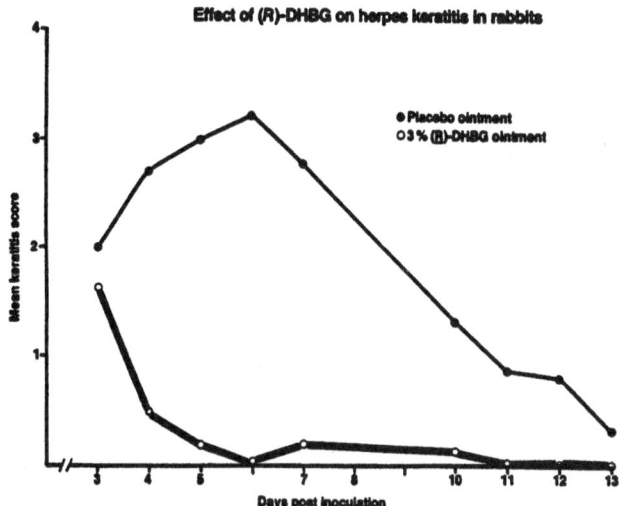

Effect of (R)-DHBG on herpes keratitis in rabbits

● Placebo ointment
○ 3 % (R)-DHBG ointment

Mean keratitis score

Days post inoculation

Herpes keratitis in rabbits was infected with HSV-1 strain C42 and
treated with 3 % (R)-DHBG ointment. Three days after virus inoculation
treatment was started. Ointment was applied in the lower fornix of each
eye four times daily for five days.

REFERENCES

1. Öberg, B. 1983. Antiviral effects of phosphonoformate (PFA, foscarnet sodium). Pharmac. Ther. 19, 387-415.
2. de Clercq, E. 1982. Comparative efficacy of antiherpes drugs in different cell lines. Antimicrob. Agents Chemother. 21, 661-663.
3. Larsson, A. and Öberg, B. 1981. Selective inhibition of herpesvirus DNA synthesis by foscarnet. Antiviral Res. 1, 55-62.
4. Stenberg, K., Skog, S., and Tribukait, B. 1983. Effects of foscarnet on the cell kinetics of Madin-Darby canine kidney cells. Biochim. Biophys. Acta 762, 31-35.
5. Stenberg, K., Skog, S., and Tribukait, B. 1983. Concentration-dependent effects of foscarnet on the cell cycle of human embryonic cells in culture. 13th Internat. Congr. Chemother.
6. Larsson, A., Alenius, S., Johansson, N.-G., and Öberg, B. 1983. Antiherpetic activity and mechanism of action of 9-(4-hydroxybutyl)-guanine. Antiviral Res. 3, 77-86.
7. Larsson, A., Öberg, B., Alenius, S., Hagberg, C.-E., Johansson, N.-G., Lindborg, B., and Stening, G. 1983. 9-(3,4-dihydroxybutyl)-guanine, a new inhibitor of herpesvirus multiplication. Antimicrob. Agents Chemother. 23, 664-670.
8. Larsson, A. and Tao, P.-Z. 1984. Phosphorylation of four acyclic guanosine analogues by Herpes simplex virus type 2 thymidine kinase. Antimicrob. Agents Chemother., in press.
9. Larsson, A., Brännström, G. and Öberg, B. 1983. Kinetic analysis in cell culture of the reversal of antiherpes activity of nucleoside analogs by thymidine. Antimicrob. Agents Chemother. 24, 819-822.

ACYCLOVIR TREATMENT IN STROMAL HERPERIC KERATITIS

R. VAN GANSWIJK, J.A. OOSTERHUIS, J. VERSTEEG

Acyclovir (Zovirax [R]) is an acyclic nucleoside possessing pronounced inhibitory activity against herpes simplex and varicella zoster virus. Contrary to other antiviral drugs topical instillation of acyclovir in the normal eye yields a marked aqueous level[1]. Because of the favourable results in dendritic keratitis[2,3], we started acyclovir treatment in those cases of stromal herpetic keratitis in which the therapeutic effect of IDU, TFT and Ara-A had proven to be inadequate.

Material and method

Thirty-five patients with long-standing deep stromal herpetic keratitis associated with mild-to-severe uveitis were treated with acyclovir ointment. Criteria of selection were:

A. Presence of deep stromal infiltration.
B. History of recurrent keratitis with typical dendritic or geographic lesions observed in one or more of the previous attacks.
C. Corneal anaesthesia.

Patients with keratitis complicated by a secondary bacterial or fungal infection were excluded from our study as were patients with keratitis of the disciform type, which responds promptly to corticosteroid therapy only. Serum antibody titers were not determined as they have not proved to be helpful in the diagnosis of recurrent or long-standing herpetic disease. No attempts were made to isolate virus from the conjunctivae as this mostly renders negative results in the absence of fresh dendritic ulceration.

Acyclovir ointment was prescribed 5 times daily until one week after all signs of inflammation had disappaered. Other antiviral and antibiotic medication at time of referral was stopped. Topical steroid therapy was continued when already used or was added three times

Maudgal, P.C. and Missotten, L., (eds.) Herpetic Eye Diseases.
© *1985, Dr W. Junk Publishers, Dordrecht/Boston/Lancaster. ISBN 978-94-010-8935-7*

daily to the acyclovir regimen, as were mydriatics and, if necessary, treatment for intraocular hypertension. Patients were examined twice weekly until signs of inflammation had diminished thereafter at longer intervals.

Results

The results in 35 patients are summarized in the figure on the next page. After four weeks of acyclovir therapy all signs of activity had disappaered in all patients. No correlation was found between the duration of the keratitis prior to acyclovir treatment and the healing time on acyclovir therapy.

Recurrence of herpetic keratitis was observed in 10 of the 35 patients. In 3 cases (1,18,24) the recurrent dendritic lesions responded well to acyclovir or TFT therapy. In 7 cases (4,5,8,12,13,26 and 30) corneal stromal oedema reappaered, presumably due to premature discontinuation of the corticosteroids.

Discussion

This investigation was carried out as an open study, since patients prior to referral had been treated without success with other antiviral drugs and most of them also with corticosteroids. In our therapeutic regimen the previously given virostatic medication was replaced by acyclovir which enabled us to use the pre-acyclovir period as control period.

No additional systemic acyclovir therapy was required. The rapid healing of deep stromal keratitis by local acyclovir may be attributed to the therapeutic level of the drug in the cornea after topical application.

The decrease of complaints of pain, photophobia and lacrimation (in 3-7 days) preceded the clinical signs of regression of the inflammation and may be considered as the first signs of therapeutic effect. No serious side effects of acyclovir were noted. Moreover, in patients with a dystrophic state of the corneal epithelium due to long term treatment with other antiviral drugs at rather high dosages replacement of the drugs by acyclovir more than once led to rapid improvement of the dystrophic cornea.

215

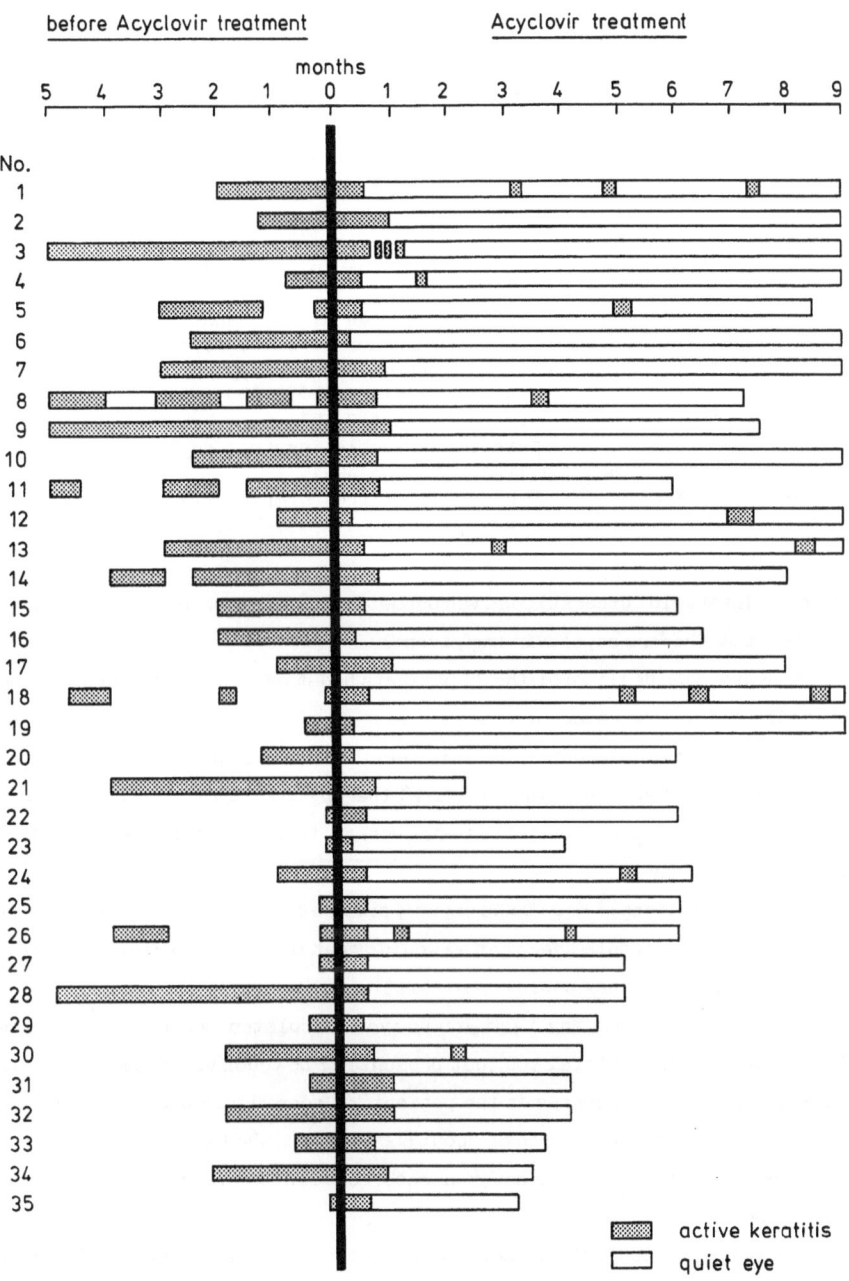

before Acyclovir treatment | Acyclovir treatment

months

active keratitis
quiet eye

Like other antiviral drugs acyclovir does not eradicate the latent
herpes infection of the trigeminal ganglion and the lacrimal glands.
In our series 3 patients developed a recidive of their dendritic keratitis. Almost all patients required low-dose corticosteroid treatment

216

for many months or even longer. Premature cessation resulted in recurrence of
stromal oedema in 7 patients, as was also reported by Kaufman[4].

Acyclovir is not only an effective, but also a safe antiviral drug in deep stromal
herpetic keratitis.

REFERENCES

1. Poirier RH, Kingham JD, Hutcherson S. Human aqueous penetration of
   topically applied acyclovir ophtalmic ointment. Am J Med 1982
   (Acyclovir Symposium); 73: 393.
2. La Lau C, Oosterhuis JA, Vertseeg J, van Rij G, Renardel de Lavalette
   JGC, Craandijk A, Lamers WRMJ, Mierlobensteyn Th. Aciclovir and trifluorothymidine in herpetic keratitis. Preliminary report of a multi-
   centered trial. Docum Ophthalmol 1981; 50: 287-290.
3. Colin J, Tournoux A, Chastel C, Renard G. Kératite herpétique superficielle. Traitement comparatif en double insu par acyclovir et idoxuridine. Nouv Press Méd 1981; 10: 2969-2975.
4. Kaufman HE, Martola EL, Dohlman CH. Herpes simplex treatment with
   IDU and corticosteroids. Tr AAOO 1963; 67: 695-701.

DISCUSSION :

O.P.van Bijsterveld (Utrecht): Dr.Van Ganswijk, do you know what the previous
treatment was before acyclovir was given ?

R.Van Ganswijk (Leiden): 24 of the 35 patients had used an antiviral drug, in most
cases TFT and in some cases IDU.

O.P.van Bijsterveld (Utrecht): There is terrible habit in Holland to taper antiviral therapy. If you taper the antiviral therapy you might actually stimulate
virus resistance. Could you tell at what dosage these patients used TFT ? Was
it five times a day ?

R.Van Ganswijk (Leiden): No, it was about 4 times a day, and often tapered down to
twice daily. When people knew that we would treat them with acyclovir, they had
2 weeks to go before they could come, sometimes they stopped it altogether.

A.Patterson (Liverpool): May I ask you how you calculated the recurrence rate
in the patients in the trial you just presented ? Do you have a recurrence rate
in herpes keratitis, perhaps in the patients in your clinic over the years ? I
worked out the recurrence rate of about 650 patients who had an attack about
every 35 years. I just wonder how your recurrence rate compares with the one
that I have.

R.Van Ganswijk (Leiden): We did not calculate the recurrence rate. In this study
3 of the 35 patients had a recurrence of dendritic keratitis while still on corticosteroids. The recurrences responded well to antiviral treatment.Stromal
edema developed in 7 other patients when corticosteroids were stopped premat-
urely.

ANTIVIRAL TREATMENT OF HERPES SIMPLEX STROMAL DISEASE

J.I. McGILL, Southampton

INTRODUCTION

Once the stroma is involved in herpes simplex corneal infection, treatment is prolonged, recurrent attacks are common, and visual loss is often profound. The exact aetiology of the stromal involvement must remain in doubt. Herpes simplex virus has been successfully grown from corneae with stromal disease removed at the time of keratoplasty (Shimeld et al. 1983). After treatment with just steroids for herpes simplex disciform keratitis there is a high incidence of corneal epithelial ulceration (Patterson and Jones, 1967), unless topical antivirals are also used as cover for the topical steroid therapy.

If herpes simplex virus corneal infection results in stromal disease experimentally there is a transient immunosuppression (Meyers-Elliott and Chitjian, 1980; Carter and Easty, 1981; Easty et al. 1981), and this could aid its intraocular dissemination. Incomplete viral particles have been seen in stromal scars (Dawson et al. 1968; Ahonen, in press), but not in stromal tissues after disciform keratitis (Ahonen et al., in press). Transient endothelial changes have been seen prior to the onset of uveitis induced by herpes simplex virus (Vannas et al. 1983). Herpes simplex virus has been isolated from the anterior chamber and could cause an endotheliitis, leading on to disciform keratitis (Sundmacher, 1981). Therefore, direct viral invasion at least plays a part in stromal disease.

Until recently the only available antiviral has been IDU, which has poor stromal penetration, but with the advent of more soluble antivirals that penetrate the deep layers of the cornea, and even the anterior chamber, in therapeutic levels, it has been possible to study the clinical effects of antivirals used alone in the treatment of herpes simplex stromal disease. Trifluorothymidine penetrates the cornea readily. Acyclovir also readily

Maudgal, P.C. and Missotten, L., (eds.) Herpetic Eye Diseases.
© *1985, Dr W. Junk Publishers, Dordrecht/Boston/Lancaster. ISBN 978-94-010-8935-7*

penetrates the corneal layer, with therapeutic and aqueous levels found after both topical and systemic administration (Poirier, 1982; Hung and Patterson, 1983).

Over the last few years at Southampton Eye Hospital we have had the chance of studying patients treated with steroids and Acyclovir together, or Acyclovir alone, in the treatment of herpes simplex stromal disease.

MATERIAL

All patients presenting to my External Diseases Clinic at the Southampton Eye Hospital between 1979 and 1981 with stromal disease following on a previous attack of herpes simplex corneal ulceration were included in this study.   At each visit the corneal signs were recorded, including the presence or absence of herpes epithelial disease, stromal infiltration and oedema, its extent and severity and duration, and the presence or absence of an associated uveitis, secondary glaucoma, or iris involvement. Record was taken of previous attacks and prior steroid administration.

Patients were divided up into those with stromal infiltration (Group I) lying beneath active corneal ulceration, and those who developed a classic disciform keratitis (Group II) some time after previous herpes simplex ulceration, with no associated epithelial involvement at the time of the attack.   Patients in Group I with infiltration beneath the ulcer were treated on a double blind basis as part of a clinical trial comparing Acyclovir with Ara-A in the treatment of herpes simplex ulceration.

RESULTS

The results show that a significant proportion of patients treated with topical Acyclovir for their initial stromal attack responded favourably (Table I and II).   Both stromal infiltration beneath an active ulcer, and disciform keratitis, responded favourably without the concomitant use of steroids.   In the comparative trial of Acyclovir and Ara-A four patients treated with Ara-A for stromal infiltration required the addition of steroids, but none of the Acyclovir group did.

Once topical steroids had been added, or if steroids had been used previously for another attack of stromal disease, then it was not possible to control the stromal disease with topical Acyclovir alone, and topical steroids had to be added to achieve a successful resolution of the disease.

Once steroids had been added, then prolonged treatment was necessary, resulting in frequent recurrences and in difficulty in weaning the patients fully off all treatment.   In many cases low dose topical steroids had to be continued for many months (Table II).

In one case prolonged stromal disease led to endothelial damage, with permanent corneal oedema resulting due to endothelial decompensation.

CONCLUSIONS

Patients presenting with their first attack of stromal involvement from their hepres simplex infection can successfully be treated with topical Acyclovir, but if treatment has to be prolonged for more than one month because of continued stromal involvement, or if the clinical signs increase during treatment, then topical steroids must be added to prevent permanent corneal endothelial damage.   The prior use of topical steroids requires topical steroids to be used for subsequent attacks.

This work lends support to the hypothesis that stromal involvement is due in part to active herpes simplex viral invasion and that disciform keratitis is due to deep stromal active viral replication.   Whether the entire clinical picture of oedema, stromal infiltration and swelling is due just to viral replication, or whether it is due to a supra-added immune response remains to be determined.

TABLE I

To show the effect of antiviral on stromal response beneath ulcer

	Number	Healed	Days to heal	Steroids required
Acyclovir	20	20	12.3	0
Ara-A	17	12	8.0	5

TABLE II

To show the effect of Acyclovir alone on herpes simplex disciform keratitis compared to that of Acyclovir and steroids

	Attacks	Healed	Days	Treatment duration	Recurrences
Acyclovir	13	13	21	41	1
Acyclovir and steroids	12	12	77	308	10

REFERENCES

1.   Shimeld C, Tullo AB, Easty DL, Tomsitt J.   1982   Isolation of
      herpes simplex virus of the cornea in chronic stromal keratitis.
      Br J Ophthalmol 66: 643-647.

2.   Patterson A, Jones BR.   1967   The management of ocular herpes.
      Trans Ophthalmol Soc UK 82: 59-84.

3.   Meyers-Elliott RH, Chitjian RA.   1981   Immunopathogenesis of
      corneal inflammation in herpes simplex virus stromal keratitis:
      Role of the polymorphnuclear leucocyte.   Invest Ophthalmol Vis
      Sci 20: 784-798.

4.   Carter C, Easty DL.   1981   Experimental ulcerative herpetic
      keratitis.   I.   Systemic immune responses and resistance to
      corneal infection.   Br J Ophthalmol 65: 77-81.

5.   Easty DL, Carter C, Funk A.   1981   Systemic immunity in herpetic
      keratitis.   Br J Ophthalmol 65: 82-88.

6.   Dawson C, Togni B, Moore TE.   1968   Structural changes in chronic
      herpetic keratitis.   Arch Ophthalmol 79: 740-747.

7.   Vannas A, Ahonen R, Makihe J.   1983   Corneal endothelium in
      herpetic keratouveitis.   Arch Ophthalmol 101: 913-915.

8.   Sundmacher R.   1981   A clinico-virologic classification of
      herpetic anterior segment disease with special reference to
      intraocular herpes.   In: Herpetische Augenerkrankungen,
      R. Sundmacher (ed.), pp 203-208, J.F. Bergmann Verlag, Munich.

9.   Poirier RH, Kingham JD, de Miranda P, Annel M.   1982   Intraocular
      antiviral penetration.   Arch Ophthalmol 100: 1964-1967.

10.   Hung SO, Patterson A, Rees PJ.   1984   Pharmacokinetics of oral
      acyclovir (Zovirax) in the eye.   Br J Ophthalmol 68: 192-195.

DISCUSSION :

L.M.T. Collum (Dublin) : I could just disagree and argue a little with James that, as I mentioned earlier, a lot of these
disease entities resolve spontaneously. I think that to run
the risk of leaving the permanent corneal damage is, perhaps
not justifiable; because a number of them, as you said, you
had to put on steroids anyway. I accept entirely the steroid
problem; but even then I think one or two of, whatever percent
it is, does not justify the claim of the efficacy of antiviral
in stromal disease. I really don't think that the evidence is
there yet that acyclovir, or indeed any antiviral, will cure
or curb the stromal reaction. You suggested it, but I am not
certain that the proof is there yet.

J.Mc.Gill (Southampton) : Yes, I think I just trying out an idea.
Its an open study on the disciform. What we must do is coded
clinical trials. The trouble is that the number of cases we
have is small. That is for first time stromal disease and coded
trials can only be carried out on first time stromal disease,
that have never had steroids before, to avoid the steroid rebound
and dependency problem.We get a lot of recurrent cases. I
think that we are managing them better now with antivirals and
steroids. Certainly, the number of my patients coming to grafting is much less than say ten years ago. This may be because
we know more, or may be because with newer antivirals, particularly trifluorothymidine or acyclovir, they penetrate better, so
you get less stromal disease. But if somebody would like to do
a coded trial we will be delighted.

P.A. Asbell (New York) : I just wanted to relate my experience
with Dr. Kaufman when we used topical and systemic
acyclovir in the treatment of stromal disease. First, I would
like to echo some of the other speakers, that one needs to be
careful in defining what you mean by stromal disease.
We looked particularly at two types of disciform edema and
necrotizing keratitis. In both groups, the epithelium was intact
and the patients had not had steroids for at least three weeks
prior to this clinical open trial. We used both topical and

systemic treatment five times a day, and used presumably enough dosage to get therapeutic aqueous levels. In the disciform edema group, the majority had no change or in fact worsened during the two week trial; when the trial was stopped and the patients converted to standard treatment (topical trifluorothymidine and corticosteroids) all of them markedly improved. In the necro- tizing keratitis, we had one patient that did do better and one that did not. Our general feeling from this admittedly uncontrol- led trial – a first experience with the systemic and topical treat- ment – is that it did not appear to be efficacious in disciform edema, and that it is certainly questionable whether it was at all effective for deep necrotizing keratitis.

J.McGill (Southampton) : Penny, did they have steroids before.

P.A. Asbell (New York) : In disciform edema, the majority had not.

J.McGill (Southampton) : But you said that they had no steroids for two to three weeks.

P.A. Asbell (New York) : Three weeks without steroids was the minimal criterion for entering the trial. With disciform edema, most of them never had had steroids. The necrotizing keratitis cases were all very difficult, and all had had steroids previously.

J.McGill (Southampton) : I shouldn't have expected any of them to get better if they had prior steroids at any time. I don't know what it is the steroids do. I have no idea. I wish that somebody can tell me the mechanism. If they had steroids ten years previously they still require them for the current attack. There is no way out of it.

V. Victoria-Troncoso (Ghent) : I would like to explain the mecha- nism of action of steroids at the cytological level. The first point is the penetration. It seems that prednisolone penetrates much better than dexamethasone, and second the steroids act by blocking the membranes. During the herpetic infections, at least in the corneal epithelium, there is a lysosomal cycle. Steroids block the lysosomes and diminish the cytolyses. That is one of the mechanisms. But how it is working together with

224

an antiviral, I don't know. The pure lysosomal cycle which
is healing spontaneously the herpes keratitis in rabbits becomes
longer when you give steroids.

J.McGill (Southampton) : Can you tell me what is the long term
effect ? What effect the steroids have on the membrane as
such, so that every time you have a recurrent attack they need
steroids ?

V.Victoria-Troncoso (Ghent) : I can tell you only on the experimental basis. In our model the cycle of the virus in the epithelium was 12 days, and the lysosomal cycle was between six
and eight days. Once you put steroids, the lysosomal cycle
becomes longer, upto 11 or 12 days.

P.C. Maudgal (Leuven) : James, when you give steroids, how long
do you give them and at what dosage ?

J.McGill (Southampton) : I have a sliding scale when I give steroids, just start off with a full dose of say Predsol which is
0,3% in our country, with full antiviral cover five times a
day, whatever antiviral I am using. When the signs have
regressed, over three week steps, I reduce my steroids by log
or semilog dilution to 0,1 and 0,03; 0,01 percent. So over
a period of two or three months, I have got them down to 0,01%
steroids, still four times a day. At that stage, I taper off
the antiviral. When we have got down to 0,001 Predsol, I
then gradually reduce the frequency. But sometime for stromal
disease, especially the disciform, in order to prevent recurrences, they have to go on maintainance dosages of steroids; say
once or twice a day of 0,001% Predsol. And those people down
to 0,001% I do not use antiviral cover, I take it off. But
everytime you try to reduce the low dose maintainance steroids,
they get a recurrence of the stromal reaction. That is what
I have found. But long term antivirals have no effect at all,
and you got all the problems of toxicity and possible resistance. So, unless you are on high dose of steroids, I don't use

antiviral cover. The following table illustrates the scheme of steroids and antiviral administration.

Steroids	Antiviral application
Predsol 0.3%	Five times a day
Predsol 0.1%	Five times a day
Predsol 0.03%	Four times a day
Predsol 0.01%	Four times a day, gradually tapered to twice a day
Predsol 0.001%	No antivirals

TREATMENT OF HERPETIC KERATO-UVEITIS : Comparative action of
Vidarabine, Trifluorothymidine and Acyclovir in combination
with corticoids.

J.COLIN, D.MAZET, C.CHASTEL, Department of ophthalmology,
BREST University Hospital, BREST, FRANCE.

Clinical trials in herpetic kerato-uveitis have been no-
toriously difficult to execute because of the variable nature of the disease, which may be mediated by inflammatory mechanisms, or by viral replication, or by both (2).

Herpes simplex virus has been demonstrated deep in the
corneal stroma, although the usefulness of topically applied
antiviral compounds alone to ameliorate stromal keratitis
has not been proven.

Klauber and Ottoway (3) reported a significantly faster
healing rate of herpetic keratitis with stromal involvement
when treated with 5-times-daily application of Acyclovir 3 %
ointment compared with Idoxuridine 0,5 % ointment. In contrast Mc Culley et al (4) found no difference between the
two drugs. In a double-masked comparison acyclovir ointment
applied 5 times daily was only successful in treating herpetic disciform keratitis when administered concomitantly with
a local corticosteroid (betamethasme 0,01 % drops) : lesions
healed in all 21 patients receiving the combined therapy and
did so at a faster rate (p < 0,004) than in those receiving
acyclovir and placebo. Lesions healed in only 11 of 19 patients treated with acyclovir and placebo (1).

The following study was designed to compare the combinations with local corticosteroids of Vidarabine, Trifluorothymidine or Acyclovir in the treatment of herpetic kerato-
uveitis. The effect of antivirals on the stromal reaction
was evaluated during treatment with a precise posology of
corticosteroids adapted in all patients to the intensity of
the inflammatory activity of the anterior segment.

Maudgal, P.C. and Missotten, L., (eds.) Herpetic Eye Diseases.
© *1985, Dr W. Junk Publishers, Dordrecht/Boston/Lancaster. ISBN 978-94-010-8935-7*

PATIENTS AND METHODS

The 73 patients included in this open comparative study
suffered from herpetic kerato-uveitis. Diagnosis was based on
the history and clinical appearance of patients. The inflammatory lesions of the stroma and uvea justified the use of
topical corticosteroids. The patients were treated with corticosteroids and either Trifluorothymidine or Vidarabine at
random for the first 46 cases and with corticosteroids and
Acyclovir for the 27 next patients. They were seen by the same two observers on days 7, 14, 21 and 28. Patient data are
given in table I. The antiviral agent was given 5 times daily.

In order to quantify the inflammation of the anterior segment, the method described by Williams et al (9) was used.
The basis for the topical corticosteroids therapy was determined according to the degree of inflammation of the anterior segment as follows :

Total score :   > 9   Dexamethasone (2 mg), one subconjuncti-
                         val injection every day and 0,25 % Pre-
                         dnisolone eyedrops administered 6 times
                         a day.

                6 - 8   0,25 % Prednisolone eyedrops administe-
                         red 6 times a day.

                3 - 5   0,25 % Prednisolone eyedrops administe-
                         red 4 times a day.

                0 - 2   No treatment.

The "total score" was determined at each consultation, and
the corticosteroid therapy adapted accordingly. 17 patients
suffering from ocular hypertension were effectively treated
with Timolol eyedrops and Acetazolamide tablets. All the patients received 1 % Homatropine drops throughout the trial.
The Kruskal-Wallis test was used to compare treatment groups
for duration of symptoms prior to treatment and initial scores. The evolution of the scores was compared between treatment groups by the t test and the Wilcoxon sum of rank test.
The population of healed patients was compared with the chi-
square test and by Fischer's exact test.

RESULTS

Demographic comparison of the treatment groups showed no significant differences except for the duration of symptoms prior to treatment. The duration was 7,5 days, 5,2 days and 4,6 days in the Trifluorothymidine, Vidarabine and Acyclovir groups, respectively. (table I).

DISTRIBUTION OF PATIENTS IN THE THREE TREATMENT GROUPS

	Trifluorothymidine and corticoids	Vidarabine and corticoids	Acyclovir and corticoids
No of patients	23	23	27
Sex M	18	13	16
F	5	10	11
Mean age	51.4	47.7	49 8
Previous herpetic keratitis	20	20	24
Duration of symptoms (median weeks)	7.6	5.3	4.6
Previous IDU therapy for current attack	23	23	27
Previous steroid therapy for current attack	3	2	5

The therapeutical combination of corticosteroids and anti-viral agent resulted in a decrease of the ocular inflammation in most patients. The mean improvement of the total score was 4,03. There was a significant difference between the TFT and Vidarabine groups (p < 0,01) and between the ACV and Vidarabine groups (p < 0,002), but not between the ACV and TFT groups (fig. 1).

During the 28 days period treatment, the number of healed patients was only four in the Vidarabine and steroids group. Nine patients healed in the TFT and steroids group ; and 20 patients healed in the ACV and steroids group. The difference was highly significant between ACV and Vidarabine (p : 0,00006), significant between ACV and TFT (p : 0,01) but not significant between TFT and Vidarabine (fig. 2).

Serious side effects were not observed in this series. Punctate corneal lesions was noted similarly in the three groups but did not need discontinuation of treatment.

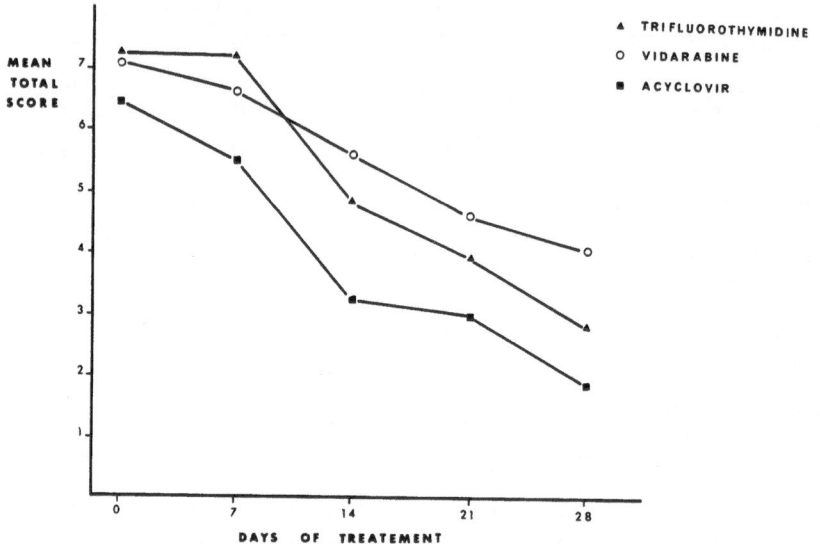

Fig. 1 : Mean total score during the therapeutical combination of corticosteroids and antiviral agent.

Fig. 2 : Cumulative healing rate for patients with herpetic kerato-uveitis.

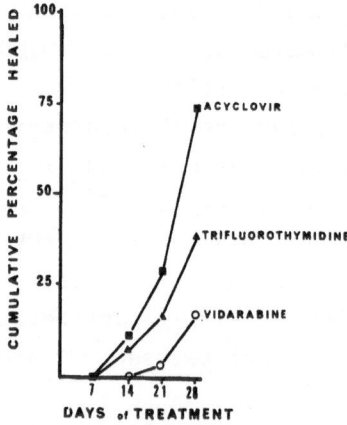

COMMENTS

The combination of antiviral agent and corticosteroid is mostly needed in the treatment of herpetic kerato-uveitis (7, 8).

Our open clinical trial has shown a difference in the ocular improvement according to the antiviral agent. This may be related to the different penetration of these drugs into the cornea and anterior chamber. Only trace amount of Vidarabine and its active metabolite Hypoxanthine arabinoside appear in the aqueous after topical administration. Therapeutic levels of TFT may appear in the aqueous of patients who have notable structural changes and altered corneal permeability (5). However, TFT could not be detected in aqueous in patients with intact cornea (6). On the other hand substancial levels of Acyclovir were detected in the aqueous humour indicating a relatively high level of penetration. When corticosteroids are needed to control the inflammatory reaction in patients with herpetic kerato-uveitis, Acyclovir appear more effective than Vidarabine and Trifluorothymidine.

We thank Dr BARTH for carrying out the statistical analysis of this clinical trial.

REFERENCES

1 - COLLUM L.M.T., LOGAN P., RAVENSCROFT T., Acyclovir (Zovirax) in herpetic disciform keratitis, Br. J. Ophthalmol. 1983, 67, 115-118.
2 - FALCON M.G., Herpes simplex virus infections of the eye and their management with acyclovir, J. Antimicrob. chemotherapy 1983, 12, 39-43.
3 - KLAUBER A., OTTOWAY E., Acyclovir and Idoxuridine treatment of herpetic keratitis - a double blind clinical study, Acta ophthalmologica 1982, 60, 838-844.
4 - Mc CULLEY J.P., BINDER P.S., KAUFMAN H.E. et al, Double blind, multicenter clinical trial of Acyclovir vs Idoxuridine for treatment of epithelial herpes simplex keratitis, Ophthalmology 1982, 89, 1195-1200.
5 - PAVAN-LANGSTON D., NELSON D.J., Intraocular penetration of Trifluridine, Am. J. Ophthalmol. 1979, 87, 814-818.
6 - POIRIER R.H., KINGHAM J.D., DE MIRANDA P. et al, Intraocular antiviral penetration, Arch. Ophthalmol. 1982, 100, 1964-1967.

232

7 - SUNDMACHER R., Use of nucleoside analogues in the treat-
    ment of herpes simplex virus eye diseases, Metabolic, Pe-
    diatric and Systemic ophthalmol. 1983, 7, 89-94.
8 - VAN GANSWIJK R., COSTERHUIS J.A., SWART-VANDENBERG M. et
    al, Acyclovir treatment in stromal herpetic keratitis,
    Doc. Ophthalmol. 1983, 55, 57-61.
9 - WILLIAMS H.P., FALCON M.G., JONES B.R., Corticosteroids
    in the management of herpetic eye disease, Trans. Oph-
    thalmol. Soc. UK 1977, 97, 341-344.

DISCUSSION :

P.C.Maudgal (Leuven): Dr.Colin, I did not catch it, I have difficulty in dignos-
ing uveitis when there is severe corneal edema. When you cann't see through
the cornea very well, how do you diagnose and grade iritis ?

J.Colin (Brest): Your comment points out one of the major criticisms of William's
scoring system to quantify the keratouveitis. In the case of corneal edema, we
have tried to evaluate the uveal inflammation but it is often difficult to
determine a precise score.

G.O.Waring (Atlanta): You managed your steroids based upon the degree of inflammation by the Willam scores. Were the three groups comparable in the amount of
inflammation ? The sense of my question is, did the acyclovir cases for example
get more steroids than the other groups, because they responded more slowly
and you have a feedback cycle then, which results in administering higher doses
of steroids. It is an important point, because if the steroids were not administered more or less equally in the three groups, then the trial looses its
impact.

J.Colin (Brest): Before treatment, there was no statistical difference between
the 3 groups in the amount of inflammation according to the total score. However, the acyclovir group had a score of 6.4 while TFT and vidarabine had respectively scores of 7.2 and 7.1. The acyclovir cases in fact were given less
steroids than the other groups.

A.Patterson (Liverpool): Your acyclovir group, before the trial started, 20% of
them had received steroids. In one of the other groups only 8% had received
steroids pretrial. Have you any comment in regard to this ?

J.Colin (Brest): This small difference may well be due to the fact that the TFT-
vidarabine study was performed before the ACV study. The patients refered to
us by the ophthalmologists during the first period were given less steroids
than now.

ORAL ACYCLOVIR (ZOVIRAX^R) IN HERPETIC KERATITIS

L.M.T. Collum, P. MacGerrtick, J. Akhtar (Royal Victoria Eye and Ear Hospital, Dublin, Ireland), P.J. Rees (Wellcome Research Laboratories, Beckenham).

SUMMARY

Twenty-nine patients with simple herpetic dendritic corneal ulceration have been entered in this double-blind, randomised comparative study of oral acyclovir and acyclovir ophthalmic ointment. Healing was achieved in all 14 patients treated with acyclovir ointment and in 14 of the 15 patients who received oral acyclovir. The mean healing time, 5.6 days, was identical for both groups of patients. The mean trough concentration of acyclovir in the tear fluid of patients receiving oral therapy was in excess of the ED_{50} of herpes simplex virus type 1. No significant local or systemic adverse effects were recorded in either group.

1. INTRODUCTION

Acyclovir has a selective antiviral effect on cells infected with herpes simplex (1,2). Since 1979, when it was first demonstrated to have a good clinical antiviral effect (3), topical application of acyclovir has been shown to be similar to (4-6) or somewhat better than (7-11) idoxuridine and adenine arabinoside and equal to trifluorothymidine (12) in the management of herpes simplex dendritic corneal ulceration.

There are a number of problems regarding the use of topical treatment in the eye. Many patients have difficulty instilling ointment, either because they are unable to do so, or because their vision becomes blurred with the presence of the ointment, or because their spectacle lenses become coated with ointment from the lashes. Elderly patients and children are particularly difficult groups. The young will frequently resist any attempt to instil anything into the eye, while the elderly, who may perhaps have a tremor or arthritis are often physically unable to apply the ointment effectively. For these reasons, any effective systemic antiviral which could be used as a substitute for topical treatment would be attractive. In many instances it is easier for patients to take 5 tablets daily than put ointment in the eye 5 times a day. A further

Maudgal, P.C. and Missotten, L., (eds.) Herpetic Eye Diseases.
© *1985, Dr W. Junk Publishers, Dordrecht/Boston/Lancaster. ISBN 978-94-010-8935-7*

potential advantage of systemic treatment is that it may provide sufficient levels deep in the eye to be helpful in the management of complicated herpetic eye disease such as uveitis or stromal inflammation.

Acyclovir has been widely used, both topically and systemically, in the treatment of herpes simplex cutaneous infections (13) and has shown a remarkably low adverse reaction profile. Anecdotal evidence suggests that both intravenous and oral acyclovir may be effective in the treatment of herpes simplex ocular infection (14-16). The intraocular penetration of orally-administered acyclovir (400 mg, 5 times daily) was determined in a recent study (17). The mean concentration of acyclovir in the aqueous humour was well in excess of the normal in vitro ED50 range for herpes simplex virus type 1.

In an open, pilot study conducted at the Royal Victoria Eye and Ear Hospital, Dublin, 8 patients with simple dendritic corneal ulceration were treated with oral acyclovir. All 8 patients healed and the only adverse effect recorded was slight nausea in one patient. In view of this apparently favourable response to oral acyclovir a larger, randomised, double-blind clinical trial was initiated to compare the efficacy of oral acyclovir and acyclovir ophthalmic ointment in the management of herpes simplex dendritic keratitis. This paper presents an interim analysis of the results from the first 29 patients admitted to the trial.

2. MATERIAL AND METHODS

Twenty-nine patients with simple dendritic ulceration and who gave their informed consent have been included in the study to date. Patients who were unable to attend regularly for follow-up, females of child-bearing age, children under 14 years of age, patients with other ocular diseases and patients who had received antiviral or steroid therapy within the previous 12 months were excluded from the study. Diagnosis was based on history and clinical appearance of the lesion. Patients were seen by the same three observers at least every 3 days and at each visit a full ocular examination was carried out.

Patients were randomly allocated to receive either 3% acyclovir ophthalmic ointment and placebo tablets or placebo ointment and acyclovir (400 mg) tablets, both to be administered five times daily. Cyclopentolate (0.5%) and eye pads were used in all patients unless contra-indicated. If the lesion remained static for 4 days, deteriorated at any time or failed to heal by 14 days the patient was withdrawn from the study and alternative medication administered. The lesion was regarded as healed when there was no staining with fluorescein. Cystic disturbance or slight irregularity of the epithelial cells was ignored in order to standardise the healing criteria. Patients' symptoms were noted at each visit and a record was made of any adverse effects. All patients had blood samples taken before commencing treatment and at the end of therapy for haematological and biochemical analysis. In addition, blood and tear fluid samples were collected from all patients 48 hours after starting treatment for measurement of acyclovir concentrations. The specimens were collected 4·hours following the previous dose of acyclovir in order to standardise the measurements at approximately the trough levels. Acyclovir concentrations were determined by radioimmunoassay conducted by the Department of Clinical Pharmacology, Wellcome Research Laboratories.

3.   RESULTS

Fourteen patients were treated with acyclovir ophthalmic ointment and 15 received oral acyclovir. All 14 patients treated with the ointment healed in a mean time of 5.6 days (range 2 to 13 days). Fourteen of the 15 recipients of oral acyclovir healed in an identical mean time of 5.6 days (range 3 to 12 days). There was no alteration in haematological parameters or blood chemistry in either group and no patient reported any untoward side effects. The only possible adverse effect noted by the observers was minimal superficial punctate epitheliopathy in 3 patients receiving acyclovir ophthalmic ointment. One of these patients suffered from Sjogren's Syndrome.

Samples for determination of plasma levels of acyclovir were obtained from 14 patients receiving acyclovir ointment and from 14 patients receiving oral therapy. Samples of tear fluid were obtained from 13 patients treated with acyclovir ophthalmic ointment and from 14 patients who received oral drug. The results of the drug assays are summarised in Table 1. Plasma levels of acyclovir in all patients treated with ophthalmic ointment were below the limit of detection of the assay (<0.01 µM) while concentrations of the drug in the tear fluid of these patients ranged from 1.87 µM to greater than 130 µM. It is likely that the wide variation in tear fluid levels of acyclovir and the high concentrations of drug seen in the samples obtained from some patients are due to contamination of the specimens by residual acyclovir ointment in the eye. Oral administration of acyclovir resulted in trough plasma levels of the drug ranging from 0.96 µM to 6.87 µM (mean 3.6 µM) and concentrations in the tear fluid ranging from 0.16 µM to 1.45 µM.

Table 1 Concentrations of drug in the plasma and tear fluid of patients receiving oral acyclovir (400 mg 5 times daily) or 3% acyclovir ophthalmic ointment (5 times daily)

ORAL ACYCLOVIR			ACYCLOVIR OPHTHALMIC OINTMENT		
Patient Number	Acyclovir concentration (μM)		Patient Number	Acyclovir concentration (μM)	
	Plasma	Tears		Plasma	Tears
1	0.96	<0.01	3	<0.01	>5.0
2	6.62	<0.01	4	<0.01	>11.0
6	1.83	0.16	5	<0.01	>9.0
8	1.39	0.28	7	<0.01	>3.0
9	6.08	0.36	10	<0.01	3.73
12	2.06	1.01	11	<0.01	42.7
14	2.23	0.43	13	<0.01	-
15	-	-	17	<0.01	34.3
16	4.28	1.28	18	<0.01	9.71
19	3.32	0.92	20	<0.01	>130
22	3.03	0.22	21	<0.01	1.87
23	6.62	1.08	24	<0.01	108.32
25	3.16	0.27	26	<0.01	42.84
27	1.78	0.25	28	<0.01	78.43
29	6.87	1.45			

Drug levels in the tear fluid of the first two patients treated with oral acyclovir fell below the limit of detection of the assay (<0.01 μM) due to low sample volumes and technical problems in conducting the assay. Excluding these two patients, the mean concentration of acyclovir in the tear fluid following oral administration was 0.64 μM.

4.   DISCUSSION

There is now a considerable body of evidence demonstrating the efficacy of topical acyclovir in the treatment of superficial herpes simplex keratitis (see Introduction). The results available to date in this study show that oral acyclovir compares favourably with topical application in both time to healing and the proportion of patients healed.

A previous study (17) has demonstrated good penetration of orally-administered acyclovir into the aqueous humour but this is the first study in which concentrations of acyclovir in the tear fluid have been determined following oral therapy. For the treatment of superficial herpetic eye infection determination of drug concentrations in the tear fluid may be a more appropriate measure of potential efficacy.

Mean trough plasma levels of acyclovir in the study patients who received oral drug are similar to those reported previously (18, 19). They are considerably lower than the concentrations of drug routinely achieved by intravenous administration (20) and therefore well within tolerance limits. Both the mean tear fluid concentration of acyclovir (0.64 µM) and the lowest individual value (0.16 µM) recorded in patients taking oral drug are similar to or greater than the mean ED_{50}s of 0.15 µM and 0.18 µM reported for clinical isolates of herpes simplex virus type 1 (21, 22). Drug levels in the tear fluid were determined four hours following the previous dose of acyclovir and therefore represent trough concentrations.

The results available to date in this study suggest that potentially therapeutic concentrations of acyclovir may be achieved in the tear fluid following oral administration of 400 mg 5 times daily. This suggestion is further substantiated by the available efficacy data. However, larger numbers of patients may be required before firm conclusions can be made regarding the relative efficacy of oral and topical acyclovir in controlling herpes simplex dendritic keratitis. Patient recruitment to the present study is continuing.

ACKNOWLEDGEMENT

The authors wish to express their gratitude to Mr. S. Jeal and Mrs. J. Fox of the Clinical Pharmacology Department, Wellcome Research Laboratories for their excellent assistance in conducting the acyclovir assays.

REFERENCES

1. Elion GB, Furman PA, Fyfe JA, de Miranda P, Beauchamp L and Schaeffer HJ (1977) Selectivity of action of an antiherpetic agent, 9-(2-hydroxyethoxymethyl)guanine. Proc. Natl. Acad. Sci. USA 74, 5716-5720.
2. Schaeffer HJ, Beauchamp L, de Miranda P, Elion GB, Bauer DJ and Collins P (1978) 9-(2-hydroxyethoxymethyl) guanine activity against viruses of the herpes group. Nature 272, 583-585.
3. Jones BR, Coster DJ, Fison PN, Thompson GM, Cobo LM and Falcon MG (1979) Efficacy of acycloguanosine (Wellcome 248U) against herpes simplex corneal ulcers. Lancet i, 243-244.
4. Coster DJ, Wilhelmus KR, Michaud R and Jones BR (1980) A comparison of acyclovir and idoxuridine as treatment for ulcerative herpetic keratitis. Br. J. Ophthalmol. 64, 763-765.

5.   McCulley JP, Binder PS, Kaufman HE, O'Day DM and Poirier RH (1982) A double-blind multicenter clinical trial of acyclovir vs. idoxuridine for treatment of epithelial herpes simplex keratitis.   Ophthalmol. 89, 1195-1200.

6.   Laibson PR, Pavan-Langston D, Yeakley WR and Lass J (1982) Acyclovir and vidarabine for the treatment of herpes simplex keratitis. Am. J. Med. 73, 281-285.

7.   Collum LMT, Benedict-Smith A and Hillary IB (1980) Randomised double-blind trial of acyclovir and idoxuridine in dendritic corneal ulceration. Br. J. Ophthalmol. 64, 766-769.

8.   Colin J, Tournoux A, Chastel C and Renard G (1981) Superficial herpes simplex keratitis.   Double-blind comparative trial of acyclovir and idoxuridine. Nouv. Presse Med. 10, 2969-2975.

9.   Klauber A and Ottovay E (1982) Acyclovir and idoxuridine treatment of herpes simplex keratitis - a double blind clinical study. Acta Ophthalmol. 60, 838-844.

10. McGill J, Tormey P and Walker CB (1981) Comparative trial of acyclovir and adenine arabinoside in the treatment of herpes simplex corneal ulcers. Br. J. Ophthalmol. 65, 610-613.

11. Young BJ, Patterson A and Ravenscroft T (1982) A randomised double-blind clinical trial of acyclovir (Zovirax) and adenine arabinoside in herpes simplex corneal ulceration. Br. J. Ophthalmol. 66, 361-363.

12. La Lau C, Oosterhuis JA, Versteeg J, van Rij G, Renardel de Lavalette JGC, Craandijk A and Lamers WPMA (1982) Acyclovir and trifluorothymidine in herpetic keratitis: a multicentre trial. Br. J. Ophthalmol. 66, 506-508.

13. Proceedings of the second international acyclovir symposium, London 15-18 May, 1983. Eds. Field HJ, Phillips I.   J. Antimicrob. Chemother. 12B.

14. Van Der Meer JWM and Versteeg J (1982) Acyclovir in severe herpes virus infections. Am. J. Med. 73(1A), 271-274.

15. Sundmacher R (1983) Oral acyclovir therapy for virologically proven intraocular herpes simplex virus disease.   Klin. Mbl. Augenheilk. 183, 246-250.

16. Grutzmacher RD, Henderson D, McDonald PJ and Coster DJ (1983) Herpes simplex chorioretinitis in a healthy adult. Am. J. Ophthalmol. 96, 788-796.

17. Hung SO, Patterson A and Rees PJ (1984) Pharmacokinetics of oral acyclovir (Zovirax) in the eye. Br. J. Ophthalmol. 68, 192-195.

18. de Miranda P, Whitley RJ, Barton N et al. (1982) Systemic absorption and pharmacokinetics of acyclovir (ACV) (Zovirax) capsules in immunocompromised patients with herpesvirus infections.   22nd Intersci. Conf. Antimicrob. Agents Chemother. Abs. 418.

19. Van Dyke R, Straube R, Large K, Hintz M, Spector S and Connor JD (1982) Pharmacokinetics of increased dose oral acyclovir.   22nd Intersci. Conf. Antimicrob. Agents Chemother. Abs. 414.

20. Whitley RJ, Blum, MR, Barton N and de Miranda P (1982) Pharmacokinetics of acyclovir in humans following intravenous administration. A model for the development of parenteral antivirals. Am. J. Med. 73, 165-171.

21. Crumpacker CS, Schnipper LE, Zaia JA and Levin MJ (1979) Growth inhibition by acycloguanosine of herpesviruses isolated from human infections. Antimicrob. Agents Chemother. 15, 642-645.

22. De Clerq E, Descamps J, Verhelst G et al. (1980) Comparative efficacy of antiherpes drugs against different strains of herpes simplex virus.   J. Infect. Dis. 141, 563-574.

DISCUSSION :

H.J. Field (Cambridge) : You did not mention whether the treatment
failure was related to the acquisition of resistance.

L.M.T. Collum (Dublin) : I have no information about that. The
patient that failed to respond had developed a peripheral
indolent lesion, which probably was not actively herpetic at
that time. Because the epithelium was broken, we couldn't
assume that that was not the case. We did not do virological
studies as such. We didn't design it to fit into the trial. It
would be a thing perhaps one should consider.

J.McGill (Southampton) : Louis, how did you suck up the tears ?

L.M.T. Collum (Dublin) : We used a micropipette and a microtube
which were sterilized for each patient. On the slitlamp we
could see tears coming on the top of the glass rod. When
that was filled, we emptied it into our little tube, filled it two
or three or more times as we went along. Now, I am not quite
sure where the question is leading ! I wondered myself about
this method, but it works.

J. McGill (Southampton) : How do you get the suction ?

L.M.T. Collum (Dublin) : Suck it up orally.

J. McGill (Southampton) : Weren't you worried about inhaling ?

L.M.T. Collum (Dublin) : I think this is a reasonable point. We
did think about it, and perhaps we should be using a syringe
or some other form of aspirator.

J. McGill (Southampton) : Could you not use micropipette and use
capillary action to suck up the fluid ?

L.M.T. Collum (Dublin) : We tried that. It does not work effectively enough. We get drops, but we don't get the volume that
we need.

J. McGill (Southampton) : The next point is that if you take it
up in the pipette and pour it into the micropot, what about
the evaporation you get from the pot ?

L.M.T. Collum (Dublin) : Well, I would hope we are not getting
much evaporation. We seal the tubes and deep freez them
straightaway. We are very careful in every patient as not
to use local anaesthetic, or do not aspirate when we have used
fluorescein or rose bengal or anything like that.

J. McGill (Southampton) : You do get evaporation unless you are very careful. We found that in our patients. Also what was the binding of the drug to the side of the pot ?

L.M.T. Collum (Dublin) : I cann't answer that.

J. McGill (Southampton) : A lot of immunoglobulins will bind to the side of the glass pot, and you are going to measure the wrong concentration.

L.M.T. Collum (Dublin) : You mean high or low ?

J. McGill (Southampton) : Low.

L.M.T. Collum (Dublin) : Yes, perhaps ?

E. De Clercq (Leuven) : It was a very fascinating talk and I congratulate you with your study. First of all I have a technical question. I am not sure about the correlation between the drug levels in plasma and tears. Did you try to calculate a correlation coefficient for the plasma levels and tear levels ?

L.M.T.Collum (Dublin) : No, we didn't. I stress that it is a preliminary study and we are only half way through. I had hoped it to be much more advanced for this meeting, but for one reason or another it isn't.

E. De Clercq (Leuven) : Then I have one more question. In evaluating the advantages of oral versus topical treatment, you forgot one factor, that is the cost of treatment.

L.M.T Collum (Dublin) : I look at it in terms of being a physician. I am there to do the best I can for the patient. At this stage the cost would be perhaps irrelevant, because we are looking for information. We let the Minister for Health worry about the cost later on, when we prove that it works.

P.A.Asbell (New York) : Did you find any difference in the post-treatment clinical course in either of these groups in terms of the incidence of either recurrence and/or stromal disease ?

L.M.T. Collum (Dublin) : In that group, in a period of a little more than three months, we had two recurrences. One patient developed classical stromal edema and another patient developed a fresh dendrite, well after they had healed. So there is no question of the oral treatment with acyclovir preventing or reducing recurrences.

A DOUBLE-BLIND, DUAL-CENTRE COMPARATIVE TRIAL OF ACYCLOVIR (ZOVIRAX[R]) AND ADENINE ARABINOSIDE IN THE TREATMENT OF HERPES SIMPLEX AMOEBOID ULCERS

S.O. Hung, A. Patterson, (St. Paul's Eye Hospital, Liverpool, England.) L.M.T. Collum, P. Logan, (Royal Victoria Eye and Ear Hospital, Dublin), P. Rees (Wellcome Research Laboratories, Kent, England)

SUMMARY

Thirty eight patients were included in this dual-centre, double-blind comparative study of acyclovir and adenine arabinoside in the treatment of herpetic amoeboid corneal ulceration. Eighteen of the 19 acyclovir recipients healed in a mean time of 11.7 days and 18 of the 19 patients treated with adenine arabinoside healed in a mean time of 11.2 days. There was no statistically significant difference between the two groups in terms of healing. The only adverse reaction seen was superficial punctate keratopathy in 2 acyclovir and 3 adenine arabinoside recipients.

1.   INTRODUCTION

Acyclovir is a new antiherpes agent having selective antiviral activity and low toxicity to normal host cells (1). Double-blind comparative clinical trials in the treatment of herpes simplex dendritic keratitis have shown acyclovir to be at least as effective as (2-4) or superior to (5-9) idoxuridine and adenine arabinoside, and generally equivalent to trifluorothymidine (10).

Amoeboid corneal ulceration is a more complicated type of herpes simplex infection with a tendency to involve the stroma with associated uveitis (11). Trifluorothymidine (TFT) was found to be superior to adenine arabinoside (12) in the treatment of amoeboid ulcers, possibly due to the increased solubility of TFT which may have allowed greater stromal uptake. Topical acyclovir has good corneal penetration (13). This paper examines the role of acyclovir in the management of herpetic amoeboid corneal ulcerations in comparison with adenine arabinoside.

Maudgal, P.C. and Missotten, L., (eds.) Herpetic Eye Diseases.
© *1985, Dr W. Junk Publishers, Dordrecht/Boston/Lancaster. ISBN 978-94-010-8935-7*

2.   MATERIALS AND METHODS

Patients presenting with an amoeboid ulcer and who gave their informed consent were included in the study. Patients who had been receiving antiviral agents or were unable to attend regularly for assessment were excluded.

The amoeboid ulcers were stained with Rose Bengal and examined by slit lamp microscopy. The size of the ulcer, extent of stromal reaction and severity of uveitis were recorded on first presentation and at subsequent follow up. Duration and severity of symptoms were noted.

Patients were randomly assigned to either 3% acyclovir (ACV) or 3% adenine arabinoside (Ara A) ointment to be applied topically 5 times daily. The patients were seen for assessment of healing of the ulcers at least twice weekly or more frequently if necessary. Healing was defined as absence of Rose Bengal staining over the original site of the amoeboid ulcer. Patients were withdrawn from the study if the ulcer increased in size over 3 days or remained static for more than 10 days.

Any adverse symptoms, allergic or toxic responses were recorded. Patients receiving topical steroids at entry were gradually weaned off over 2 weeks.

3.   RESULTS

Thirty-eight patients were included in the study, 19 were treated with acyclovir and 19 with adenine arabinoside. Patients characteristics at entry are summarised in Table 1.

Table 1 Summary of patient characteristics at entry.

		Ara A	ACV
Sex	Males	7	11
	Females	12	8
Ulcer size	Small	14	5
	Large	5	14
% with previous attacks		42%	42%
Median age (years)		61	45
Median symptom duration (days)		11	7
Mean severity of symptoms (score)		2.0	1.9
Mean stromal infiltration (score)		1.3	1.0
Mean uveitis (score)		0.7	0.9

Age, duration and severity of symptoms, stromal infiltration and uveitis were compared using Mann-Whitney tests and distribution of sex, occurrence of previous attacks and previous therapy with topical steroids or antibiotics were compared using chi-squared tests. No significiant differences were found between the 2 groups for these parameters. However, the acyclovir group did have a significantly higher proportion of patients with large ulcers ($p<0.05$, chi-squared test). Nine patients were receiving topical steroid at presentation (Table 2).

Table 2 Previous therapy

	Ara A	ACV
Steroids	6	3
Antibiotic	3	8

One patient from each group was withdrawn from the trial as the ulcer had remained static for 10 days. Two ulcers in each group took more than 20 days to heal. Healing times for the two treatment groups were compared by logrank analysis and no significant difference was found (Fig. 1).

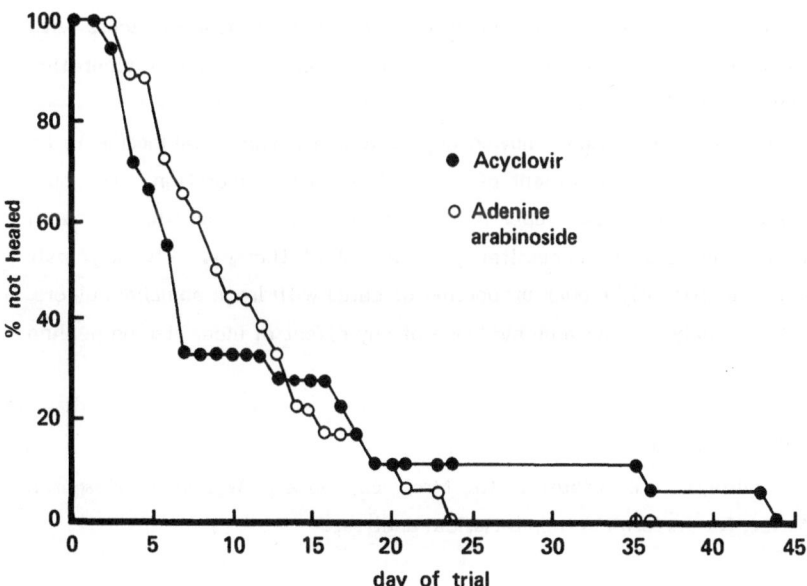

FIGURE 1. Cumulative frequency distribution of time taken to heal

Stromal disease regressed and settled in all but two patients receiving adenine arabinoside who required further treatment with prednisolone 0.05% eye drops after the ulcers had healed. The only adverse reactions seen were superficial punctate keratopathy in 2 patients receiving acyclovir and 3 receiving adenine arabinoside.

4.   DISCUSSION

Amoeboid corneal ulceration is a more severe form of herpetic infection with associated stromal involvement and uveitis, particularly if the ulcers are steroid enhanced. A study in 1967 showed that 92% of amoeboid ulcers were steroid enhanced (14). In 1979, another study reported a lower incidence of 53%. In this trial 29% of the patients had been treated with topical steroid for dendritic ulceration.   This downward trend may reflect increasing awareness among general medical practitioners of the potential problems in prescribing topical steroid.

Amoeboid ulcers have a high incidence of complications such as anterior stromal scarring, descemetocoele, secondary glaucoma, recurrent epithelial keratitis and metaherpetic ulceration (14). It is therefore important to treat such ulcers with an effective and relatively non-toxic antiviral agent. Idoxuridine has been shown to successfully heal 73% of amoeboid ulcers (14) but it is known that prolonged use of idoxuridine in the treatment of ulcers with severe stromal involvement can cause toxicity leading to indolent ulceration which may take weeks to heal.

The results of this study showed acyclovir and adenine arabinoside to be equally effective in the treatment of amoeboid herpetic ulceration. The only adverse reaction noted was superficial punctate keratopathy which cleared spontaneously and did not necessitate withdrawal of therapy. The acyclovir group had a significantly higher proportion of cases with large amoeboid ulcers, but a separate analysis showed no evidence of any effect of ulcer size on healing time.

ACKNOWLEDGEMENT

The authors are grateful to Mrs. C. Burke, Wellcome Research Laboratories, for performing the statistical analyses.

REFERENCES

1. Elion GB, Furman PA, Fyfe JA et al. (1977) Selective action of an antiherpetic agent, 9-(2-hydroxyethoxymethyl)guanine. Proc. Natl. Acad. Sci. U.S.A. 74, 5716-5720.

2. Coster DJ, Wilhelmus KR, Michaud R and Jones BR (1980) A comparison of acyclovir and idoxuridine as treatment for ulcerative herpetic keratitis. Br. J. Ophthalmol. 64, 763-765.

3. McCulley JP, Binder PS, Kaufman HE et al. (1982) A double-blind, multicenter clinical trial of acyclovir vs idoxuridine for treatment of epithelial herpes simplex keratitis. Ophthalmology 89, 1195-1200.

4. Laibson PR, Pavan-Langston D, Yeakley WR and Lass J. (1982) Acyclovir and vidarabine for the treatment of herpes simplex keratitis. Am. J. Med. 73, 281-285.

5. Collum LMT, Benedict-Smith A and Hillary IB (1980) Randomised double-blind trial of acyclovir and idoxuridine in dendritic corneal ulceration. Br. J. Ophthalmol. 64, 766-769.

6. Colin J, Tournoux A, Chastel C and Renard G (1981) Superficial herpes simplex keratitis. Double blind comparative trial of acyclovir and idoxuridine. Nouv. Presse Med. 10, 2969-2975.

7. Klauber A and Ottovay E (1982) Acyclovir and idoxuridine treatment of herpes simplex keratitis - a double blind clinical study. Acta Ophthalmol. 60, 838-844.

8. McGill J, Tormey P and Walker CB (1981) Comparative trial of acyclovir and adenine arabinoside in the treatment of herpes simplex corneal ulcers. Br. J. Ophthalmol. 65, 610-613.

9. Young BJ, Patterson A and Ravenscroft T (1982) A randomised double-blind clinical trial of acyclovir (Zovirax) and adenine arabinoside in herpes simplex corneal ulceration. Br. J. Ophthalmol. 66, 361-363.

10. La Lau C, Oosterhuis JA, Versteeg J et al. (1982) Acyclovir and trifluorothymidine in herpetic keratitis: a multicentre trial. Br. J. Ophthalmol. 66, 506-508.

11. Thygeson P and Kimura SJ (1957) Deep forms of herpetic keratitis. Am. J. Ophthalmol. 43, 109.

12. Coster DJ, Jones BR and McGill J (1979) Treatment of amoeboid herpetic ulcers with adenine arabinoside or trifluorothymidine. Br. J. Ophthalmol. 63, 418-421.

13. Poirier RH, Kingham JD, de Miranda P and Annel M (1982) Intraocular antiviral penetration. Arch. Ophthalmol. 100, 1964-1967.

14. Patterson A and Jones BR (1967) The management of ocular herpes. Trans. Ophthal. Soc. U.K. 87, 59-83.

DISCUSSION :

J.McGill (Southampton) : Three questions. How many patients were atopic ? Because if there was uneven distribution, this would bias your results.

S.O. Hung (Liverpool) : I have not got the data.

J.McGill (Southampton) : Secondly, I would suggest that your groups were not similar because six in ara-A group had steroids and only three in the acyclovir group. It may be important in the small numbers you have as withdrawal of steroids would lead to an exacerbation of the stromal disease and if there were more steroid treated patients in one group, this would bias the results.

S.O. Hung (Liverpool) : It has been analysed that small number of patients with previous steroid therapy has no statistically significant difference in the two groups.

J.McGill (Southampton) : Fine. The other problem is that why did you use ara-A and not trifluorothymidine. Trifluorothymi-dine has been shown to be better for amoeboid ulcer.

S.O.Hung (Liverpool) : This is a part of a series of studies that we have performed in Liverpool. We have done the study com-paring acyclovir with ara-A in simple dendritic ulcers. This is a continuation of that study.

C.R. Dawson (San Francisco) : How do you think this would compare with gentle wiping debridement ? Do you have a com-parable study in which the time to healing with debridement was evaluated ?

A. Patterson (Liverpool) : Could I answer to Dr.Dawson Mr. Chair-man ? In previous trial we found debridement cured 33% of amoeboid-dendritic ulcers and 90% of simple dendritic ulcers. However because of the extensive area you have to apply the cautery or carbolic acid, the succes rate is very much reduced. So, in our series it is about 33% cured with cautery.

TOPICAL BROMOVINYLDEOXYURIDINE TREATMENT OF HERPES SIMPLEX KERATITIS

P.C. MAUDGAL[1], M. DIELTIENS[1], E. DE CLERCQ[2] and L. MISSOTTEN[1]

[1]Eye Research Laboratory of the Ophthalmology Clinic, and [2]Rega Institute for Medical Research, Katholieke Universiteit Leuven, B-3000 Leuven, Belgium.

1. INTRODUCTION

Bromovinyldeoxyuridine $\big($(E)-5-(2-bromovinyl)-2'-deoxyuridine, BVDU$\big)$ is a newly synthesized thymidine analogue (1), structurally related to the classical antiherpes agents idoxuridine (5-iodo-2'-deoxyuridine, IDU) and trifluridine (5-trifluoromethyl-2'-deoxyuridine, TFT). These compounds are 5-substituted analogues of 2'-deoxythymidine (dThd), the natural precursor of DNA synthesis.

In cell culture, BVDU exceeds IDU, TFT, and various other antiherpes compounds such as foscarnet (phosphonoformate), vidarabine (9-β-D-arabinofuranosyladenine, ara-A, Vira-A) and acyclovir $\big($9-(2-hydroxyethoxymethyl)guanine, acycloguanosine, Zovirax$\big)$ in potency and selectivity against herpes simplex virus type 1 (HSV-1) (2-4).

BVDU inhibits the replication of HSV-1 (2-4) and varicella-zoster virus (VZV) (5,6) at a concentration of $0.002 - 0.01$ µg/ml, whereas drug concentrations up to $50 - 100$ µg/ml are required to affect normal cell metabolism. This selective antiherpetic activity of BVDU is attributed to a specific phosphorylation by the HSV-1- or VZV-encoded dThd kinase (7,8). In its 5'-triphosphate form, BVDU competitively inhibits the utilization of 2'-deoxythymidine triphosphate (dTTP) by the viral DNA polymerases, because BVDU 5'-triphosphate (BVDUTP) has a greater affinity for the HSV-1 DNA polymerase than for the cellular DNA polymerases α, β and γ (9). Furthermore, BVDUTP can serve as an alternate substrate of DNA polymerase (10) and be incorporated as BVDU 5'-monophosphate into viral DNA (11). The extent of viral yield reduction is closely related to the amount of BVDU incorporated into the viral DNA (11). HSV-2-encoded dThd kinase is less efficient in phosphorylating BVDU (8,12), which makes this compound less active against HSV-2. BVDU is ineffective against dThd kinase-deficient (TK⁻) HSV mutants.

We have previously reported that BVDU is superior to IDU in the

Maudgal, P.C. and Missotten, L., (eds.) Herpetic Eye Diseases.
© *1985, Dr W. Junk Publishers, Dordrecht/Boston/Lancaster. ISBN 978-94-010-8935-7*

prevention of HSV-1 epithelial keratitis in rabbits, and BVDU also promotes significantly greater healing of established keratitis, whether both drugs are used as eye ointments or eyedrops (13,14). When applied to rabbit eyes as 0.1 % or 0.5 % eyedrops, BVDU proved superior to 1 % TFT eyedrops in suppressing the development of stromal keratitis (15). In another set of rabbit experiments, in which keratitis and iritis were produced by inoculation of HSV-1 into the anterior chamber, 0.5 % BVDU eyedrops had a significantly greater healing effect on keratitis and iritis than 1 % TFT eyedrops (16). Using a radiolabeled analogue of BVDU, $\left(^{125}I\right)$IVDU, as eyedrops, we detected three- to nine-fold higher concentrations of the compound in the aqueous humor of rabbits than the concentrations required for inhibition of virus replication in cell culture (17).

Oral administration of BVDU to rabbits as capsules at 10 mg/kg/day or 100 mg/kg/day for 4 days significantly reduced the severity of keratitis and iritis in comparison to placebo treatment (16).

Our previous clinical studies (18,19) have shown that BVDU is a safe and efficacious drug for the treatment of herpes simplex keratitis in patients. In this paper, we report the results of our follow-up observations on a larger group of patients over a more extended time period.

2. DENDRITIC CORNEAL ULCERS

Sixty-nine patients who presented with dendritic keratitis were treated with 0.1 % BVDU eyedrops, one drop of the drug being administered into the eye 9 times a day at 1-hour intervals. Three patients were lost to follow-up. Sixty-six patients have been followed for an average period of 37 months (from 2.5 to 56 months) (Table 1).

At the start of BVDU treatment half of the patients had been treated, albeit unsuccessfully, with other antiviral compounds (IDU, TFT, Vira-A) for at least 10 days. Dendritic keratitis was associated with stromal disease in 49 patients. Twenty-eight patients were using topical corticosteroids along with antiviral drugs. Two patients were on oral prednisolone after a kidney transplantation. Topical corticosteroid therapy was stopped in all patients when they were put on BVDU eyedrops. Corticosteroids were reinstituted in 13 patients as their stromal disease worsened.

In 47 patients the duration of the acute keratitis episode before BVDU treatment was 1 month or less (average : 9.34 days). These patients healed in an average time of 8.3 days on BVDU medication (Table 1). Eleven patients whose duration of symptoms was for more than 1 month but less than 1 year (average : 2.83 months) healed on BVDU therapy in an average time of 9 days. Two patients who had a history of recurrent keratitis for 1.5 years, without being free of symptoms at any time, healed in an average time of 12 days. Those patients who had failed to respond to other antivirals also responded promptly to BVDU treatment (Table 4). Dendritic keratitis recurred in 20 patients (30.3 %) during the follow-up period. Before BVDU treatment 28 patients (40.5 %) had suffered recurrences. The recurrent disease responded to BVDU therapy as quickly as did the initial episodes.

Table 1. Topical BVDU treatment in patients with dendritic corneal ulcers

Treatment regimen : BVDU 0.1 % eyedrops 5-9 x per day, up to 3 weeks.
Number of patients : 69 (3 lost to follow-up).
Follow-up period : Average 37 months (2.5 - 56 months).
Number of patients with clinical resistance to IDU, TFT and/or Vira-A : 34.
Average duration of symptoms before BVDU treatment versus healing time on
  BVDU therapy :

Duration of symptoms		Average healing	No. of
Total period	Average	time	patients
< 1 month	9.34 months	8.3 days	47
1 month – 1 year	2.83 months	9 days	17
> 1 year	1.5 years	12 days	2

Recurrences before BVDU treatment : 28 patients (40.5 %).
Recurrences after BVDU treatment : 20 patients (30.3 %).

Of the 13 patients with dendritic keratitis and stromal disease where we had to re-install topical corticosteroids, 10 patients became corticosteroid-dependent. In these patients corticosteroids were weaned off over a prolonged period under BVDU cover. Bullous keratopathy developed in 2 patients, dry eye condition was observed in 4 patients and lower canaliculitis in one patient. One patient showed local hypersensitivity to topical BVDU application.

3. GEOGRAPHIC CORNEAL ULCERS

Twenty-seven patients who presented with geographic corneal ulcers associated with stromal keratitis were treated with 0.1 % BVDU eyedrops (Table 2). Thirteen patients also had keratic precipitates. Eighteen patients had been using either IDU, TFT, Vira-A or Zovirax without any beneficial effect, before their treatment was switched to BVDU. Fifteen patients were using topical corticosteroids along with antiviral drugs. All patients, whether their duration of symptoms before BVDU therapy was less or more than 1 month, healed with an average time of 11 to 12 days (Table 2) on 0.1 % BVDU eyedrops. Topical corticosteroids, however, had to be reinstalled in 12 patients for their stromal disease as these patients turned out to be corticosteroid-dependent. Other complications observed in this group were bullous keratopathy (2 patients), aseptic epithelium defect (2 patients), dry eye (7 patients) and contact allergy to BVDU eyedrops (4 patients).

During an average follow-up period of 33.6 months (from 25–54 months) recurrence of dendritic, geographic or stromal keratitis occurred in 13 patients (48.1 %), whereas 19 patients (70.4 %) had suffered recurrences before BVDU treatment.

Table 2. Topical BVDU treatment in patients with geographic corneal ulcers

Treatment regimen : BVDU 0.1 % eyedrops 5 – 9 x per day, up to 7 weeks.
Number of patients : 27.
Follow-up period : 33.6 months (2.5 – 54 months).
Number of patients with clinical resistance to IDU, TFT, Zovirax and/or
 Vira-A : 18.
Average duration of symptoms before BVDU treatment versus healing time on
 BVDU therapy :

Duration of symptoms		Average healing	No. of
Total period	Average	time	patients
< 1 month	9.2 days	11.2 days	14
> 1 month	2.7 months	12.3 days	13

Recurrences before BVDU treatment : 19 patients (70.4 %).
Recurrences after BVDU treatment : 13 patients (48.1 %).

4. STROMAL KERATITIS

Twenty-nine patients who presented with stromal keratitis were treated with 0.1 % BVDU eyedrops (Table 3). These patients did not have epithelial ulcerations. Twenty patients had been using either IDU or TFT without any relief. Except for 7 patients, all other patients were using topical corti-

costeroids. As in the dendritic and geographic keratitis groups, topical
corticosteroids were stopped at the time antiviral therapy was switched to
BVDU. One patient was lost to follow-up. Stromal disease became quiscent
in 5 patients without concomitant instillation of topical corticosteroids.
For the other patients, we had to prescribe topical corticosteroids along
with BVDU eyedrops, as their ocular condition either did not improve suf-
ficiently fast or became worse. Fifteen patients became corticosteroid-
dependent. Three patients developed dry eye, and 2 patients became allergic to topical BVDU application. One patient, whose stromal disease had
resolved, developed a severe iritis one week after BVDU treatment was
stopped. This patient was treated successfully with topical BVDU eyedrops,
corticosteroids and mydriatics.

In the group of patients with stromal keratitis there was no correlation between the duration of disease before treatment and the healing time
under BVDU therapy (Table 3). Nine patients who had stromal keratitis for
less than 1 month (average : 11 days) healed in an average· time of 34
days. Fifteen patients with symptoms for more than 1 month but less than 1
year (average : 2.7 months) healed in an average time of 31 days. Five patients with stromal disease for more than 1 year (average : 3.5 years)
healed in an average time of 20.6 days. During an average follow-up period
of 29.5 months (range : 2.5 - 54 months) 14 patients (50 %) developed recurrence of herpetic corneal disease. The recurrence rate before BVDU
treatment was 72.4 % (21 patients).

Table 3. Topical BVDU treatment in patients with stromal keratitis

Treatment regimen : BVDU (0.1 % eyedrops 5 - 9 x day, up to 6 months.
Number of patients : 29 (1 lost to follow-up).
Follow-up period : average 29.5 months (2.5 - 54 months).
Number of patients with clinical resistance to IDU and/or TFT = 19.
Average duration of symptoms before BVDU treatment versus healing time on
  BVDU therapy :

| Duration of symptoms | | Average healing | No. of |
Total period	Average	time	patients
< 1 month	11 days	34 days	9
1 month - 1 year	2.7 months	31 days	15
> 1 year	3.5 years	20.6 days	5

Recurrences before BVDU treatment : 21 patients (72.4 %).
Recurrences after BVDU treatment : 14 patients (50 %).

5. COMMENTS

This long-term follow-up study in 125 patients confirms our previous results on the efficacy and safety of topical 0.1 % BVDU eyedrops in the treatment of herpes simplex dendritic and geographic corneal ulcers and stromal keratitis (18-20). All patients responded to BVDU, including those 71 patients that had been treated unsuccessfully with other antiviral drugs, i.e. IDU, TFT, Vira-A and, in once case, Zovirax (Table 4).

Table 4. Analysis of data on patients clinically resistant to other anti- viral drugs

Keratitis	Antiviral agent used before BVDU treatment	No. of patients[a]	Average healing time by BVDU therapy
Dendritic corneal ulcers	IDU	25	9.4 days[b]
	TFT	12 (4 patients also resistant to IDU)	8.9 days[b]
	Vira-A	1 (also resistant to IDU)	5 days
Geographic corneal ulcers	IDU	13	10.4 days
	TFT	8 (3 patients also resistant to IDU)	10.3 days
	Ara-A	3 (also resistant to IDU)	11.3 days
	Zovirax	1 (also resistant to TFT)	7 days
Stromal keratitis	IDU	18	30 days
	TFT	7 (5 patients also resistant to IDU)	38.1 days

[a] Patients clinically resistant to more than one antiviral drug were coun- ted separately for each drug.
[b] One patient lost to follow-up.

Except for contact allergy to BVDU in 6 patients, no other local or systemic toxic effects of the drug were observed. Complications like bul- lous keratopathy, aseptic epithelium defect and dry eye, as observed in some patients, were not drug-related, as they are known sequelae of the disease itself. When administered to rabbits as 0.1 % or 0.5 % eyedrops, BVDU does not retard the regeneration of the corneal epithelium (21).

Because of the efficient corneal penetration of topically applied BVDU (17), this drug can be used for the topical treatment of stromal ke- ratitis and iritis. However, treatment of stromal disease may require con- comitant use of topical corticosteroids (22-24) because of the immune reaction initiated by the HSV antigens. In the present study, 49 patients in the dendritic keratitis group had associated stromal disease and 28 of

them were using topical corticosteroids along with other antivirals. Once
BVDU treatment was initiated, we had to re-install topical corticosteroids
only in 13 patients, and 10 of these became corticosteroid-dependent.
Similarly, in the geographic keratitis group all 27 patients had associated stromal disease of variable severity and 15 of them were using topical
corticosteroids before BVDU therapy was initiated. Except for 12 patients
who were corticosteroid-dependent, all others healed on 0.1 % BVDU eyedrops
alone. In the stromal keratitis group, again, 5 of the 29 patients healed
without the use of topical corticosteroids and 15 patients became corticosteroid-dependent. This does not imply that BVDU did not affect the severity
of keratitis in those patients in whom we had to re-install corticosteroids
or those who became corticosteroid-dependent, because all these patients
were using other topical antiviral drugs without any beneficial effect before they were put on BVDU eyedrops. Since these patients had not responded
to IDU, TFT, Vira-A or Zovirax, in combination with topical corticosteroids, we believe that BVDU was instrumental in arresting the virus replication cycle in the corneal stroma that would otherwise have lead to the
release of virus-specific antigens needed to initiate or maintain the immunologic reaction that is characteristic of stromal disease (22-24).

REFERENCES

1. Jones AS, Verhelst G, Walker RT. 1979. The synthesis of the potent antiherpes virus agent, E-5-(2-bromovinyl)-2'-deoxyuridine and related
   compounds. Tetrahedron Lett., 4415-4418.
2. De Clercq E, Descamps J, Barr PJ, Jones AS, Serafinowski P, Walker RT,
   Huang GF, Torrence PF, Schmidt CL, Mertes MP, Kulikowski T, Shugar D.
   1979. Comparative study of the potency and selectivity of anti-herpes
   compounds. In: Antimetabolites in Biochemistry, Biology and Medicine.
   Skoda J, Langen P (eds.), Pergamon Press, Oxford, pp. 275-285.
3. De Clercq E, Descamps J, De Somer P, Barr PJ, Jones AS, Walker RT.
   1979. (E)-5-(2-Bromovinyl)-2'-deoxyuridine : a potent and selective
   anti-herpes agent. Proc. Natl. Acad. Sci. USA 76, 2947-2951.
4. De Clercq E, Descamps J, Maudgal PC, Missotten L, Leyten R, Verhelst
   G, Jones AS, Walker RT, Busson R, Vanderhaeghe H, De Somer P. 1980.
   Selective anti-herpes activity of 5-(2-halogenovinyl)-2'-deoxyuridines
   and -2'-deoxycytidines. In: Developments in Antiviral Therapy. Collier
   LH, Oxford J (eds.), Academic Press, London, pp. 21-42.
5. De Clercq E, Descamps J, Ogata M, Shigeta S. 1982. In vitro susceptibility of varicella-zoster to E-5-(2-bromovinyl)-2'-deoxyuridine and
   related compounds. Antimicrob. Agents Chemother. 21, 33-38.
6. Shigeta S, Yokota T, Iwabuchi T, Baba M, Konno K, Ogata M, De Clercq
   E. 1983. Comparative efficacy of antiherpes drugs against various
   strains of varicella-zoster virus. J. Infect. Dis. 147, 576-584.

7. Cheng Y-C, Dutschman G, De Clercq E, Jones AS, Rahim SG, Verhelst G, Walker RT. 1981. Differential affinities of 5-(2-halogenovinyl)-2'-deoxyuridines for deoxythymidine kinases of various origins. Mol. Pharmacol. 20, 230-233.

8. Descamps J, De Clercq E. 1981. Specific phosphorylation of E-5-(2-iodovinyl)-2'-deoxyuridine by herpes simplex virus-infected cells. J. Biol. Chem. 256, 5973-5976.

9. Allaudeen HS, Kozarich JW, Bertino JR, De Clercq E. 1981. On the mechanism of selective inhibition of herpesvirus replication by (E)-5-(2-bromovinyl)-2'-deoxyuridine. Proc. Natl. Acad. Sci. USA 78, 2698-2702.

10. Allaudeen HS, Chen MS, Lee JJ, De Clercq E, Prusoff WH. 1982. Incorporation of E-5-(2-halovinyl)-2'-deoxyuridines into deoxyribonucleic acids of herpes simplex virus type-1 infected cells. J. Biol. Chem. 257, 603-606.

11. Mancini WR, De Clercq E, Prusoff WH. 1983. The relationship between incorporation of E-5-(2-bromovinyl)-2'-deoxyuridine into herpes simplex virus type 1 DNA with virus infectivity and DNA integrity. J. Biol. Chem. 258, 792-795.

12. Fyfe JA. 1982. Differential phosphorylation of (E)-5-(2-bromovinyl)-2'-deoxyuridine monophosphate by thymidylate kinases from herpes simplex viruses types 1 and 2 and varicella zoster virus. Mol. Pharmacol. 21, 432-437.

13. Maudgal PC, De Clercq E, Descamps J, Missotten L, De Somer P, Busson R, Vanderhaeghe H, Verhelst G, Walker RT, Jones AS. 1980. (E)-5-(2-Bromovinyl)-2'-deoxyuridine in the treatment of experimental herpes simplex keratitis. Antimicrob. Agents Chemother. 17, 8-12.

14. Maudgal PC, De Clercq E, Descamps J, Missotten L. 1979. Comparative evaluation of BVDU ((E)-5-(2-bromovinyl)-2'-deoxyuridine) and IDU (5-iodo-2'-deoxyuridine) in the treatment of experimental herpes simplex keratitis in rabbits. Bull. Soc. Belge Ophtalmol. 186, 109-118.

15. Maudgal PC, De Clercq E, Descamps J, Missotten L, Wijnhoven J. 1982. Experimental stromal herpes simplex keratitis. Influence of treatment with topical bromovinyldeoxyuridine and trifluridine. Arch. Ophthalmol. 100, 653-656.

16. Maudgal PC, Uyttebroeck W, De Clercq E, Missotten L. 1982. Oral and topical treatment of experimental herpes simplex iritis with bromovinyldeoxyuridine. Arch. Ophthalmol. 100, 1337-1340.

17. Maudgal PC, Verbruggen AM, De Clercq E, Busson R, Bernaerts R, de Roo M, Ameye C, Missotten L. 1985. Ocular penetration of (^{125}I)IVDU, a radiolabeled analogue of bromovinyldeoxyuridine. Invest. Ophthalmol. Vis. Sci., in press.

18. Maudgal PC, Missotten L, De Clercq E, Descamps J, De Meuter E. 1981. Efficacy of (E)-5-(2-bromovinyl)-2'-deoxyuridine in the topical treatment of herpes simplex keratitis. Albrecht von Graefes Arch. Klin. Ophthalmol. 216, 261-268.

19. Maudgal PC, De Clercq E, Descamps J, Missotten L. 1981. Efficacy of E-5-(2-bromovinyl)-2'-deoxyuridine in the topical treatment of herpetic keratitis in rabbits and man. In: Herpetische Augenerkrankungen. Sundmacher R (ed.), J.F. Bergmann Verlag, München, pp. 339-341.

20. Maudgal PC, De Clercq E, Missotten L. 1984. Efficacy of bromovinyl-deoxyuridine in the treatment of herpes simplex virus and varicella-zoster virus eye infections. Antiviral Res. 4, 281-291.

21. Maudgal PC, De Kimpe N, De Clercq E, Descamps J, Missotten L, Geysen A. 1982. Influence of (E)-5-(2-bromovinyl)-2'-deoxyuridine on corneal epithelium healing. Graefe's Arch. Clin. Exp. Ophthalmol. 218, 275-281.

22. Metcalf JF, Kaufman HE. 1976. Herpetic stromal keratitis : evidence for cell mediated immunopathogenesis. Am. J. Ophthalmol. 82, 827-834.
23. Meyers RL, Chitjian PA, Fiorello P. 1979. Studies on the immunopatho-genesis of chronic and recurrent herpes simplex virus keratitis in man : immunoperoxidase antibody study. In: Proceedings of the 23rd International Congress of Ophthalmology. Shimizu K, Oosterhuis JA (eds.), Excerpta Medica, Amsterdam, pp. 1739-1743.
24. Meyers-Elliott RH, Pettit TH, Maxwell WA. 1980. Viral antigens in the immune ring of herpes simplex stromal keratitis. Arch. Ophthalmol. 98, 897-904.

DISCUSSION :

E. De Clerq (Leuven) : I have a problem with the interpretation of clinical resistance. How long do you treat the patient before you decide that the patient is "clinically resistant" ? Is this after days, weeks or months ?

P.C.Maudgal (Leuven) : There are no hard and fast rules. If the ocular condition deteriorates during therapy, either the disease is resistant to treatment or the patient is not com-plying. If the compliance is good there is at least some impro-vement in symptoms. In those cases, for epithelial disease, I would roughly wait for one week to judge the effect of medica-tion. If the disease does not respond or partially responds and then the improvement stops, I interpret it as "clinical resistan-ce". It happens very often that during the first three or four days there is progress, and then either the ulcer does not heal further or the condition starts deteriorating despite antiviral therapy. If you then change the antiviral, improvement general-ly follows.

A. Pathak (Ghent) : As a clinician I would like to share the ex-periences of my colleagues who have been very well busy with herpetic diseases. Mostly we associate antiviral drugs with antibiotics. It is not a practice in our university clinic only but I believe with many other clinicians too. Is it worthwhile to associate the two drugs or it is not necessary ?

P.C. Maudgal (Leuven) : I know that it is a common practice in this country but I don't give antibiotics to these patients. There is a simple reason to that. Any compound you put into the eye is foreign to body. In addition, all ophthalmic preparations contain preservatives that damage the epithelium cells and even retard healing. It has been shown that benzalkonium chloride for example disturbs the tear film, which causes other problems. Yesterday, it was remarked that the dry eye problems may deteriorate the epithelial herpetic keratitis. Finally, antibiotics are not indicated for the treatment of herpetic disease. Of course, if you have basis to suspect associated bacterial infection on clinical grounds, or if you are dealing with a laboratory proven associated bacterial infection, you have to use appropriate antibiotics alongwith antiherpes compounds.

A. Pathak (Ghent) : Even in the cases of epithelial keratitis, don't you associate, for the initial few days, with antibiotics, or you go purely on antiviral drugs.

P.C. Maudgal (Leuven) : We use only antiviral drugs right from the beginning.

L.M.T. Collum (Dublin) : Apropos your saying that the virus has become resistant and ....

P.C. Maudgal (Leuven) : Excuse me for interruption. I did not say that the "virus" became resistant. I understand very well that the laboratory proven "resistance" and "clinical resistance" are two separate enteties.

L.M.T. Collum (Dublin) : I just wanted to clarify that. Because I think that some of those ulcers that stop responding, the virus is probably no longer active, and you are dealing with unhealty epithelium trying to go across the basement membrane which is probably damaged. So, this is just a subtle distinction there.

P.C.Maudgal (Leuven) : Yes, I agree with you. That happens in some cases.

PERMEABILITY OF THE CORNEA TO (^{125}I)IVDU, AN ANALOGUE OF BROMOVINYLDEOXY-URIDINE

A.M. VERBRUGGEN[1], E. DE CLERCQ[2], P.C. MAUDGAL[3], C. AMEYE[3], R. BUSSON[2], R. BERNAERTS[2], M. DE ROO[1] and L. MISSOTTEN[3]

[1]Laboratory of Nuclear Medicine and Radiopharmacy, [2]Rega Institute for Medical Research, and [3]Eye Research Laboratory, Ophthalmology Clinic, Katholieke Universiteit Leuven, B-3000 Leuven, Belgium.

1. INTRODUCTION

Bromovinyldeoxyuridine ((E)-5-(2-bromovinyl)-2'-deoxyuridine, BVDU) is a highly potent and selective antiherpes drug. It inhibits the replication of herpes simplex virus type 1 (HSV-1) (1,2) and varicella-zoster virus (VZV) (3,4) at a concentration of about 0.01 µg/ml, whereas concentrations up to 50 - 100 µg/ml are required to affect normal host cell functions.

In animal models, BVDU was found to be effective in the topical and systemic treatment of HSV-1 skin infections (5,6), orofacial lesions (7), genital herpes (8) and encephalitis (9,10). In rabbits topically applied BVDU was significantly superior to idoxuridine (5-iodo-2'-deoxyuridine, IDU) in the treatment of HSV-1 epithelial keratitis (11,12), and also significantly better than trifluridine (5-trifluoromethyl-2'-deoxyuridine, TFT) in promoting the healing of deep stromal keratitis (13) and iritis (14).

BVDU 0.1 % eyedrops have been found to be safe and effective for the treatment of patients with dendritic or geographic corneal ulcers and stromal disease (16,17).

2. CORNEAL PERMEABILITY

We investigated the corneal permeability of BVDU by using its radio-labeled analogue, (^{125}I)IVDU {(E)-5-(2-(^{125}I)iodovinyl)-2'-deoxyuridine} which has been used in the past to determine the mechanism of antiviral action of (E)-5-(2-halogenovinyl)-2'-deoxyuridine. (^{125}I)IVDU is phosphorylated in HSV-1-infected cells by the virus-encoded thymidine kinase (18), incorporated into HSV-1 DNA (19), but not incorporated into DNA of uninfected cells (20).

(^{125}I)IVDU was synthesized according to a procedure described pre-

Maudgal, P.C. and Missotten, L., (eds.) Herpetic Eye Diseases.
© *1985, Dr W. Junk Publishers, Dordrecht/Boston/Lancaster. ISBN 978-94-010-8935-7*

viously (21). With a micropipette, 5 µl of either 0.2 % or 0.5 % (^{125}I)IVDU
were instilled into each eye of four rabbits at one hour intervals. In each
dosage group, one rabbit was killed one hour after the first, second, third
and fourth application of the drug. Blood samples were obtained from the
ear vein before killing the animals, and aqueous samples were aspirated
from the anterior chamber, using a tuberculine syringe, immediately after
the death of the animals. The (^{125}I)IVDU content in the aqueous and plasma
samples was determined by comparison with the radioactivity measured for a
standard (^{125}I)IVDU solution and the antiviral activity of the aqueous
fluid was assayed by incubating serial dilutions of the samples on HSV-1-
infected primary rabbit kidney cells. Both aqueous and plasma samples were
subjected to chromatographic analysis to detect degradation products of
(^{125}I)IVDU.

After instillation of 0.5 % (^{125}I)IVDU eyedrops, concentrations of
the compound in the aqueous fluid ranged from 90 ng/ml one hour after a
single application to 222 ng/ml one hour after the four consecutive applications of (^{125}I)IVDU at an hourly interval. Drug concentration in the
anterior chamber fluid was lower after instillation of 0.2 % (^{125}I)IVDU
eyedrops, ranging from 37 ng/ml one hour after a single administration to
92 ng/ml one hour after four consecutive applications at one hour intervals. At both dosage regimens, the drug levels gradually increased in the
aqueous with the number of applications. Similarly, (^{125}I)IVDU concentrations in the plasma increased after repeated applications of the compound,
but the plasma drug levels remained lower than those achieved in the
aqueous.

Since the minimum antiviral concentration of iodovinyldeoxyuridine is
10 ng/ml, the drug levels achieved in the aqueous humor after topical application of 0.2 % (^{125}I)IVDU eyedrops exceeded its minimum antiviral concentration by three- to nine-fold. Furthermore, all samples exhibited an
antiviral activity up to a dilution of 1:6, which is consistent with the
radioactivity data.

The radioactive material found in the aqueous samples upon instillation of topical (^{125}I)IVDU eyedrops consisted mainly of intact (^{125}I)IVDU
and, as minor components, $\underline{(E)}$-5-$(2-(^{125}I)$iodovinyl$)$uracil$)$ $((^{125}I)$IVU$)$ and
free (^{125}I)iodide. The release of free iodide must be attributed to the
action of a deiodinase, and the release of (^{125}I)IVU is most probably due
to the action of thymidine phosphorylase (22) or pyrimidine nucleoside

phosphorylases in general. These enzymes are assumed to be present in peripheral tissues.

3. COMMENT

To exert a healing effect on HSV stromal keratitis or iritis, the topically administered antiviral compounds must be able to penetrate the cornea. Our experiments show that $(^{125}I)IVDU$, a radiolabeled analogue of BVDU, when given topically as 0.2 % eyedrops, achieves drug levels in the aqueous humor which are three- to nine-fold higher than its minimum antiviral concentration in cell culture. Still higher drug levels were detected in the anterior chamber fluid when 0.5 % $(^{125}I)IVDU$ eyedrops were used. Most of the radioactive material detected in the samples consisted of intact $(^{125}I)IVDU$. This would explain our previous observations on the efficacy of 0.5 % BVDU eyedrops in the topical treatment of HSV-1 stromal keratitis (13) and iritis (14) in rabbits. The pronounced healing effect of BVDU eyedrops on herpetic stromal disease in patients (16,17) can also be attributed to an efficient penetration in the cornea.

REFERENCES

1. De Clercq E, Descamps J, De Somer P, Barr PJ, Jones AS, Walker RT. 1979. (E)-5-(2-Bromovinyl)-2'-deoxyuridine : a potent and selective anti-herpes agent. Proc. Natl. Acad. Sci. USA 76, 2947-2951.
2. De Clercq E, Descamps J, Verhelst G, Walker RT, Jones AS, Torrence PF, Shugar D. 1980. Comparative efficacy of antiherpes drugs against different strains of herpes simplex virus. J. Infect. Dis. 141, 563-574.
3. De Clercq E, Descamps J, Ogata M, Shigeta S. 1982. In vitro susceptibility of varicella-zoster virus to E-5-(2-bromovinyl)-2'-deoxyuridine and related compounds. Antimicrob. Agents Chemother. 21, 33-38.
4. Shigeta S, Yokota T, Iwabuchi T, Baba M, Konno K, Ogata M, De Clercq E. 1983. Comparative efficacy of antiherpes drugs against various strains of varicella-zoster virus. J. Infect. Dis. 147, 576-584.
5. De Clercq E, Zhang Z-X, Descamps J, Huygen K. 1981. E-5-(2-Bromovinyl)-2'-deoxyuridine vs. interferon in the systemic treatment of infection with herpes simplex virus of athymic nude mice. J. Infect. Dis. 143, 846-852.
6. De Clercq E. 1984. Topical treatment of cutaneous herpes simplex virus infection in hairless mice with (E)-5-(2-bromovinyl)-2'-deoxyuridine and related compounds. Antimicrob. Agents Chemother. 26, 155-159.
7. Park N-H, Pavan-Langston D, Boisjoly HM, De Clercq E. 1982. Chemotherapeutic efficacy of E-5-(2-bromovinyl)-2'-deoxyuridine for orofacial infection with herpes simplex virus type 1 in mice. J. Infect. Dis. 145, 909-913.
8. Sim IS. 1984. Oral and topical treatment of experimental HSV-1 genital herpes with (E)-5-(2-bromovinyl)-2'-deoxyuridine. J. Antimicrob. Chemother. 14 (Suppl. A), 111-118.

9. De Clercq E, Zhang Z-X, Sim IS. 1982. Treatment of experimental herpes simplex virus encephalitis with (E)-5-(2-bromovinyl)-2'-deoxyuridine in mice. Antimicrob. Agents Chemother. 22, 421-425.

10. Park N-H, Pavan-Langston D, De Clercq E. 1983. Efficacy of (E)-5-(2-bromovinyl)-2'-deoxyuridine in the treatment of experimental herpes simplex virus encephalitis in mice. Antiviral Res. 3, 7-15.

11. Maudgal PC, De Clercq E, Descamps J, Missotten L. 1979. Comparative evaluation of BVDU ((E)-5-(2-bromovinyl)-2'-deoxyuridine) and IDU (5-iodo-2'-deoxyuridine) in the treatment of experimental herpes simplex keratitis in rabbits. Bull. Soc. belge Ophtal. 186, 109-118.

12. Maudgal PC, De Clercq E, Descamps J, Missotten L, De Somer P, Busson R, Vanderhaeghe H, Verhelst G, Walker RT, Jones AS. 1980. (E)-5-(2-Bromovinyl)-2'-deoxyuridine in the treatment of experimental herpes simplex keratitis. Antimicrob. Agents Chemother. 17, 8-12.

13. Maudgal PC, De Clercq E, Descamps J, Missotten L, Wijnhoven J. 1982. Experimental stromal herpes simplex keratitis. Influence of treatment with topical bromovinyldeoxyuridine and trifluridine. Arch. Ophthalmol. 100, 653-656.

14. Maudgal PC, Uyttebroeck W, De Clercq E, Missotten L. 1982. Oral and topical treatment of experimental herpes simplex iritis with bromovinyldeoxyuridine. Arch. Ophthalmol. 100, 1337-1340.

15. Boisjoly HM, Park N-H, Pavan-Langston D, De Clercq E. 1983. Herpes simplex acyclovir-resistant mutant in experimental keratouveitis. Arch. Ophthalmol. 101, 1782-1786.

16. Maudgal PC, Missotten L, De Clercq E, Descamps J, De Meuter E. 1981. Efficacy of (E)-5-(2-bromovinyl)-2'-deoxyuridine in the topical treatment of herpes simplex keratitis. Albrecht von Graefes Arch. Klin. Ophthalmol. 216, 261-268.

17. Maudgal PC, De Clercq E, Missotten L. 1984. Efficacy of bromovinyldeoxyuridine in the treatment of herpes simplex virus and varicella-zoster virus eye infections. Antiviral Res. 4, 281-291.

18. Descamps J, De Clercq E. 1981. Specific phosphorylation of E-5-(2-iodovinyl)-2'-deoxyuridine by herpes simplex virus-infected cells. J. Biol. Chem. 256, 5973-5976.

19. Mancini WR, De Clercq E, Prusoff WH. 1983. The relationship between incorporation of E-5-(2-bromovinyl)-2'-deoxyuridine into herpes simplex virus type 1 DNA with virus infectivity and DNA integrity. J. Biol. Chem. 258, 792-795.

20. De Clercq E, Heremans H, Descamps J, Verhelst G, De Ley M, Billiau A. 1981. Effects of E-5-(2-bromovinyl)-2'-deoxyuridine and other selective anti-herpes compounds on the induction of retrovirus particles in mouse BALB/3T3 cells. Mol. Pharmacol. 19, 122-129.

21. Maudgal PC, Verbruggen AM, De Clercq E, Busson R, Bernaerts R, De Roo M, Ameye C, Missotten L. 1985. Ocular penetration of ([125I])IVDU, a radiolabeled analogue of bromovinyldeoxyuridine. Invest. Ophthalmol. Vis. Sci., in press.

22. Desgranges C, Razaka G, Rabaud M, Bricaud H, Balzarini J, De Clercq E. 1983. Phosphorolysis of (E)-5-(2-bromovinyl)-2'-deoxyuridine (BVDU) and other 5-substituted-2'-deoxyuridines by purified human thymidine phosphorylase and intact blood platelets. Biochem. Pharmacol. 32, 3583-3590.

DISCUSSION :

V. Victoria-Troncoso (Ghent) : The methods like radiochromato-
graphy will be replaced in future by analytical electron microscopy. With this method one will be able to follow some ions.
Could you tell me how the molecule, that you have used, splits
once it enters into the epithelium. It is a technical question
for me.

A.M. Verbruggen (Leuven) : We know that there is deiodination
as for all iodinated molecules in which iodine is bound to a
double bond. So there is a gradual release of iodine in the
form of iodide. Secondly, we have also observed a gradual
release of IVU as the molecule is split.

E. De Clercq (Leuven) : When you said "split", do you mean at
the level of the N-glycosidic linkage between the sugar and
the pyrimidine base ?

V. Victoria-Troncoso (Ghent) : Yes.

E. De Clercq (Leuven) : This cleavage is catalyzed by pyrimidine
nucleoside phosphorylases. As a matter of fact the expert on
phosphorolysis, Dr. C. Desgranges, is just sitting next to you.
Claude, could you perhaps comment on this matter ?

V. Victoria-Troncoso (Ghent) : That's in order to follow, you know.

E. De Clercq (Leuven) : Well, let us say that the levels of that
enzyme vary widely from one tissue to another, especially the
liver is very rich in this enzyme. In cell cultures we only
have small amounts of pyrimidine nucleoside phosphorylases.
I wonder how much phosphorylase activity is present in the
corneal epithelium cells ! It is an interesting question that
should be resolved.

USE OF ARA-A IN HERPETIC EYE DISEASES : A REVIEW

C. AMEYE

Ophthalmology Clinic, U.Z. St.-Rafaël, Kapucijenvoer 7

B-3000 Leuven, Belgium.

Ara-A or vidarabine is a non-halogenated purine analogue with a poor water solubility. It was originally synthesized as a potential anticancer drug[1], but its greatest clinical value is as an antiviral agent.

1. Activity in vitro

In vitro, ara-A demonstrates a broad-spectrum activity against DNA-viruses and generally little or no activity against non-oncogenic RNA viruses[2]. As shown in table 1[3-13], ara-A inhibits the replication of herpes simplex virus (HSV) types 1 and 2, varicella zoster virus (VZV), cytomegalovirus (CMV) and vaccinia virus (VV). Ara-A was also effective against HSV-strains with biochemical resistance to idoxuridine (IDU)[14]. Ara-A is inactive against adenoviruses.

When tested against HSV (HF strain) in human (HEp-2)cell culture, ara-A produced a 75 to 90% reduction in viral plaques at concentrations of 10 g/ml (an activity comparable to that of IDU and ara-C)[8]. Against VZV in human embryonic lung (WI-38) cell culture[2], ara-A provoked 50 to 100% inhibition of cytopathogenic effects at concentrations ranging from 5 to 53 g/ml[2]. Both in HEp-2 and WI-38 cell culture, the cytotoxic concentration of ara-A has approximately 170 g/ml.

A comparative study on the susceptibilities of HSV types 1 and 2, VZV and CMV to ara-A, ara-C and IDU in WI-38 cells indicated that on a weight basis, ara-C is more active than ara-A and IDU[15].

Ara-A inhibits the viral DNA-synthesis with a limited selectivity[16,17]. The exact mechanism of action is not clear. Different hypotheses for the antiviral action of ara-A and/or its metabolites are shown in table II[18]. According to De Clercq et al[19], the selectivity index of ara-A is 5, when measured as the ratio of

Maudgal, P.C. and Missotten, L., (eds.) Herpetic Eye Diseases.
© *1985, Dr W. Junk Publishers, Dordrecht/Boston/Lancaster. ISBN 978-94-010-8935-7*

264

Table 1 : Activity of ara-A against viruses in cell culture.

Virus	Cell culture	Activity*
DNA-viruses		
Herpes viruses		
HSV_1-HSV_2	human (HeLa; WI-38)	$+$[3,4]
VZV	human (HEL; WI-38)	$+$[5]
CMV	human (WI-38)	$+$[6]
Poxviruses		
VV	human (HeLa); avian (primary chick embryo)	$+$[3,7]
Adenoviruses		
Adeno 3	human (Hep-2; KB)	$+$[5,8]; $-$[9,10,11]
RNA-viruses		
Oncornaviruses		
Rous sarcoma	avian (primary chick embryo)	$+$[5,8]
Rhabdoviruses		
Rabies	rodent (BHK-21)	$+$[12]
Vesicular stomatitis	bovine (MDBK)	$+$[13]

*Antiviral activity in cell culture measured with one or more in vitro test procedures (plaque reduction, inhibition of cytopathogenicity, reduction of titratable virus or hemagglutimation).

Table II : POSSIBLE MECHANISMS OF ANTIVIRAL ACTION OF ARA-A.

1. Inhibition of DNA polymerase
2. Incorporation into DNA
3. Inhibition of m RNA polyadenylation
4. Inhibition of ribonucleotide reductase
5. Inhibition of S-adenosylhomocysteine hydrolase

antimetabolic activity to its antiviral activity. This is comparable to the selectivity of IDU, and exeeds the selectivity of ara-C and F_3T.

2. Animal studies.

In a large number of animal studies, ara-A demonstrated the same broad spectrum of anti-DNA virus activity as in vitro. It was proven to be active against HSV and VV in ophthalmic, cutaneous, intraperitoneal and central nervous system infections[20].

2.1. In several animal studies, ara-A was compared to IDU for the treatment of superficial HSV-keratitis. When the antiviral agents were applied topically as a 0,5% to 20% suspension or as a 0,3% to 20% ointment, ara-A was equally or more effective than IDU in the treatment of the corneal herpes disease inrabbits[14], [21-24] and hamsters[25]. Topical ara-A application (3,3% ointment) was also effective in the treatment of experimental herpetic keratitis in rabbits produced by IDU-resistant strains[14]. Furthermore ara-A was effective in the treatment of superficial herpetic keratitis in rabbits when administered subcutaneously (250mg/kg/day[21]; 90-750mg/kg/day[20]). In hamster HSV keratitis, oral administration of ara-A, even in high doses (up to 500mg/kg/day), did not decrease the mortality rate, although it significantly increased the life span of the ara-A treated hamsters as compared to non treated animals[20].

Topical ara-A (5% suspension) was also found to be superior to IDU (0,1% in distilled water) in the treatment of vaccinial keratitis in rabbits[26].

2.2. In monkeys and rabbits, the subconjunctival injection of ara-A (as a 5% suspension, daily or every 2 or 4 days) was successful in the treatment of experimental herpetic keratouveitis, although this caused irritation and conjunctival granuloma formation[21]. Topical ara-A was moderately[27] or not[28] active in the treatment of HSV keratouveitis in rabbits.

2.3. Treatment of intracerebral HSV and VV infections in rodents by the intraperitoneal (HSV infections : 250-1000 mg/kg/day[29-31]; VV infections : 30-500 mg/kg/day[32,33]), oral (HSV infections : 2000 mg/kg/day[30]; VV infections : 1000 mg/kg/day[33]), subcutaneous

(HSV infections : 1000^{31}, $2000^{30,31,34}$ or $3000^{30,34,35}$ mg/kg in 1 day) and percutaneous (VV infections : 250-1000 mg/kg/day[38]) administration of ara-A caused a statistically significant increase in both the number of survivors and the mean survival time for the treated animals that succumbed. In mice ara-A was also active against intracerebral HSV infections when administered intra-venously[20], and against intracerebral HSV and VV infections after intracerebral administration[36]. In the latter experiment its activity was equal or superior to that of F_3T, and markedly superior to that of ara-C, where as IDU was totally inactive in this assay[36].

2.4. An important observation in these animal studies was that ara-A in therapeutic doses did not demonstrate hematological or myelosuppressive toxicity. Also it did not suppress the immune system of the host; to the contrary, ara-A might stimulate the immunity development[25,30,32-34].

Extensive toxicity studies were conducted in animals[37]. Topical administration of ara-A (as 3,3% or 10% ointment, or as 20% sus-pension) to the eyes or to the entire mid-portion of the body skin of rabbits for 7 to 28 days, and the intravenous administration of 15mg/kg/day for 28 days in rhesus monkeys were well tolerated without significant clinical, histopathological or laboratory signs of toxicity.

When 170 to 3000mg ara-A/kg/day was given orally to mice for 28 days, the highest dose provoked a marked weight loss; this effect tapered off to no loss of body weight at the lowest dose. The prolonged oral administration of the high doses of ara-A also caused variable livermalfunction, hepatomegalocytosis gonadal atrophy and a discrete tendency toward neutrocytosis and lympho-penia. The clinical and laboratory abnormalities did not reverse during 2 weeks of drug-free diet. The gonads recovered completely after 6 weeks and the hepatomegalocytosis (observed only in rats and mice) normalized after 1 year. The oral LD_{50} (50% lethal dose) in mice and rats was above 5020mg/kg.

The intramuscular injection of ara-A caused local toxicity : local swelling and tenderness with inflammation and necrosis, followed by granulomatous changes. The extent and duration of damage are related directly to the dose of the suspension injected. The systemic toxicity of a daily intramuscular administration (for 28 days) of a 20% suspension of ara-A was studied in rats, dogs and rhesus monkeys : dogs tolerated doses up to 50mg/kg/day (higher doses were not used) and rats showed a reversible suppression of weight gain at doses above 150mg/kg/day; the rhesus monkeys were the most sensitive animals with neurotoxic manifestations (visual disturbances, tremor, weakness, incoordination, somnolence, convulsions after stimuli) appearing at doses above 25mg/kg/day.   Otherwise the intramuscular administration caused no biochemical, hematological or histopathological abnormalities in animals.

The acute LD_{50} in mice on intraperitoneal injection was about 4700mg/kg.

Ara-A was found to be teratogenic in rats and rabbits, but apparently not in rhesus monkeys[38].   The rabbits were most sensitive : a daily intramuscular injection of 5mg ara-A/kg/day during the period of organogenesis provoked teratogenic effects. These were also observed after topical administration, during the period of organogenesis, of a 10% ara-A ointment covering an area in excess of 5% of the total body surface. Daily instillations of 10% ara-A gels into the vaginas of pregnant rats during late pregnancy had no effect on the offspring.

Under chronic ara-A treatment (30 or 50 mg/kg/day intramusculary for 5 months) an increased incidence of tumors in the kidney and liver was seen in rodents[37].

3.   Clinical studies :

3.1.   A large number of double blind studies in patients were conducted to compare the therapeutic efficacy of ara-A and IDU in the treatment of superficial HSV keratitis.   From this multitude of studies[39-48], following conclusions can be drawn :

1. Ara-A and IDU (mostly administered as a 3% ointment and a 0,5% ointment respectively, 5 times a day) have a comparable antiviral activity in the treatment of epithelial HSV keratitis.   The effect of both drugs is approximately the same in improvement of symptoms and in percentage and duration of corneal reepithelialisation.   In these studies 60 to 95% of the herpetic lesions healed

in 2 to 4 weeks of treatment, and the mean time for corneal reepithelialisation, mostly between 5 and 9 days, ranged from 3 to 12,5 days, depending on the patient group submitted to investigation (Different factors influenced the healing rates : the preceding history and therapy,the mean size of the lesions at start of therapy and the type of lesions e.g., the geographic and dendritogeographic lesions showing a lower percentage and rate of healing in comparison to the dendritic ulcers).

2. With Ara-A treatment significantly more patients had improved distant visual acuity (50%) than with IDU treatment (30 to 43,5 %)[45,46]. This could be explained by a significantly better quality of regenerating epithelium under ara-A treatment[49,50]

3. The toxic reactions to ara-A were similar to those to IDU, but generally they were less frequent.

In a series of open clinical studies[39,40,42,46,51-57], patients suffering from superficial herpetic keratitis, who were clinically resistant to IDU or had shown toxicity or allergy to IDU, were treated by Ara-A. Fifty to 90 % of the patients showed complete corneal reepithelialisation within 2 to 4 weeks of treatment (average reepithelialisation period varied from 6,5 to 12 days). In one of these studies[46], where globally 80 % of the IDU resistant or intolerant patients were treated successfully with ara-A, 95 % of the dendritic lesions and 60 % of the geographic ulcers reepithelialized within 4 weeks.

In several double blind studies[42,58-61] the healing rate of epithelial keratitis under ara-A and F_3T treatment was comparable, but a trend emerged suggesting that F_3T may be more effective than ara-A in the treatment of the amoeboid ulcers. Also with F_3T, generally less failures of therapy occurred, the difference being increased when steroid treatment was given simultaneously. In cases of F_3T allergy, treatment with ara-A was succesful[42,45]. In comparison to newer antiviral agents, ara-A was mostly less active and less specific.

3.2 Ara-A was also tested in the treatment of herpetic stromal disease and keratouveitis in patients. Topical ara-A was reported to have some beneficial effect in keratouveitis, but only when the corneal epithelium was unhealthy or disrupted.[62] This beneficial effect of the drug may be limited to its effect on the epithelial lesions : when these heal, the rest of the inflammation improves to a certain extent[63].

Investigations on the corneal and intraocular penetration of ara-A[62,64-67] via topical and subconjunctival routes in rabbits and human or during in vitro corneal perfusion revealed that ara-A penetrates the intact epithelium very poorly (this penetration improving when the epithelium is damaged or removed), and that ara-A is deaminated in the cornea to ara-Hx (ara-hypoxanthine), a 10 times more watersoluble metabolite that better penetrates the anterior chamber, but unfortunately has much less antiviral activity[24,68]. Therefore, after topical or subconjunctival administration of ara-A in rabbits, significant levels of ara-Hx and hardly or no detectable levels of ara-A were found in the aqueous humor[62]. After topical administration of clinical doses of ara-A to humans with normal corneas, only ara-Hx was found in the aqueous in trace amounts (0,04-0,28 g/ml)[64]. These studies show that because of its inadequate corneal penetration topically administered ara-A is not useful for the treatment of deeper herpetic ocular infections.

Subcutaneous (5 mg/kg/day for 10 days)[69] and intravenous (20 mg/kg/day for 7 days)[70] administration of ara-A was reported to cause improvement in herpetic stromal disease and keratouveitis in humans.

3.3 Significant reduction of mortality and morbidity was reported with intravenous administration of ara-A in the treatment of herpetic encephalitis (15 mg/kg/day for 10 days)[71-72], neonatal herpetic infections (15 mg/kg/day for 10 days)[73] and VZV infections in immunosuppressed patients (10 mg/kg/day for 5 days)[74,75]. In these studies the importance of early drug administration in the course of the disease was emphasized.

3.4 In many of the above mentioned studies, adverse reactions on ara-A were reported. By topical treatment, the local toxicity (burning, irritation, pain, lacrimation, injection, etc.) was usually mild and reversible. Many of the complaints could be considered concurrent conditions associated with the underlying disease, or a manifestation of drug failure to prevent stromal disease. Among the toxicity that can be attributed to ara-A a punctate epitheliopathy of the cornea and conjunctiva[42,44,76] can be metioned. It appears in 3 to 10% of cases, generally 1 to 7 weeks after the onset of treatment, and clears (in 2-3 weeks) after withdrawal of the drug. Reversible punctal occlusion[41] was also reported. After topical administration of therapeutical doses of ara-A, no adverse systemic (hematologic, renal or hepatic) side effects were detected[39,45].

Intramuscular administration has caused pain at the injection site[77]. In a study where different doses of ara-A (10-15-20-30 mg/kg/day, 7 days) were administered intravenously to patients treated for complicated infection with VZV or HSV, 6 types of reversible adverse reactions to ara-A were observed[78] : 1 transient and moderate anorexia, nausea and/or vomiting; 2. weight loss, 3. weakness, usually with impaired ambulation; 4. megaloblastosis in the erythroid series in the bone marrow (with normal peripheral bloodcell counts); 5. generalized tremors (associated in 1 case with abnormal electroencephalogram activity) and 6. thrombophlebitis at the intravenous injection site. These toxic effects predominated in patients given 20 mg of ara-A/kg/day.

Acute neurologic (ataxia, tremor, myoclonus) and gastrointestinal toxicity has been observed with ara-A in patients with impaired renal function or chronic hepatitis[79,80].

Clinical doses of intravenous ara-A have been reported to cause erhythematous skin rash[72,75], diarrhea[72,75,81], myalgia[70], confusion and hallucinations[75,81]. The transient leukopenia, thrombocytopenia and decreased hemoglobin levels that were reported[70,72,75,82,83] can possibly be influenced by the necessitated large amounts of intravenous fluid administration. Generally, with clinically used doses, no significant adverse effects of vidarabine were demonstrated on the renal functions, the liver or the bone marrow, even in previously compromised patients[69,73,75,81]. However, when the dose of ara-A was increased to 30 mg/kg/per day, significant bone marrow depression might result[84]. Systemic administration of ara-A at antiviral concentrations, does not reduce the cellmediated immune response[85] or the antibody response of the host[86].

Conclusions

Ara-A has two serious drawbacks that limit its usefulness : first
its poor solubility in aqueous medium (0,5 mg/ml H_2O) which ne-
cessitates a large fluid load of several liters for intravenous administration, and second, its rapid deamination to the much less
active ara-hypoxanthine.

The first problem may be circumvented by using ara-AMP (ara-A-
5'-monophosphate)[87-90] which is markedly more soluble than ara-A,
and is readily converted to the parent compound in biological
fluids. The clinical potential of ara-AMP is under investigation.
The second problem could be overcome by cyclaradine[91], the carbo-
cyclic analogue of ara-A, which is as active as ara-A in vitro,
but is resistant to deamination by the adenosine deaminase.

The clinical usefulness of ara-A may be summarized
as follows :

1. topical treatment of superficial herpetic keratitis : as 3% ointment, ara-A is a useful alternative drug for the treatment of
   epithelial herpetic infections. Its efficacy as a topical antiviral agent is comparable to that of the other available drugs,
   and it can be successfully used in many patients who develop
   toxicitiy, allergy or resistance to other antiviral compounds.

2. Since the systemic toxicity of ara-A is relatively low when used
   at the therapeutic doses, it can be administered intravenously
   in the treatment of life-threatening DNA viral disease :
   -HSV encephalitis (15 mg/kg/day for 10 days)
   -neonatal herpetic infections (15 mg/kg/day for 10 days)
   -VZV infection in immunodeficient patients (10 mg/kg/day for
    5 days)

REFRENCES

1. LEE, W.W., BENITEZ, A., GOODMAN, L. and BAKER, B.R.
   J.Am.Chem.Soc. 82 : 2648-2649, 1960.

2. SHANNON, W.M. In Pavan-Langston D, Buchanan R.A. and
   Alford C.A. Jr (eds.) : Adenine Arabinoside : An Antiviral
   Agent. Raven Press, New York, 1975, pp. 1-43.

3. PRIVAT DE GARILHE, M. and RUDDER J.DE.C.R. Acad. Sci. 259
   2725-2728, 1964.

4. PERSON, D.A., SHERIDAN, P.J. and HERRMANN, E.C.Jr. Infect.
   Immun. 2 : 815-820, 1970.

5. SCHABEL, F.M. Jr. Chemotherapy 13 : 321-338, 1968.

6. SIDWELL, R.W., ARNETT, G. and DIXON, G.J. Intensci. Conf.
   Antimicrob. AgentsChemother., 7 : 64, 1967.

7. FREEMAN, G., KUEHN, A. and SULTANIAN, I.Ann. N.Y. Acad.
   Sci. 130 : 330-342, 1965.

8. MILLER, F.A., DIXON, G.J., EHRLICH, J., SLOAN B.J. and
McLEAN, I.W.Jr.Antimicrob. Agents Chemother. 8 : 136- 147, 1968.

9. SMITH, C.W., SIDWELL, R.W., ROBINS, R.K. and TOLMAN, R.L.J.
   Med. Chem. 15 : 883-887, 1972.

10.SIDWELL, R.W., ALLEN, L.B., HUFFMAN, J.H., KHWAJA, T.A.,
   TOLMAN, R.L. and ROBINS R.K.Chemotherapy, 19 : 325-340, 1973.

11.MIYAI, K., ALLEN, L.B., HUFFMAN, J.H., SIDWELL, R.W. and
   TOLMAN, R.L.J.Med. Chem., 17 : 242-244, 1974.

12.JANIS, B. and HARMON, M.W.Intersci. Conf. Antimicrob. Agents
   Chemether. 14 : Abstr. 242, 1974.

13.GRANT, J.A. and SABINA, L.R.Antimicrob. Agents Chemother. 2
   201-205, 1972.

14.NESBURN, A.B., ROBINSON, C., DICKINSON, R.Invest. Opthalmol.
   13(4) : 302-304, 1974.

15. FIALA M., CHOW A.W., MIYASAKI K. and GUZE L.B. J. Infect.
   Dis. 129 : 82-85, 1974.

16. SCHWARTZ P.M., SHIPMAN C. Jr. and DRACH J.C.Intersci. Conf.
   Antimicrob. Agents Chemother., 14 : 33, 1974.

17. SCHWARTZ P.M., SANDBERG J.N., SHIPMAN C. Jr. and DRACH
   J.C.Intersci. Conf. Antimicrob. Agents Chemother., 15 : 357,
   1975.

18. DRACH J.C. In De Clercq E. and Walker R.T. (ed.) : Targets
    for the Designof Antiviral Agents. Plenum Pren,
    New York, 1984, pp 234-240.

19. DE CLERCQ E., DESCAMPS J., BARR P.J. et al. In Skoda J. and
    Langen P. (ed.) : Antimetabolitesin Biochemistry,
    Biology and Medicine. Pergamon Press, Oxford and New York,
1979,
    pp.275-285.

20. SLOAN B.J.In Pavan-Langston D., Buchanan R.A. and Alford
    C.A. Jr. (ed.) : Adenine arabinoside : an antiviral agent.
    Raven Press, New York, 1975, pp 45-94.

21. KAUFMAN H.E., ELLISON E.D. and TOWNSEND W.M. : Arch.
    Ophthalmol. 84 : 783-787, 1970.

22. OKUMOTO M., HYNDIUK R.A., VALENTON M., SMOLIN G. and
    BOHIGIAN G. : Invest. Ophthalmol. 9 :980, 1970.

23. NESBURN A.B., FRIEDMAN R.D., ZINITI P. and CRAVY T. :
    Invest. Ophthalmol. 9 980, 1970.

24. PAVAN-LANGSTON D., LANGSTON R.H.S. and GEARY P.A. : Arch.
    Ophthalmol. 92 : 417-421, 1974.

25. SIDWELL R.W., DIXON G.J., SCHABEL F.M.Jr. and KAUMP D.H.
    Antimicrob. Agents Chemother. 8 : 148-154, 1968.

26. HYNDIUK, R.A., OKUMOTO, M., DAMIANO, R.A., VALENTON, M.
    and SMOLIN, G. : Arch. Ophthalmol. 94 : 1363-1364, 1976.

27. PAVAN-LANGSTON D., LASS J. and CAMPBELL R. : Arch. Ophthal-
    mol. 97 : 1132-1135, 1979.

28. KAUFMAN H.E. : Int. Ophthal. Clin. 15 : 163-169, 1975.

29. SCHARDEIN J.L. and SIDWELL R.W. : Antimicrob. Agents Chemo-
    ther. 8 : 155-160, 1968.

30. SLOAN B.J., MILLER F.A., EHRLICH J., Mc.LEAN I.W. and
    MACHAMER H.E. : Antimicrob. Agents Chemother. 8 161-171, 1968.

31. SCHMIDT-RUPPIN R.H. : Chemotherapy 16 : 130-143, 1971.

32. SIDWELL R.W., DIXON G.J., SELLERS S.M. and SCHABEL F.M.Jr.:
    Appl. Microbiol.16 : 370-392, 1968.

33. DIXON G.J., SIDWELL R.W., MILLER F.A. and SLOAN B.J. : Anti-
    microb. Agents Chemother. 8 : 172-179, 1968.

34. SLOAN B.J., MILLER F.A. and MCLEAN I.W.Jr. : Antimicrob.
    Agents Chemother. 10 : 74-80, 1970.

35. MILLER F.A., SLOAN B.J. and SILVERMAN C.A. : Antimicrob. Agents Chemother. 9 : 192–195, 1969.

36. ALLEN L.B. and SIDWELL R.W. : Antimicrob. Agents Chemother. 2 : 229–233, 1972.

37. KURTZ S.M. : In Pavan–Langston D., Buchanan R.A. and Alford C.A. Jr. : Adenine arabinoside : An Antiviral Agent. Raven Press, New York, 1975, pp. 145–157.

38. SCHARDEIN J.L., HENTZ D.L., PETRERE J.A., FITZGERALD I.E. and KURTZ S.M. : Teratology, 15 : 231–242, 1977.

39. PAVAN–LANGSTON D. and DOHLMAN C.H. : Am. J. Ophthalmol. 74,1 : 81–88, 1972.

40. DRESNER A.J. and SEAMANS M.L. : In Pavan–Langston D., Buchanan R.A. and Alford C.A. Jr (ed.). : Adenine Arabinoside : An Antiviral Agent. Raven Press, New York, 1975, pp. 381–392.

41. HYNDIUK R.A., SCHULTZ R.O. and HULL D.S. : In Pavan Langston D., Buchanan R.A. and Alford C.A.Jr.(eds.) : Adenine Arabinoside : An antiviral Agent. Raven Press, New York, 1975 pp. 331–335.

42. JONES B.R., McGILL J.L., McKINNON J.R., HOLT–WILSON A.D. and WILLIAMS H.P. : In Pavan–Langston D., Buchanan R.A. and Aford C.A. Jr.(eds.) : Adenine Arabinoside : An Antiviral Agent. Raven Press, New York, 1975 pp 411–416.

43. LAIBSON P.R., HYNDIUK R., KRACHMER J.H. and SCHULTZ R.O.: Invest. Ophthalmol. 14 (10) : 762–763, 1975.

44. LAIBSON P.R. and KRACHMER J.H. : In Pavan–Langston D., Buchanan R.A. and Alford C.A. Jr. (ed.) : Adenine Arabinoside : An Antiviral Agent. Raven Press, New York, 1975, pp 323–330.

45. PAVAN–LANGSTON D. : Am. J. Ophthalmol. 80 : 495–502, 1975.

46. PAVAN–LANGSTON D. and BUCHANAN R.A. : Tr. Am. Acad. Opht. Otol. 81 : OP813–OP825, 1976.

47. MARKHAM R.H.C., CARTER C., SCOBIE M.A., METCALF C. and EASTY D.L. : Trans. Ophthalmol. Soc. U.K. 97 : 333–340, 1977.

48. CHIN G.N. : Ann. Ophthalmol. : 10,9 : 1171–1174, 1978.

49. LANGSTON R.H.S., PAVAN–LANGSTON D. and DOHLMAN C.H. : Arch. Ophthalmol. 92 : 509–513, 1974.

50. DESBORDES J.M., THOMPSON P., GIRAUD J., DENIS J. and POULIQUEN Y. : J. Fr. Ophthalmol. 4, 12 : 797-804, 1981.

51. CHIN G.N., HYNDIUK R.A. and SCHULTZ R.O. : Presented at the Association for Research in Vision and Ophthalmology, spring meeting, Sarasota, Florida, May 5, 1973.

52. HYNDIUK R.A., HULL D.S., SCHULTZ R.O., CHIN G.N., LAIBSON P.R. and KRACHMER J.H. : Am. J. Ophthalmol. 79(4) : 655-658, 1975

53. JONES D.B. : In Pavan-Langston D., Buchanan R.A. and Alford C.A. Jr. (eds.) : Adenine Arabinoside : An Antiviral Agent. Raven Press, New York, 1975 pp. 371-379.

54. O'DAY D.M., POIRIER R.H., JONES D.B. and ELLIOTT J.H. : Am. J. Ophthalmol. 81(5) : 642-649, 1976.

55. COLIN J., BAIKOFF G., CHASTEL C. and RENARD G. : J. Fr. Ophtalmol. 2,3 : 205-208, 1979.

56. COLIN J., FILY J., RENARD G. and CHASTEL C. : Bull. Soc. Ophtalmol. Fr., 1981.

57. McGILL J.I., WILLIAMS H.P., McKINNON J.R., HOLT-WILSON A.D. and JONES B.R. : Trans. Ophthal. Soc. U.K. 94 : 542-552, 1974.

58. McKINNON J.R., McGILL J.I. and JONES B.R. : In Pavan-Langston D., Buchanan R.A. and Alford C.A.Jr.(eds.) : Adenine Arabinoside : An Antiviral Agent. Raven Press, New York, 1975 pp. 401-410.

59. COSTER D.J., McKINNON J.R., McGILL J.I., JONES B.R. and FRAUNFELDER F.T. : J. Infect. Dis. 133 (suppl) : 173-177, 1976.

60. COSTER D.J., JONES B.R. and McGILL J.I. :Br.J. Ophthalmol. 63, 418-421, 1979.

61. VAN BIJSTERVELD O.P. and POST H. : Br. J. Ophthalmol. 64, 33-36, 1980.

62. PAVAN-LANGSTON D., DOHLMAN C.H., GEARY P. and SULZEWSKI D. : In Pavan-Langston D., Buchanan R.A. and Alford C.A. Jr. (eds.) : Adenine Arabinoside : An Antiviral Agent. Raven Press, New York, 1975, pp.293-306.

63. KAUFMAN H.E. : J. Infec. Dis. 133 (suppl.) A 96-A 100, 1976.

64. POIRIER R.H., KINKEL A.W., ELLISON A.C. and LEWIS R. :
    In Pavan-Langston D., Buchanan R.A. and Alford C.A. Jr
    (eds.) : Adenine Arabinoside : An Antiviral Agent. Raven
    Press, New York, 1975, pp. 307-312.

65. O'BRIEN W.J. and EDELHAUSER H.F. : Invest. Ophthalmol.
    Visual Sci. : 16, 12 : 1093-1103, 1977.

66. PAVAN-LANGSTON D., NORTH D., GEARY P.A. et al. : Arch.
    Ophtalmol. 94 : 1585-1588, 1976.

67. POIRIER R.H., KINGHAM D., DE MIRANDA P. and ANNEL M.
    Arch. Ophtalmol. 100 : 1964-1967, 1982.

68. CONNOR J.D., SWEETMAN L., CAREY S., STUCKEY M.A. and
    BUCHANAN R. : In Pavan-Langston D., Buchanan R.A. and
    Alford C.A. Jr (eds.) : Adenine Arabinoside : An Antiviral
    Agent. Raven Press, New York, 1975, pp. 177-196.

69. BRIGHTBILL F.S. and KAUFMAN H.E. : Ann. Ophtalmol. 6 :
    25-32, 1974.

70. ABEL R. Jr., KAUFMAN H.E. and SUGAR J. : Am.J. Ophalmol.
    79(4) 659-664, 1975.

71. WHITLEY R.J., SOONG S.J., DOLIN R. et al. : N. Eng. J. med.
    297,6 : 289-294, 1977.

72. WHITLEY R.J., SOONG S.J., HIRSCH M.S. et al. : N. Eng. J.
    Med. 304,6 : 313-318, 1981.

73. WHITLEY R.J., NAHMIAS A.J., SOONG S.J.et al. : Pediatrics 66,4
    : 495-501, 1980.

74. LUBY J.P., JOHNSON M.T., BUCHANAN R. et al. : In Pavan-
    Langston D., Buchanan R.A. and Alford C.A. Jr (eds.) :
    Adenine Arabinoside : An Antiviral Agent. Raven Press, New
    York, 1975, pp. 237-245.

75. WHITLEY R.J., CH'IEN L.T., DOLIN R. et al. : N. Eng. J.
    Med. 294,22 : 1193-1199, 1976.

76. FALCON M.G., JONES B.R., WILLIAMS H.P., WILHELMUS K. and
    COSTER D.J. : In Sundmacher R. (ed.) : Herpetische
    Augenerkrankungen. J.F. Bergmann Verlag, München, 1981, pp
    263-268.

77. CH'IEN L.T., GLAZKO A.J., BUCHANAN R.A., ALFORD C.A. Jr.
    Intersci. Conf. Antimicrob. Agents Chemother., 11, p. 47, 1971.

78. ROSS A.H., JULIA A. and BALAKRISHNAN C. : J. Infect. Dis.
    133 (Suppl.) : A 192–A198, 1976.

79. MARKER S.G., HOWARD R.J., GROTH K.E. et al. : Arch. Intern.
    Med. : 140 : 1441–1444, 1980.

80. SACHS S.L., SMITH J.L., POLLARD R.B. et al. : JAMA : 241,
    28, 1979.

81. KEEN R.E. : In Pavan-Langston D., Buchanan R.A. and Alford
    C.A. jr (eds) : Adenine Arabinoside : An Antiviral Agent.
    Raven Press, New York, 1975, pp. 265–273.

82. CH'IEN L.T., SCHABEL F.M. Jr. and ALFORD C.A. Jr. : In
    Carter W.A. (ed.) : Selective inhibitors of viral function.
    Cleveland, CRS Press, 1973, pp. 227–256.

83. LAUTER C.B., BAILEY E.J., WILSON F.M. and LERNER A.M. : J.
    Clin. Invest. 52 : 50a, 1973.

84. BODEY, G.P., GOTTLIEB, J., McCREDIE, K.B. et al. : In
    Pavan-Langston, D., Buchanan, R.A. and Alford, C.A. Jr.
    (eds) : Adenine Arabinoside : An Antiviral Agent. Raven
    Press, New York, 1975, pp. 281–285.

85. STEELE, R.W., CHAPA, I.A., VINCENT, M.M., HENSEN, S.A. and
    KEENEY, R.E. : Antimicrob. Agents Chemother. 7 : 203–207,
    1975.

86. ZAM, Z.S., CENTIFANTO, Y.M. and KAUFMAN, H.E. : Intersci.
    Conf. Antimicrob. Agents Chemother. 14 : 139, 1974.

87. SIDWELL, R.W., ALLEN, L.B., HUFFMAN, J.H., REVANKAR, G.R.,
    ROBINS, R.K. and TOLMAN, R.L. : Antimicrob. Agents
    Chemother. 8(4) : 463–467, 1975.

88. TROBE, J.D., CENTIFANTO, Y., ZAM, Z.S., VARNELL, E.D. and
    KAUFMAN, H.E. : Invest. Ophthalmol. 15(3) : 196–199, 1976.

89. KAUFMAN, H.E. and VARNELL, E.D. : Antimicrob. Agents
    Chemother. 10(6) : 885–888, 1976.

90. FALCON, M.G. and JONES, B.R. : J.Gen.Virol. 36 : 199–202,
    1977.

91. VINCE, R., DALUGE, S. : J. Med. Chem. 20 : 612–613, 1977.

TRIFLURIDINE INDUCED CORNEAL EPITHELIUM DYSPLASIA

P.C. MAUDGAL[1], B. VAN DAMME[2], and L. MISSOTTEN[1].

[1] Eye Research Laboratory of the Ophthalmology Clinic and
[2] Pathology Department, Katholieke Universiteit Leuven,
B-3000 Leuven, Belgium.

Trifluridine (5-trifluoromethyl-2'-deoxyuridine, TFT), as 1% eye-drops, is used for the topical treatment of herpes simplex virus keratitis. Hypersensitivity and toxic reactions to the drug, i.e., punctate epithelial keratopathy, filamentary keratitis, epithelial and stromal edema, lacrimal punctum stenosis, and conjunctival acute ischemic reaction have been reported.[1-3]. We have previous-ly described the development of corneal epithelium dysplasia caused by TFT in three patients[4]. In the meantime we have seen a similar complication in an additional patient.

SUBJECTS AND METHODS

Four elderly male patients, aged between 67 and 70 years, who consulted us for their herpes simplex virus keratitis have been using TFT 1% eyedrops from 1 to 10 months. The ocular disease had started either as a typical dendritic corneal ulcer or as kera-touveitis.

All patients had a gelatinous appearing, slightly raised corneal epithelium lesion. The involved epitheliuml had a ground-glass appearance and exhibited opaque cells, edema and elongated sur-face cells.

In one patient the origin of the lesion was actually observed at

Maudgal, P.C. and Missotten, L., (eds.) Herpetic Eye Diseases.
© *1985, Dr W. Junk Publishers, Dordrecht/Boston/Lancaster. ISBN 978-94-010-8935-7*

the superior limbus when he was referred to us for advice. We stopped TFT eyedrops and instead prescribed BVDU 0.1% ((E)-5-2-(bromovinyl)-2'-deoxyuridine, bromovinyldeoxyuridine) eyedrops. However, the referring ophthalmologist again reinstituted TFT treatment. This patient came back to us with the epithelial lesion covering the upper-third of the cornea. In two other patients the epithelial lesions were present in the upper half of cornea when we first saw them, and the fourth patient had the total corneal surface involvement. In three patients with upper corneal involvement, the epithelial lesions were sharply demarcated from the lower normal cornea. These lesions progressively extended downwards. The conjunctival blood vessels were markedly dilated in these eyes. No herpetic corneal lesions were observed in any of the patients.

We scraped the corneal epithelium for histopathological examination. In two patients a corneal replica was made before scraping[5]. The epithelium regenerated in about one week, but it was edematous and possessed some diffusely scattered opaque cells. Edema gradually subsided and opaque cells migrated to the center of the cornea before disappearing in 3 to 4 months.

HISTOPATHOLOGY

Corneal replicas revealed elongated surface cells, oriented with their long axis from the libmus to the lower border of the lesion. Punctate areas of cell degeneration and partly detached cells were present. The nuclei were generally small and perinuclear vacuoles and cytoplasmic granules were seen in some cells.

281

Histopathological examination of the scraped epithelium revealed changes suggestive of moderate to severe epithelium dysplasia, i.e., cellular atypism, loss of cell polarity, dyskeratosis, parkaratosis and a few mitotic figures. No histological changes suggestive of herpes simplex virus infection were seen.

COMMENT

Dysplastic eye lesions are cnaracterized by a disturbance in the normal maturation of surface epithelium, associated with cellular atypism and loss of cell polarity[6]. The histological changes detected in our patients indicate that these patients had developed dysplastic lesions. It is difficult to state whether these lesions were non-neoplastic or a true precarcinomatous condition[7,8]. Our patients were between 67 and 70 years of age. Intraepithelial epitheliomas (Bowens' disease) have been reported in patients around 60 years age[9]. In our patients there was no history of exposure to arsenicals or beryllium. All patients had used TFT eyedrops for the treatment of herpes simplex keratitis. We believe that dysplastic change in our patients was induced by TFT used at recommended dosage i.e. one drop of the drug instilled 6 times a day. This complication should be kept in mind when evaluating herpes simplex keratitis patients treated by TFT. For a detailed discussion of the TFT toxicity and epithelium dysplasia the reader is referred to our previous report on corneal epithelium dysplasia after trifluridine use[4].

REFERENCES

1. COSTER DJ, McKINNON JR, McGILL JI, JONES BR, FRAUNFELDER FT 1976. Clinical evaluation of adenine arabinoside and tri-fluorthymidine in the treatment of corneal ulcers caused by herpes simplex virus. J Infect Dis. 113 (Suppl. 1), A 173-A 177.

2. FALCON MG, JONES BR, WILLIAMS HP, COSTER DJ 1977. Management of herpetic eye disease. Trans Ophthalmol Soc UK 97,-345-349.

3. FALCON MG, JONES BR, WILLIAMS HP, WILHELMUS K, COSTER DJ 1981. Adverse reactions in the eye from topical therapy with idoxuridine, adenine arabinoside and trifluorthymidine. In : Sundmacher R (ed), Herpetic Eye Diseases, München, J.F. Bergman Verlag.

4. MAUDGAL PC, VAN DAMME B and MISSOTTEN L. 1983. Corneal epithelium dysplasia after trifluridine use. Graefes' Arch Clin Exp Ophthalmol, 220, 6-12.

5. MAUDGAL PC. 1976. The epithelial response in keratitis sicca and keratitis herpetica (an experimental and clinical study). Doctoral thesis, University of Leuven. Doc Ophthalmol 45,223-327, 1978.

6. CRAWFORD JB. 1981. Conjunctival tumors. In : Duane TD (ed) : Clinical Ophthalmology, vol. 4, Philadelphia, Harper and Row.

7. ZIMMERMAN LE. 1964. Squamous cell carcinoma and related lesions of the bulbar conjunctiva. In : Boniuk M (ed), Ocular and Adnexal Tumors. New and Controversial Aspects. St. Louis. C.V. Mosby Co.

8. ZIMMERMAN LE. 1969. The cancerous, precancerous and pseudo-cancerous lesions of the cornea and conjunctiva. In : Raycroft PV (ed), Corneoplastic Surgery, Oxford, Pergamon Press.

9. PIZZARELLO LD, JAKOBIEC FA. 1978. Bowen's disease of the conjunctiva : a misnomer. In Jakobiec FA (ed), Aesculapius Publishing Co. Ocular and Adnexal Tumors, Birmingham.

DISCUSSION :

E. De Clercq (Leuven) : Is it known that you can get dysplasia of the corneal epithelium ? I am asking this question as a non-ophthalmologist.

P.C. Maudgal (Leuven) : Yes, it is known. Elderly people who have been exposed to berylium, arsenic etc. during their career are prone to develop this condition. It has also been referred to as Bown's disease.

E. De Clercq (Leuven) : Was this observed after a long exposure to TFT ? Was it perhaps misused in the sense that it was administered for a longer time than it was necessary ?

P.C. Maudgal (Leuven) : Your question could be the starting point for a good discussion on the management of herpetic corneal diseases. One may ask that for how long stromal keratitis should be treated. The simple answer is that as long as the disease has not resolved completely. However, if the ophthalmologist fails to detect the dysplastic change and thinks that it is a post herpetic condition, and continues to administer the antiviral drug, then you may call it the misuse of the antiviral. That is precisely what happened in these patients.

H.J.M.Völker-Dieben (Leiden) : Do you remember that Dr. Witmer advised as prophylaxis after keratoplasty for three months to one year TFT eyedrops ? It might be of interest to enquire about his patients.

P.C. Maudgal (Leuven) : If I remember correctly, at Freiburg meeting he advised two or three drops of TFT per day.

H.J.M. Völker-Dieben (Leiden) : It was not reported in the article, the dosage varied from patient to patient.

P.C. Maudgal (Leuven) : I hope he has read my paper. As I pointed out earlier, one should not interpret this change as a postherpetic condition. Looking at Dr. Witmer's patients could give us information on the question whether less frequent administration of TFT for long periods would also induce corneal epithelium dysplasia.

M.G. Falcon (London) : Certainly I very much agree that trifluorothymidine is toxic. Do you think there is any chance that any
of those problems could be due to breakdown products of TFT,
since it is very unstable in the solution.

P.C. Maudgal (Leuven) : I think Professor De Clercq is more quali-
fied to answer this question.

E. De Clercq (Leuven) : What do you mean by the breakdown products of trifluridine ?

M.G. Falcon (London) : I am no chemist or pharmacologist, but
I believe that very unpleasant fluorine compounds are produced
by the spontaneous breakdown of TFT. Perhaps there is a
chemist who can provide more information.

E. De Clercq (Leuven) : I am not sure whether TFT gives rise
to the release of free fluorine atoms, but we should not forget
that TFT is a powerful inhibitor of thymidylate synthetase,
and, to some extent, it can also be incorporated into the host
cell DNA. Thymidylate synthetase is a crucial enzyme for the
synthesis of DNA and normal cell growth. Of all compounds
that are being used in the treatment of herpetic keratitis, TFT
is the only one that is such a potent inhibitor of this crucial
enzyme. This may be the reason, or one of the reasons, for
toxic side effects, which you see with TFT and not with the
other compounds because they are not particularly inhibitory
to thymidylate synthetase.

P. Wright (London) : In the Exernal Diseases Clinic of Moorfields
we have certainly seen epithelial dysplasia from all the antivirals. I don't think it is in particular due to TFT, by any
means. I am more impressed by the pattern of the epithelial
dysplasia you showed here, which is exactly like the one we
see with the organic mercurials, thiomersal preservative in particular. I have no explanation that why it should be in this
particular distribution with the organic mercurials. Just wonder what preservative is in your TFT drops !

P.C.Maudgal (Leuven) : It is benzalkonium chloride.

E. De Clercq (Leuven) : Have you observed epithelium dysplasia
only with TFT, or also with other antivirals ?

P.C.Maudgal (Leuven) : Only with TFT.

V. Victoria-Troncoso (Ghent) : The case you have presented is a purely iatrogenic problem, isn't it ? That is one part of the question. If it is, would you not expect superficial punctate keratitis or something like that ?

P.C.Maudgal (Leuven) : It is certainly iatrogenic, as you said. It is not a viral problem. Toxic punctate keratopathy due to TFT is very frequent, but there you don't have this distribution of the dysplastic lesion, and the lesion is not raised like here. It is important to distinguish between the two, as in the presence of punctate keratopathy you may continue to administer the antiviral, but in the presence of dysplastic change, one should stop the antiviral immediately. In our patients the lesions continued to enlarge, if we waited. We gave topical BVDU and corticosteroids to one patient in the hope that the dysplastic lesion will resolve, but it continued to progress. It does not appear that BVDU contributed to this enlargment of the dysplastic lesion, as in another patient a recurrence of dendritic keratitis was succesfully treated with topical BVDU eyedrops, without any complications. So, it seems that the epithelium dysplasia due to TFT is not easily reversible, where as the punctate keratopathy is reversible upon cessation of TFT treatment.

STEROID ADDICTION: A COMPLICATION OF USE AND ABUSE OF
STEROIDS IN HERPES SIMPLEX KERATITIS

I.S.JAIN, AMOD GUPTA AND M.R. DOGRA (DEPARTMENT OF
OPHTHALMOLOGY, POSTGRADUATE INSTITUTE OF MEDICAL EDUCATION
AND RESEARCH, CHANDIGARH, INDIA

1.INTRODUCTION

Herpes simplex virus (HSV) is said to be the most frequent
cause of corneal blindness in western countries.(Duke-Elder
S, 1965). In our country not much attention has been paid to
HSV keratitis due to widely prevalent malnutrition, trachoma
and other external ocular diseases. With the changing socio-
economic conditions, a change in the pattern of corneal
blindness is emerging in our part of the country. HSV keratitis now accounts for more than 50% of all corneal affections
(un-published data) and 0.57% of all ophthalmic out patients.
(Chakraborty, G.S. et al., 1979). Many of these patients are
first seen by general practitioners and exposed to topical
or systemic steroids. It is well established that unjudicio-
us use of steroids in HSV keratitis may lead to severe ocular
complications. (Thygeson,1977). In this study we have outli-
ned various indications and complications of use and abuse of
steroids in HSV keratitis.

2.MATERIAL AND METHODS

One hundred and ninety four patients of herpes simplex ocular
disease who attended the corneal clinic of the department of
Ophthalmology, PGIMER, Chandigarh during the period from
January 1977 to July 1982, were the subjects of this study.
The criteria for diagnosing HSV keratitis were mainly clinical history of keratitis in the past, number of recurrences
and history of any previous treatment. Visual acuity record-
ing, fluorescein staining of corneal lesions and biomicroscopic examination was done in each patient.

Maudgal, P.C. and Missotten, L., (eds.) Herpetic Eye Diseases.
© *1985, Dr W. Junk Publishers, Dordrecht/Boston/Lancaster. ISBN 978-94-010-8935-7*

288

3.OBSERVATIONS

There were 156 men and 38 women. Of these 123 (63.4%) patients were seen between the age of 21 and 40 years.One hundred and thirty patients were affected in one eye and 58 in both eyes. Thus a total of 252 eyes were available for the study. Various corneal lesions seen in these eyes are shown in Table 1. Nearly one third of the eyes had healed lesions of HSV keratitis.

Table 1. Corneal lesions in HSV keratitis

Corneal lesions	No. of eyes.
Dendritic	41
Geographic	29
Stromal Keratitis	45
Keratouveitis	25
Perforation with phthisis bulbi	4
Indolent ulcer	3
Healed kerato-uveitis	11
Corneal opacity	88
Adherent Leucoma	6
Total	252

3.1 Use and abuse of steroids

One hundred and fourteen of the 252 eyes had been exposed to steroids. Thirty-six of these had been treated elsewhere and steroids had been misused. In 23 of these 36 eyes there was a change in the ulcer pattern (Table 2.), non healing ulcer in 8 eyes and four eyes had perforation of globe. Seventeen eyes required diluted steroids in order to control keratitis in this group. In 78 eyes use of the topical steroids was indicated due to keratouveitis or stromal keratitis without epithelial involvement. Most frequent complication noted in this group was corneal thinning in 8 eyes (Table 3). Four eyes in the former and 16 eyes in the latter group became addicted to the use of topical steroids and developed recurrence whenever steroids were stopped.

Table 2. Abuse of steroidsin HSV keratitis (36 eyes).

Complications	No. of eyes
Change in ulcer pattern	23
Nonhealing ulcer	8
Perforation	4
Secondary infection	3
Hypopyon	1
Phthisis bulbi	1
Recurrence	16
Steroid addiction	4

Table 3. Use of steroids in HSV keratitis (78 eyes).

Indications of steroid therapy	No. of eyes
Keratouveitis	20
Stromal keratitis	50
Vascularised scars	8
Complications	
Corneal thinning	8
Secondary glaucoma	2
Steroid addiction	16
Recurrence	19

3.2 Recurrent HSV keratitis

One hundred and twenty-six eyes had recurrent HSV keratitis Nearly 3/4th of the eyes with multiple recurrences had been exposed to steroids or had to be put on steroids subsequently (Table 4). A total of 63.8% of the eyes treated with steroids had either stromal keratitis or keratouveitis (Table 5).

Table 4. Recurrent HSV keratitis.

Recurrences	Steroid exposed	Non-steroid exposed	Total No.of eyes
One recurrence	23	14	37
Two recurrence	10	13	23
Three or more rec.	50	16	66
Total	83	43	126

Table 5. Corneal lesions in recurrent HSV keratitis.

Corneal lesions	Steroid exposed	Non-steroid exposed
Epithelial	6	24
Epithelial with stromal infiltration	13	3
Stromal keratitis	31	3
Keratouveitis	22	3
Corneal opacity	11	10
Total	83	43

Complications like deeper infiltration, secondary infection and perforation due to use of steroids were almost universal in the group of recurrent epithelial lesions and epithelial lesions with stromal infiltration(Table 6). In contrast none of the eyes in recurrent HSV keratitis not exposed to steroids developed any of these complications. Nine of the 83 eyes with recurrent HSV keratitis exposed to steroids became steroid dependent.

Table 6. Complications of steroid theraphy in recurrent HSV keratitis (83 eyes).

Complications	Epithelial (6)	Epithelial with stromal (13)	Stromal (31)	Kerato-uveitis (22)	Corneal opacity (11)
Deepinfilt.	–	4	1	–	–
Sec.infection	1	–	1	–	–
Keratolysis	1	1	–	–	–
Perforation	1	1	–	1	–
Recurrence	–	–	–	1	–
Steroid addiction	–	5	2	1	1
Non-healing ulcer	2	2	1	–	–
Total	5	12	3	3	1

4.DISCUSSION

HSV keratitis is emerging as one of the commonest cause of blindness in our part of the country. Hence we wish to emphasize the magnitude of problems posed by use and abuse of steroids in the management of these cases. Use of topical or systemic steroids in epithelial lesions of HSV keratitis is absolutely contraindicated as we found that complications were universal in this group.

Role of steroids in epithelial lesions with stromal infiltration is controversial. Esposure to steroids may lead to deeper infiltration, keratolysis, peforation and steroid addiction. However, experimental evidence has been presented that diluted topical steroids can be safely administered under cover of antiviral therapy for such cases (Carter A and Easty DL, 1981). Topical steroids in dilution are mostly used for stromal keratitis and keratouveitis, where the improvement in keratitis and visual acuity is tremendous. However, steroid addiction is seen frequently in these eyes and they have to be kept on diluted steroids for several months to years.

5.SUMMARY

In a study of 194 (252 eyes) of HSV keratitis over a period of 5½ Years seen in the Corneal Clinic, we found misuse of steroids in 36 eyes which led to serious ocular complications like non-healing ulcers, perforation and superadded infections. In 78 eyes of keratouveitis and stromal keratitis use of topical steroids lead to complications like stromal thinning (eight eyes) and steroid addiction (16 eyes). In recurrent HSV keratitis, none of the eyes not exposed to steroids developed any of these complications.

REFERENCES

Duke-Elder S(1965) System of Opthalmology,Vol.III Part I,307
Chakraborty GS,Jain IS,Choudhry S,and Pal SR(1979) Bull
PGI, 13, 3, 146-152
Thygeson P (1977) Controversy in Ophthalmology Ed.
Brochurst RJ et al, Phil. W.B. Saunders Co.,450-469.
Carter A and Easty DL (1981) Brit.J. Ophthalmol. 65, 392.

MANAGEMENT OF HERPETIC KERATITIS BY INSTILLATION OF

CITREOUS HONEY.

Prof. Dr. Mohamed H. EMARAH, F.R.C.S.

Head of Department of Ophthalmology

University of Mansoura, Egypt

In recent years, new potent antiherpes agents have been introduced for the treatment of herpetic keratitis. However these agents are not absolutely free of toxic side effects such as punctate keratopathy, conjunctival hyperaemia and edema.

The purpose of this paper is to present a natural line of treatment for acute and chronic stromal herpetic keratitis by instillation of citreous honey in the inferior conjunctival fornix four times daily.

MATERIALS

Honeys are classified according to the principal sources from which the bees gather the nectar. In Egypt, we have three types of honeys depending on the nectars of flowers gathered by bees (Apis mellifera lamarckii) from the fields and gardens around the breading site : citreous, clover or cotton. Each type of honey has its own colour, viscosity and biological effects. Citreous honey is a pale amber colour, low viscosity and proved by the author, on purely clinical grounds, to have a good antiviral effect.

In the present study citreous honey is used dispensed for ophthalmic use in 15 ml. self-dropper plastic bottles.

SUBJECTS AND METHODS

Patients presenting with active stromal herpetic keratitis without epithelial ulceration or with metaherpetic ulceration were included in the study.

Maudgal, P.C. and Missotten, L., (eds.) Herpetic Eye Diseases.
© *1985, Dr W. Junk Publishers, Dordrecht/Boston/Lancaster. ISBN 978-94-010-8935-7*

All patients were examined with slit-lamp and positive clinical findings were recorded. Each odd-numbered patient (Group
I) received a bottle of citreous honey and was instructed to
instill one drop in the inferior conjunctival fornix four times
daily. Each even-numbered patient (Group II) was given the
conventional treatment of steroids and IDU drops mixture five
times daily as a control. Emarah (1978) proved clinically that
mixing steroids and IDU drops in one and the same bottle for
simultaneous instillation was safer and more effective than instilling them separtately. Ancillary treatment in the form of
atropine drops 1% four times daily was prescribed as long as the
inflammation remained active.

Patients were asked to return for clinical check-up on
study days 3, 7, 14 and 28 and then once monthly for six
months. The condition was judged to be improved, unchanged or
worse in comparison with the signs and symptoms noted at the
previous attendance. The treatment was stopped when either the
stromal keratitis became quiescent and no staining with rose
bengal was obtained or when dendritic ulceration supervened and
another line of treatment was recommended.

TABLE I : Results of Treatment with Honey and IDU/Steroid Mixture

Patient Groups	N°.of Patients *ST.KT	*M.KT.	N°.Ptts. Improved	N°Ptts. Worse	*M.D.T. Days	Rec. Ulcer	Glauc.
Group I: Honey	25	9	32(94.1%)	2(5.9%)	32	2	0
Group II: IDU/Steroid	28	6	26(76.5%)	8(23.5%)	46	7	1

*ST. KT = Stromal Keratitis.   *M. KT. = Metaherpetic Ulceration
*M.D.T. = Mean Duration of Treatment in Days.

RESULTS

Sixty-eight patients (49 males and 19 females) were treated. Fifty three patients had active stromal herpetic keratitis (25 in Group I and 28 in Group II) while 15 patients had metaherpetic ulceration (9 in Group I and 6 in Group II). Thirty two patients out of 34 (94.1%) treated with honey showed improvement of vision and quiescence of keratitis in an average of 32 days treatment (Table I). Only 2 patients developed dendritic ulcer and none showed glaucoma in the honey treated group, but 7 patients developed dendritic ulcer and one glaucoma in conventionally treated group during the six months follow-up period.

DISCUSSION.

Although today medicinal use of honey is largely confined to folk medicine, there are occasional reports in the modern medical literature describing its value in treatment of wounds, burns, infections and other disorders. An antibacterial effect (inhibine) was reported by Dold et al. (1937) and the identity of the inhibine effect was explained later by White et al (1963). The biological effects of honey were recently studied by Smith et al (1969) in an attempt to verify them. Blomfield (1973) stated that honey dressings surpassed any other local applications for the treatment of decubitus ulcer. Emarah (1982) demonstrated the therapeutic effect of honey in some ocular conditions.

The mode of action of honey in the resolution of inflammatory reaction is very intriguing. Clinical experience convinced me that citreous honey has a therapeutic effect, an observation which has to be verified by further biological studies.

SUMMARY.

In a controlled study on 68 patients the therapeutic effect of honey in the topical treatment of stromal herpetic keratitis and metaherpetic ulceration is presented. Quiescence of keratitis and improvement of vision in an average of 32 days occured in 94% of patients treated with citreous honey. Treatment by IDU and corticosteroids was less effective, quiescence was obtained in 76.5% after 46 days.

REFERENCES

Blomfield, M.B. (1973) : J. Amer. Med. Assoc., 224, 905.

Dold H., Du D.H., Dziao S.T. (1937) : Z. Hyg.Infectionskr., 120, 155.

Emarah, M.H. (1978) : XXIII Concilium Ophthalmologicum, Kyoto, 1751.

Emarah, M.H. (1982) : Bull.Ophtalmol. Soc. Egypt. 75, 199.

Smith, M.R., McCaughey, W.F. and Kemmerer, A.R. (1969) : J.Apic. Res., 88, 99.

White, J.W. Jr., Subers, M.H. and Schepartz, A.I. (1963) : Biochem. Biophys. Acta, 73, 57.

SEVERE HERPES SIMPLEX KERATITIS, FREQUENCY OF COMPLICATING CATARACT,
RESULTS OF CORNEAL GRAFTING.

MATS RYDBERG, M.D. (EYE DEPARTMENT, MEDICAL CENTER HOSPITAL, ÖREBRO,
SWEDEN

1.   INTRODUCTION

During the last decades the pattern of ocular infections has changed.
Formerly bacterial infections dominated, while viral infections were
more uncommon or perhaps not so often diagnosed. Thanks to all the antibacterial drugs, the bacterial infections have been more easy to treat
and diminished in importance, while virus infections seem to have
increased and have been a rising problem. Perhaps we have changed the
ecology of microorganisms through the frequent use of antibiotics and
thus made the environment more suitable for virus, and I then especially think of Herpes Simplex (H.S.).

The different ways of treating H.S. keratitis and the progresses in antiviral therapy are carefully examined at this symposium, why I shall
not touch upon this subject.

Sometimes the infection becomes so serious, that surgery, i.e. corneal
grafting, is indicated. The purpose of this paper is mainly to emphasize the fact, that in these serious cases, where grafting has been
necessary, there is a frequent presence of lens opacities. I will also
mention a little about the results of grafting, although this is much
better covered by others.

In most materials of corneal grafting, complications in form of lens
opacities are not mentioned at all or only accidentally. Thygeson -
Kimura (1957) relate presence of cataract in severe H.S. keratitis
and Hogan (1957) has found it in at least 50% of those cases.

The results of grafting have been better with more advanced technics,
better instruments and microsurgery, although there are still complica-

Maudgal, P.C. and Missotten, L., (eds.) Herpetic Eye Diseases.
© 1985, Dr W. Junk Publishers, Dordrecht/Boston/Lancaster. ISBN 978-94-010-8935-7

tions, graft reactions, secondary infections and recurrences. It is anyhow difficult to compare results from the papers 20 to 30 years ago with
results of today, early materials were often small and the indications
more limited. Some results are presented in tab. 1.

Hogan 1957	I	63%	(n=8)
	II	36%	(n=11)
Fine 1958	I	53%	(n=15)
	II	39%	(n=23)
Langstone & Al 1975	I	65%	(n=45)
	II	58%	(n=15)
Cobo & Al 1980	I	69%	
	II	44%	(n=132)
Wittmer 1981		82%	(n c:a 10)
Pouliquen 1981	I	67%	(n=47)
	II	45%	(n=51)

Tab. 1. Clear grafts in some materials of H.S. -keratitis. The
figures I and II refer to the art of keratitis. I means healed
keratitis, with no symptoms during the last six months, II means
chronic ulcers, stromal keratitis, corneal perforations.

The effect of the grafting is related to the percentage of clear grafts.
Result as to vision is not so reliable. Signs of success are also the
frequency of regrafts and recurrences of H.S. infections (Tab. 2)

Number of regrafts	Between 15 and 32% in different materials, in occasional reports 0%
Numer of recurrences	Between 16 and 32%

Tab. 2   Number of regrafts and recurrences of H.S.- keratitis in different reports.

2.   Material and methods

The material is quite small and inhomogenous, because the patients have
come from very different places and the infections have lasted for

different times. Also the number of relapses have varied.

The diagnos has been stated clinically, in only a few cases virus isolation has been possible.

The patients are mostly operated on during a ten year period until 1979
and have had no recurrences since then. Many of the patients have had
their first H.S. infection long ago.

The number of patients is 30, 17 men and 13 women. The number of eyes is
31, 17 resp. 14. (Tab 3).

		Men	Women
Number of patients with corneal grafts	30	17	13
Number of eyes grafted	31	17	14

Age at surgery years	4-84	Mean 45
Time between debut and surgery years	1-74	Mean 26
Number of recurrences before surgery	0-at last 6	Mean 3

Tab. 3. Own material of grafted H.S.-keratitis.

Age at grafting varies from 4 to 84 years, mean 45 years and the time
between debut and surgery is 1 to 74 years, mean 26 years.

3.   Results
3.1 The definite results have given 67% clear grafts in cases grade I,
but only 16% in group II. (Tab. 4)

In 9 cases a regraft has been necessary, i.e. 29% and in 12 cases, there
has been recurrens in the graft (32%).

Clear grafts	I	67%
	II	16%
Number of regrafts		9 (29%)
Number of recurrences		12 (32%)

Tab. 4 Results of grafted H.S.-keratitis in Örebro.

3.2. Complicating cataract

Many times it has been impossible to examine the lens accordingly, because of the corneal opacity, and the findings of lens opacities have been stated after the grafting, when cornea has been clear enough.

In 5 cases (16%) lens opacities have been found before surgery, while in 18 cases (58%) the lens has been impossible to examine. In 8 cases (26%) the lens has been clear.

Opacities of the lens seen before surgery	5	16%
Opacities of the lens not possible to see before surgery	18	58%
No opacities before surgery	8	26%
Opacities of the lens seen after surgery	22	70%
Simultaneous presence of cataract in the fellow eye	2	6%

Tab. 5. Presence of complicating lens opacities in severe H.S.-keratitis.

After surgery lens opacities have been found in 22 eyes (70%) and a simultaneous cataract in the fellow eye has only been present in 2 cases (6%). (Tab. 5).

4. Discussion

Severe H.S.-keratitis is always combined with a more or less pronounced uveitis, and if the course is protracted or there has been several recurrences, there are conditions for complicating cataract. Another cause for complicating lens opacities is an intense and protracted treatment with steroids, that is usual and often necessary in deep H.S.-keratitis.

Anyhow, complicating cataract may be the consequence of either of this causes or perhaps a combination of both. As long as the infection is superficial and the anterior part of the eye is possible to examine, one can wait and see as long as the media are clear, and use drug therapy. The cause of surgery has as a rule been therapeutic, and the result concerning vision has been a secondary aim. Naturally a good vision is desirable and I think a better follow up, that is possible nowadays, and grafting at the right moment will give better results, both concerning the fate of the graft and the possibilities to keep the lens clear. Consequently we can also get a better visual result.

REFERENCES

1. Cobo M., Coster J., Rice N.S.C., Jones B.R.(1980)Prognosis and management of corneal transplantation for herpetic keratitis. Arch Ophth. (Chic) 98, 1755.
2. Coelin H.B., Abelson M.B. (1976) Herpes simplex virus in human cornea, retrocorneal fibrous membrane and vitreous. Arch. Ophth. (Chic) 94, 1726.
3. Cohen E.J.& al. (1983) Corneal transplantation for herpes simplex keratitis. Am. J. Ophth. 645, 95.
4. Fine M. (1958) Treatment of herpetic keratitis by corneal transplantation. Am.J. Ophth. 46, 671.
5. Hogan M.J. Corneal transplantation in the treatment of herpetic disease of the cornea. (1957) Am.J. Ophth. 43, 147.
6. Langston R,H.S., Pavan-Langston D.,Dohlman C.H. (1975) Penetrating keratoplasty for herpetic keratitis-Prognostic and therapeutic determinants. Trans. Am.Acad. Ophth. and Otolaryng. 79, 577.
7. Pouliquen Y., Petroutsos G., Goichot E. L., Giraud J. P. (1981) Eléments du pronostic des kératoplasties sur kératites herpétiques. J.Fr. Ophth. 4, 825.
8. Sundmacher R., Neumann-Haefelin D. (1979) Herpes Simplex Virus-Isolierung aus dem Kammerwasser bei fokaler Iritis and langdauernder Keratitis Disciformis mit Sekundärglaukom. Kl. Monatsbl. Augheilk. 175, 488.
9. Thygeson Ph., Kimura S.J. (1957) Deep forms of herpetic keratitis. Am. J. Ophth. 43, 109.
10. WitmerR. (1981) Keratoplastik. Kl. Monatsbl. Augheilk. 178, 296.

DISCUSSION :

G.O. Waring (Atlanta) : Since most of these cases are unilateral, and if you take the cataract out, either at the time of surgery or afterwards, then you have an unilateral aphake. Since you had 30% recurrence of herpes, contact lens wearing is going to be much more complicated in these cases. They can not wear spectacles. How do you correct aphakia ?

M.V. Rydberg (Örebro) : The first surgery was done in sixties, during the period before we had started intraocular lense implants. So we did not have that possibility, correction with contact lenses is impossible. These patients often have good vision in their fellow eye.

G.O. Waring (Atlanta) : We have similar experience as you have. Cataract is commonly present in these eyes. It is advisable to do a keratoplasty when the eye is quiet, and then do a triple procedure and place a posterior chamber lens after extracapsular extraction. If we are able to get a quiet eye, it is very satisfactory way to correct the aphakia. I think, the patient then does have vision on that side.

M.V. Rydberg (Örebro) : Yes, that is the possibility. But you can never be sure that there will not be a herpes simplex recurrence even if you have a clear graft. It may come several years after the surgery.

PENETRATING KERATOPLASTY IN HERPETIC CORNEAL DISEASES WITH PERFORATION OR
SEVERE STROMAL KERATITIS

E.G. WEIDLE, H.-J. THIEL and W. LISCH
Univeristy Eye Clinical of Tübingen, Tübingen, F.R.G.

1. INTRODUCTION

Keratoplasty is employed in 2 different situations for herpetic corneal diseases : 1. In the inactive stage of corneal scarring. The indication is based on optical considerations and prognosis is generally good
(3-6). 2. In the active stage of corneal inflammation. Franceschetti (7)
calls this procedure keratoplasty "à chaud". Here the indication is based
on tectonic considerations when a corneal perforation occurs or is impen-
ding (descemetocele) and on therapeutic considerations when a persistent
inflammatory disease cannot be controlled with a conservative treatment.
The prognosis in these situations is questionable (1,2,6).

We performed 33 keratoplasties à chaud in the acute inflamed phase
of herpetic corneal disease between October 1980 and December 1983. The
following is a report on the results.

2. MATERIAL AND METHODS

The study is based on 16 males and 17 females (2 of whom were pregnant) ranging in age from 16 to 81 years with a mean age of 51 years.
Among those under 40 years of age, women predominated by a factor of 8 to
2. All patients had suffered from recurrent eye inflammations for
1/2 to 40 years, with a mean of 14 years. In 3 cases a perforation or descemetocele had occurred in a graft following previous keratoplasty due to
recurrent inflammatory conditions. Vision was reduced in all cases to perception of light direction or at most 0.1.

Table 1 shows the preoperative ocular status. Perforation occurred 14
times, descemetocele 9 times and necrotising stromal keratitis 10 times;
the latter was twice connected with a concomitant bacterial infection.
Many corneas displayed pronounced vascularisation. This was rated (1) as
minimal when only 1 or 2 quadrants were superficially affected, (2) as moderate when 3 or 4 quadrants were superficially affected or 1 deeply,

Maudgal, P.C. and Missotten, L., (eds.) Herpetic Eye Diseases.
© *1985, Dr W. Junk Publishers, Dordrecht/Boston/Lancaster. ISBN 978-94-010-8935-7*

304

Table 1 PREOPERATIVE OCULAR STATUS

Variable	No.	%
Perforation	14	(42)
Descemetocele	9	(27)
Necrotizing Stroma Keratitis	10	(30)
Degree of vascularization		
No (0)	7	(21)
Minimal (1)	5	(15)
Moderate (2)	15	(45)
Maximal (3)	6	(18)
Previous transplant	3	(9)
Rosacea Keratitis	1	(3)
Multiple allergies	2	(6)

and (3) as maximal when both superficial and deep manifestations were present. All the excised buttons showed signs of florid interstitial keratitis with dense leucocytic and lymphocytic infiltration of the stroma and extensive necroses, sometimes with a granulomatous reaction against Descemet's membrane.

The operative procedure corresponds to that described in our earlier publications (8,9). Freshyl removed donor corneas were transplanted together with the epithelial layers. The size of the graft ranged from 6 to 8 mm. A combined cataract extraction was performed 2 times, once intra- and once extracapsularly. When necessary, exsudates in the anterior chamber were removed instrumentally or by irrigation; synechias were separated and the chamber angle was reconstituted with HEALON[R]. A maximal hyperemia combined with fibrinous exsudation occurred in all cases. For this reason we did without iridotomy or iridectomy. The graft was fixed in place with 10-0 nylon thread. This was done with single sutures when there was corneal vascularisation or malacia, otherwise with a running suture. A drastic pupil dilatation is obligatory at the end of the operation together with local and systemic steroids and local antibiotics. A prophylactic antiviral therapy with TFT or Acyclovir was administered in 3 cases of interstitial keratitis, otherwise only in herpetic recurrences or when it was not clear whether we were dealing with an immunological reaction or a recurrence.

The follow-up time was 1/2 - 3 1/2 years with an average of 19 months.

3. RESULTS

Penetrating keratoplasty restored the integrity of the perforated, ulcerated and acutely inflamed cornea in all cases (Fig. 1A, B). The inflammations receded with astonishing speed.

The operative complications consisted of one instance of vitreal loss and subsequent retinal detachment in the simultaneous i.c. cataract extraction. The other simultaneous (e.c.) cataract extraction was performed without complications. In a further patient, who was referred to us for enucleation, a keratoplasty was done successfully and the anterior chamber reconstituted itself, but massive haemorrhaging into the eye occurred a week later.

Table 2 shows the postoperative development. Perforated corneas required an additional separation of synechias in the first week after operation in 8 of 14 cases. The lens opacities increased in 8 cases - this was always to be expected in patients over 50 years of age - and made extraction necessary 3 times within the first year after operation. In 2 cases there was an early graft failure. An immunological transplant reaction appeared 5 times, an additional herpetic recurrence 2 times. However, a total of 8 out of 14 patients retained clear grafts.

Table 2 DEVELOPMENT AFTER KERATOPLASTY IN ACTIVE HERPETIC CORNEAL DISEASE

Postoperative FINDINGS	No.	with PERFORATION	with DESCEMETOCELE	with NECROTIZING INTERSTITIAL KERATITIS	and ADDITIONAL BACTERIAL ABSCESS
	33	14	9	8	2
SYNECHIAL LYSIS	10	8	1	0	1
PROGRESSIVE CATARACT	9	8	1	0	0
(POSTOP. EXTRACTION)	(3)	(3)	0	0	0
EARLY GRAFT FAILURE	2	2	0	0	0
TRANSPLANT REACTION	14	5	3	4	2
(PERMANENT)	(8)	(4)	(1)	(1)	(2)
RECURRENT HERPES	3	2	0	0	1
TRANSPLANT EXCHANGE	4	2	1	0	1
CLEAR TRANSPLANT	22	8	7	7	0
OPAQUE TRANSPLANT	11	6	2	1	2

306

The situation was similar in descemetocele and interstitial keratitis regarding immunological reactions, but significantly better for synechias and cataracts. The additional bacterial inflammation of the corneal stroma led in both situations to a permanent immunological reaction, with a recurrence of herpes in 1 case. 4 graft exchanges were performed; none of these resulted in a permanently clear second transplant.

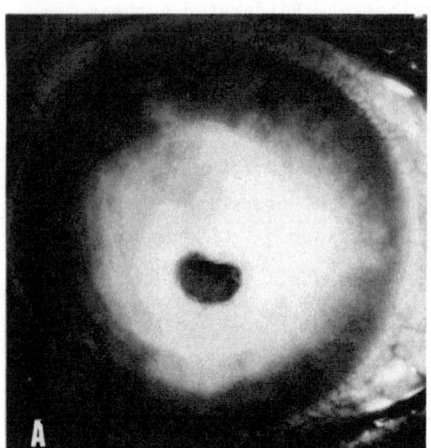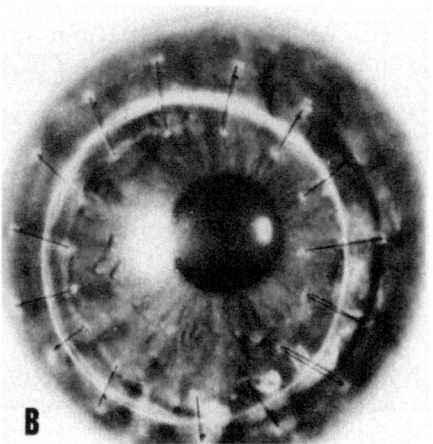

Fig. 1A. Perforated herpetic corneal ulcer. B. 7 months after keratoplasty à chaud (a loosened single suture has already been removed). Vision 0.6.

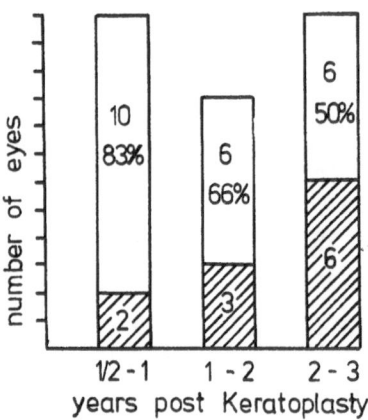

Fig. 2. Life tables for survival of clear graft after keratoplasty à chaud.
clear grafts
opaque grafts

Altogether two thirds of the grafts were clear. Follow-ups of 1/2 to 1 year after operation have shown a rate of 83 %, 1 to 2 years 66 %, and 2 to 3 years 50 % (Fig. 2).

The more pronounced the preoperative vascularisation, the less frequent was a clear graft (Table 3). Vision depended chiefly on graft clarity and whether or not a cataract was involved. In 60 % the final vision ranged from useable to excellent (Table 4).

Table 3 RELATIONSHIP OF PREOPERATIVE VASCU-
LARIZATION AND POSTOPERATIVE GRAFT CLARITY

postop. findings	preop. Vascularization 0	1	2	3
No of all grafts	7	5	15	6
No of clear grafts	5	4	10	3
%	71	80	66	50

Table 4 VISUAL OUTCOME

Visual Acuity	No.	%
0,5 - 1,0	9	27
0,1 - 0,4	11	33
< 0,1	13	39

4. DISCUSSION

Our results are comparable to the success rates of Cobo and associates (3), who worked with an identical number of patients similar to ours. At the end of 2 years they found 44 % clear grafts with a significant correlation to the degree of vascularisation. Foster and Duncan (6) on the other hand registered only 15 % clear transplants in 53 such cases 2 years following operation, and never after perforation. In contrast, these authors found 85 % clear transplants when the acute stage of the perforation could be controlled with tissue adhesion or lamellar patch grafting and the penetrating keratoplasty was done a half to a full year later during a quiet phase. Precisely in herpetic stromal defects, however, these procedures can be problematic. Weiss and his associates (10) for instance recently found over 50 % failures after tissue adhesion. On the other hand there is danger of epithelial downgrowth into the anterior chamber after patch grafting (11). We are unanimous in our opinion that keratoplasty is best done in a quiet phase during herpetic corneal disease. The fact remains, however, that keratoplasty à chaud is well suited to restore the structural integrity of the cornea after perforation or descemetocele. It can likewise arrest the development of a perforation or a total vascularisation in therapy-resistant, necrotising stromal keratitis and can last but not least quickly relieve the patient of his intense, punishing discomfort. The functional results are, considering the severity of the affliction, thoroughly

encouraging. However, the chief threats in the first few years after operation arise from graft reactions (3,6) and later from herpetic recurrences
(5). Regular supervision and carefully dosed local therapy with steroids
and in some cases antiviral medication is absolutely necessary. Should
optical rehabilitation require a renewed operation - this is true about
50 % of the time - tissue adapted donor material is to be preferred because
of the presensibilisation due to the first transplant and the frequent
presence of vascularisation.

REFERENCES

1. Beekhuis WH, Renardel de Lavalette JGC, Van Rij G, Schaap GJP (1983)
   Therapeutic keratoplasty for active herpetic corneal disease : viral
   culture and prognosis. Doc. Ophthalmol. 55, 31-35.
2. Böke W, Thiel HJ (1974) Tektonische und kurative Keratoplastik nach
   perforierender herpetischer Keratitis. Zugleich ein Beitrag zur Ver-
   wendbarkeit lyophilisierter Kornea zur Nottransplantation. Klin. Mbl.
   Augenheilk. 165, 153-159.
3. Cobo LM, Coster DJ, Rice NSC, Jones BR (1980) Prognosis and management of corneal transplantation for herpetic keratitis. Arch. Ophthalmol. 98, 1755-1759.
4. Cohen EJ, Laibson PR, Arentsen JJ (1983) Corneal transplantation for
   herpes simplex keratitis. Am. J. Ophthalmol. 95, 645-650.
5. Fine M, Cignetti FE (1977) Penetrating keratoplasty in herpes simplex
   keratitis. Recurrence in grafts. Arch. Ophthalmol. 95, 613-616.
6. Foster CF, Duncan J (1981) Penetrating keratoplasty for herpes simplex
   keratitis. Am. J. Ophthalmol. 92, 336-343.
7. Fransceschetti A, Doret M (1950) Hornhauttransplantation "à chaud".
   Klin. Mbl. Augenheilk. 117, 449-458.
8. Thiel HJ (1978) Keratoplastik bei akuten infektiösen Hornhautprozes-
   sen. Klin. Mbl. Augenheilk. 173, 171-181.
9. Weidle EG, Thiel HJ (1984) Keratoplastik à chaud als therapeutische
   Massname bei akuten Hornhautinfektionen. Klin. Mbl. Augenheilk. 184,
   in press.
10. Weiss JL, Williams P, Lindstrom RL, Doughman DJ (1983) The use of tis-
    sue adhesive in corneal perforations. Ophthalmology 90, 610-615.
11. Winter R, Püllhorn G (1978) Hornhautaufnähung bei ulzerativer Kerati-
    tis : Klinische und histologische Befunde. Klin. Mbl. Augenheilk.
    173, 237-243.

DISCUSSION :

F. Lagoutte (Bordeaux) : Have you ever tried to treat perforated
    eyes with cyanoacrylate glue before keratoplasty as Dr. Foster
    tried to convince us some years ago ?

E.G. Weidle (Tübingen) : Occasionally we use cyanoacrylate tissue
    adhesive to plug the perforated ulcers before operation, so
    that the anterior chamber is reformed which facilitates trephina-
    tion. We do not use tissue adhesive for therapy.

H.J. Thiel (Tübingen) : There are many additional problems with
    cyanoacrylate adhesives. We used histoacryl for some years
    and we observed much necrosis under this treatment after one
    or two days, and in one case ingrowth of epithelial cells into
    the anterior chamber. Therefore we no longer use histoacryl
    as therapy. We have done some experiments which were descri-
    bed in 1976. (Klin. Mbl. Augenheilk. 173, 237, 1976).

H.J.M. Völker-Dieben (Leiden) : We have used this glue as well,
    but we found out that the inflammation increases enormously.
    Therefore we don't use this glue anymore. We have tried a
    bandage lens and air in the anterior chamber, if no donnor
    material is available. I think that is better, than using cyano-
    acrylate glue which, in fact, increases the problems.

H.J. Thiel (Tübingen) : I agree with you completely.

M.V. Rydberg (Örebro) : We also used bandage lenses to save
    the eye or corneal surface. There is another solution; I just
    wonder if you have used hyaluronic acid. If there is a small
    perforation, you can have very good cornea to make a trephina-
    tion in it. Last year we had cases of two perforated herpes
    simplex keratitis. They have done very well with hyaluronic
    acid before grafting.

J. Colin (Brest) : Have you used acyclovir intravenously the day
    after keratoplasty " à chaud" ?

E.G. Weidle (Tübingen) : No, we have not used acyclovir in the
    early postoperative phase, and we have not seen any recurrence
    in this phase, but only two or three years later.

P.A. Asbell (New York) : Just a technical point. In eyes perfo-
    rated from whatever cause, I have found that the suction

trephine is extremely helpful for making the cut in the host. This is a disposable trephine that works by air suction. It is made by JedMed in St. Louis, Missouri, I believe. It is not a particularly fancy device, but it can make a very nice trephination, even in eyes that are perforated or otherwise very soft.

H.J. Thiel (Tübingen) : We use trephines only very superficially and then open the anterior chamber with knives and cut with scissors. I think that this is a good method; prior to trephination we fill up the anterior chamber with hyaluronic acid.

G.O. Waring (Atlanta) : Did you say that in a third of your patients you went back after the keratoplasty to break adhesions between the iris and graft and if so, would you tell us more about that ?

E.G. Weidle (Tübingen) : Especially in perforated eyes, we sometimes saw small synechias in spite of mydriasis. We avoid touching the iris during the keratoplasty "à chaud", because of hyperemia, and prefer to break adhesions in the quiet phase a week later.

H.J. Thiel (Tübingen) : As you know, it is better to perform the keratoplasty. If there are synechias you can break them after a few days. I think that it is a better approach because if you touch the iris, bleeding occurs suddenly or after one day. We have seen very good results when we break the synechias wihtin one week.

G.O. Waring (Atlanta) : You do it with Healon or with a mechanical sweep ? How do you do it ?

H.J. Thiel (Tübingen) : With a cannula, Healon is not necessary.

C.C. Kok-van Alphen (Leiden) : We break the synechia at the time of operation, because we think that it is again a major trauma for the endothelium of the graft when we do it later.

H.J. Thiel (Tübingen) : No, I don't think so. I make a small incision at the limbus and enter with a cannula and then separate the iris from the back of the cornea very very gently.

C.C. Kok-van Alphen (Leiden) : But it can be very tight !

H.J. Thiel (Tübingen) : If you have fixed it with a stitch, then yes.

KERATOPLASTY IN HERPETIC CORNEAL DISEASE

Results in 1oo patients
KNÖBEL, H.; HINZPETER, E.N.; NAUMANN, G.O.H.
University Eye Clinic Hamburg

INTRODUCTION

In general penetrating keratoplasty is considered a successful
treatment for herpetic corneal disease. Published data on postoperative complications vary considerably especially as definite
preoperative parameters are lacking. (1-6,1o)

In a previuos report we were able to demonstrate, that the preoperative slitlampmicroscopical findings did not correlate with
the histology of the corneal button removed during keratoplasty.
In one third of those cases showing inert scar tissue clinically
we found pronounced signs of diffuse chronic keratitis histologically; sometimes even a granulomatous reaction against Descemet's membrane. Since an inert scar is regarded unanimously as
the best precondition for successful keratoplasty it seemed important to us to take into account the histological findings of
the corneal specimen obtained rather than the preoperative clinical aspect, when evaluating the success of our surgery. (7)

SUBJECTS and METHODS

In the following we would like to report our results in 1oo
patients, who underwent penetrating keratoplasty because of
various forms of herpetic keratitis between 196o and 1975.
Among these patients 61 were male and 39 female. Their ages
ranged from 3 to 76 years at the time of surgery the average
being 43 years.

The postoperative course could be followed up to 1 year in 54
eyes. 16 eyes were observed within a range of 1 to 2 years, 13
eyes 2 to 3 years and in 17 eyes the postoperative observation
spanned 3 to 14 years. (Table 1)

If we regard the histological examination instead of preoperative clinical findings in 3o of 1oo cases avascular corneal scars
were found, in 21 cases vascularized corneal scars and in 43 cases
a chronic diffuse keratitis. 6 cases had a definite granulomatous reaction against Descemet's membrane. (Table 2)

Maudgal, P.C. and Missotten, L., (eds.) Herpetic Eye Diseases.
© *1985, Dr W. Junk Publishers, Dordrecht/Boston/Lancaster. ISBN 978-94-010-8935-7*

Table 1

POSTOPERATIVE EXAMINATION IN 100 EYES

		follow up	No of eyes
Group	I	up to 1 year	54
Group	II	up to 2 years	16
Group	III	up to 3 years	13
Group	IV	up to 14 years	17
			100

Table 2

HISTOLOGY OF 100 CORNEAL BUTTONS

nonvascularized stromal scar	3o
vascularized stromal scar	21
chronic diffuse keratitis	43
gran. reaction against Descemet's m.	6
	100

Table 3

VISUAL ACUITY AFTER PENETRATING KERATOPLASTY

	No of eyes	improvement	no improvement or worse
Group I up to 1 year	54	35	19
Group II up to 2 years	16	1o	6
Group III up to 3 years	13	8	5
Group IV 3 to 14 years	17	1o	7
	100	63	37

Table 4

CLINICAL RESULTS AFTER PENETRATING KERATOPLASTY

	No of eyes	clear graft	graft rejection	herpetic recurrence
Group I up to 1 year	54	33	18	3
Group II up to 2 years	16	11	5	-
Group III up to 3 years	13	6	5	2
Group IV 3 to 14 years	17	2	1o	5
	100	52	38	1o

Table 5

CORRELATION BETWEEN HISTOLOGY AND POSTOPERATIVE FINDINGS

No of eyes	state of graft	nonvascularized stromal scar	vascularized stromal scar	chronic diffuse keratitis	gran.reaction against Desc.m.
I 1 year					
54	33 clear grafts	9	8	14	2
	18 graft rejection	7	3	8	–
	3 herp.recurrence	1	–	2	–
II 2 years					
16	11 clear grafts	4	3	3	1
	5 graft rejection	2	2	–	1
	– herp.recurrence	–	–	–	–
III 3 years					
13	6 clear grafts	3	1	2	–
	5 graft rejection	1	1	2	1
	2 herp.recurrence	–	–	1	1
IV 4 years					
17	2 clear grafts	–	1	1	–
	1o graft rejection	1	1	8	–
	5 herp.recurrence	2	1	2	–
100	100	3o	21	43	6

In 1oo eyes 42 graft remained clear, and 63 eyes yielded an improved visual acuity postoperatively. This discrepancy is due to the fact that in spite of graft rejection or recurrent herpetic infection a better visual acuity was obtained. (Table 3) Since the observation period stretched over a time span from 1 to 14 years the patients were divided into 4 groups. In the last group 17 eyes were observed from 3 to 14 years. Only 2 eyes retained a clear graft. (Table 4)

It should be stressed, that the time factor is the most important parameter in judging the prognosis of keratoplasty in herpetic disease. This is important when one considers, that papers on the results of keratoplasty in herpes keratitis frequently deal with short postoperative follow up of 1 to 3 years. (6,9) FINE and CIGNETTI found a rate of postoperative herpes recurrence in 47% within an observation period of 15 years, opposed to a recurrence rate of 12% within an observation period between 1 to 3 years. (5)

There is no doubt, that clinically active metaherpetic keratitis at the time of surgery carries the poorest prognosis regarding immunological graft rejection and herpes recurrence.

In a previous paper we could show, that the preoperative clinical findings do not always correlate with the histology of the corneal specimen. (7)

In one third of all cases, in which clinically an inactive corneal scar was found, there were histological signs of a pronounced chronic keratitis. The most frequent histological finding was chronic inflammation of the corneal stroma (43%).

In these 43 eyes the grafts remained clear in 2o cases and became opaque due to corneal graft rejection in 17 cases and due to herpes recurrence in 5 cases. Most of the clear corneas belonged to group I, i.e. that means a postoperative observation period up to 1 year. In 1oo eyes 1o grafts were opaque due to herpes recurrence and 32 due to a clinically diagnosed immunological grafts rejection.

A time factor regarding herpes recurrence could not be found, even not in correlation to the local corticosteroid therapy given routinely within the first postoperative months.(Table 5)

This was also true regarding the clinically diagnosed cases of immunological graft rejection.

DISCUSSION

It should be mentioned, that all eyes, which showed a chronic diffuse keratitis histologically sufferd corneal graft rejection regardless of the postoperative observation period. The significance of this observation must of course be considered with caution as a herpes recurrence can mimic immunological graft rejection clinically. (8)

It is also possible, that herpes simplex infection can alter the character of the antigen situation of the tissue to such an extent, that an immunological corneal graft rejection is triggered. (1o)

Eyes, which showed the best results, were those, especially in the 2 year observation period, where the histology of the corneal button was an avascular inert scar. This fact confirmes our opinion, that an inert corneal scar is the best precondition for a penetrating keratoplasty. Opposed to this is the observation of FINE and CIGNETTI, that the activity of the inflammatory process at the time of surgery does not influence the prognosis of keratoplasty in any way. (5)

However these authors exclusively used the clinical preoperative findings as their criteria. It seemed more important to us to take into account the histological finding of the corneal button. (7)

In conclusion it must be emphasized again, that the most important fact in evaluating keratoplasty in herpetic disease is the time span of the postoperative period.

Also that the opafication of the graft whether due to immunological graft rejection or herpes recurrence can still occur up to 14 years following surgery. Altogether 5o% of the transplants remained clear.

REFERENCES

1. CASTROVIEJO, R.:   Keratoplastik
                                        Stuttgart: Thieme 1968

2. COLLIN, H.; ABELSON, M.:   Herpes simplex virus in
                                        human cornea
                                        Arch.Ophthal.94 1726-1729 (1976)

3. DAWSON, C.; TOGNI, B.;   Structural changes in chron.
   MOORE, T.:   herp.ker.
                                        Arch.Ophthal.79 74o-747 (1968)

4. FFOOKS, O.;   Role of penetrating grafts
   PICKERING, A.:   in herpetic keratitis
                                        Brit.J.Ophthal.55 321-33o (1971)

5. FINE, M.; CIGNETTI, F.E.:   Penetrating Keratoplasty in
                                        Herpes Simplex Keratitis
                                        Arch.Ophthal.95 613-616

6. HALLERMAN, W.:   Ergebnisse der Keratoplastik
                                        bei Herpes
                                        Klin.Mbl.Augenheilk.146 161-171
                                        (1965)

7. KNÖBEL, H.; HINZPETER,E.N.;   Keratopl.bei Herp.corn.
   NAUMANN, G.O.H.:   Sundmacher,R.: Herpet.Augen-
                                        erkrankungen.
                                        München: F.J.Bergmann, 1981

8. PFISTER, R.; RICHARDS,H.E.;   Recurrence of herpetic kera-
   DOHLMAN, C.:   titis in corneal grafts
                                        Amer.J.Ophthal.73 192-196 (1972)

9. POLACK, F.; KAUFMAN, H.E.:   Penetrating Keratoplasty in
                                        herpetic keratitis
                                        Amer.J.OPhthal.73 9o8-913 (1972)

318

DISCUSSION :

J. McGill (Southampton) : Can you tell me how do you clinically tell the difference between graft rejection from immunological point of view and graft re-invasion by herpes simplex virus ?

H. Knöbel (Hamburg) : If you see a dendritic figure on the epithelium we are speaking about recurrence of herpes. If you see edema of the transplant, we speak about graft rejection.

J. McGill (Southampton) : Herpes virus can be in the anterior chamber, it oculd be invading deep parts of the graft.

H. Knöbel (Hamburg) : I agree, but we have only this sign for herpes recurrence.

F. Lagoutte (Bordeaux) : May I comment in this connection ? When there is a special line, i.e. Khodadoust-Silverstein line, at the endothelial part of the cornea, only then we can be sure that it is a graft rejection.

H. Knöbel (Hamburg) : I agree.

H.J. Thiel (Tübingen) : I would like to ask you about the value of the histoplathologically observed granular reaction against Descemet's membrane.

H. Knöbel (Hamburg) : Pathologists are saying it is typical for herpes. Sometimes you can have it with mycotic ulcer, but we say it is pathognomonic of herpes disease.

PREVENTION AND TREATMENT OF HERPES RECURRENCE IN THE CORNEAL GRAFT WITH
ACYCLOVIR

C.C. KOK-VAN ALPHEN and H.J.M. VÖLKER-DIEBEN
Diaconessenhuis, Leiden, The Netherlands

1. INTRODUCTION

Recurrence of herpes in the corneal graft is a serious complication
which can cause clouding of the graft or even irreversible rejection. In
our extensive material of grafts, performed because of clouding of the cornea by herpes, we frequently encountered herpes recurrences.

Since in the Zürich Eye Clinic prophylaxis with T.F.T. (Sie, 1980)
seemed to be beneficial, it was thought useful to start an investigation
with acyclovir for the prevention of herpes recurrences in the corneal
graft. All patients studied had suffered from ocular herpes diseases for
a long time. At keratoplasty a large amount of herpes virus containing
tissue will be removed. Nevertheless a certain amount of herpes virus will
always stay somewhere near the patient's eye, since we know that herpes
virus has been found in the lacrimal gland and even in the ganglia. Nearly
all our patients with prolonged herpes were resistant to both I.D.U. and
T.F.T. Acyclovir offered a new opportunity. Furthermore we wanted to know
whether acyclovir is toxic to the epithelium, since most virostatics are
not atoxic. The third question we wanted to find an answer to was whether
treatment with acyclovir would be a useful therapy when a corneal graft
had been involved in a herpes recurrence.

2. MATERIALS AND METHODS

Our investigation was divided into two parts. The first part tried
to answer two questions :
1. Does acyclovir prophylaxis for 5 weeks influence the herpes recurrences in the graft ?
2. Does acyclovir therapy for 5 weeks cause epithelial damage of the
   graft ?
The second part tried to give an answer to the question whether acyclovir is a useful therapy whenever herpes occurs in the graft.

Maudgal, P.C. and Missotten, L., (eds.) Herpetic Eye Diseases.
© *1985, Dr W. Junk Publishers, Dordrecht/Boston/Lancaster. ISBN 978-94-010-8935-7*

We started a double-blind study in 20 patients who had to undergo a keratoplasty because of a clouded cornea caused by herpes. The grafted eyes were treated either with acyclovir ointment 3 times daily or with a placebo. These patients had a follow-up of six to eighteen months. In Table 1 the data of both groups are assembled.

Table 1.

	Acyclovir	Placebo
Mean Follow-up (weeks)	60·3	47·3
Mean Age (range)	60·2 (43-82)	52·5 (22-69)
Number of Grafts: First	7	5
Second	1	2
Third +	2	3
"Matched" grafts	4	7
"At Random" grafts	6	3

To answer question 2, each day of the treatment the epithelium of the graft as well as of the recipient rim was carefully examined by means of a slitlamp. Each day staining with fluoresceine was carried out.

For the answer to the second part of our investigation, which covered a period of 1 1/2 years, we treated 25 rather desperate cases with herpes recurrence in the graft with acyclovir ointment 3 times daily. For an average time of 14.3 years these patients had been suffering from herpes recurrences before keratoplasty. They were all resistant to I.D.U. as well as to T.F.T. The time lapse between grafting and the herpes recurrence varied from 1 month to 7 years. We started therapy 1-14 days after the onset of the herpes recurrence. Some patients did not visit our office immediately after their trouble began.

3. RESULTS

Prophylaxis. In the acyclovir group one patient (no. 3) had to stop treatment because of allergy. We saw 3 herpes recurrence patients, who had only one week of treatment and had to be treated further with T.F.T. Case 4 had a rejection after 64 weeks - a very late rejection - and healed after 3 weeks of resumed therapy with acyclovir. Case 7 had a recurrence

1

after 30 weeks and needed over 30 weeks of renewed treatment to heal. In the placebo group we also saw 3 recurrences, definitely earlier than in the acyclovir group. Case 10 did not well on the placebo ointment. Since we did not know whether we were treating with the placebo or with the drug, we also gave T.F.T. for the patient's benefit.

In both groups we met with 3 rejections. In the placebo group the rejections came earlier than in the acyclovir group. We will now review both groups in Figures 1 and 2.

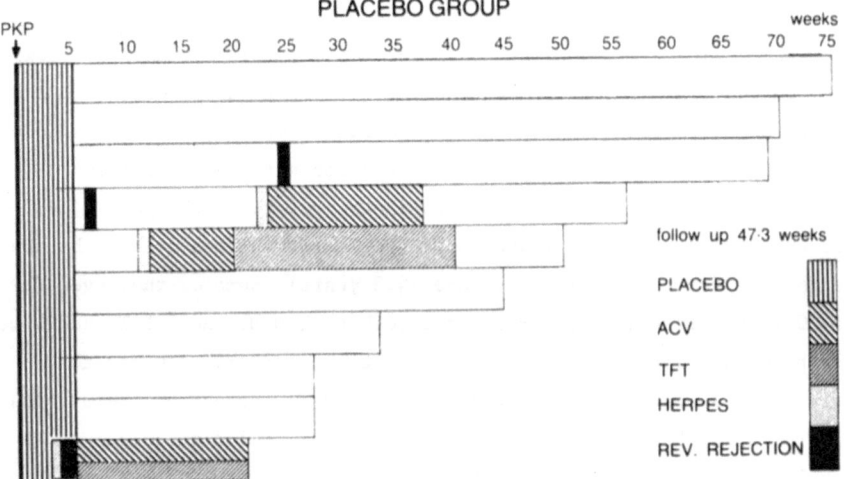

(a) Follow-up and Clinical Course in Acyclovir and Placebo Groups

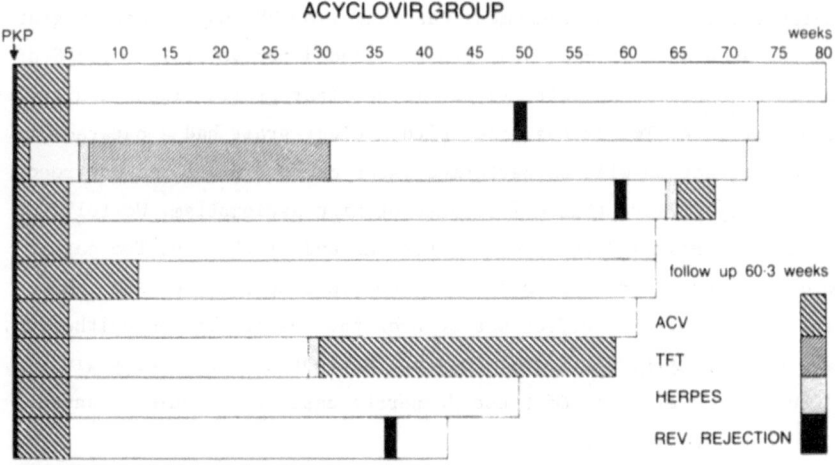

(b) Recurrence of Herpes in Corneal Grafts

Figures 1 (above) and 2 (below).

321

Comparing these two groups, we see no significant difference and can only state that herpes recurrences and rejections manifested themselves earlier in the placebo group. Case 10 of the placebo group had a rejection which was triggered by the herpes. We often see this phenomenon and would stress that corticosteroid therapy is always needed after keratoplasty and should never be stopped in cases of herpes recurrence. Conclusion : acyclovir does not seem to influence herpes recurrence in the corneal graft.

Toxicity of acyclovir in the epithelium . The healing of the epithelium of the graft was quite normal in both groups. We conclude that treatment with acyclovir for 5 weeks after keratoplasty did not have any toxic effect on the regrowth of the endothelium. We saw no toxic effect in the patients who were treated for a longer period after the recurrence.

The second part of our investigation deals with the usefulness of acyclovir treatment when herpes occurs in the graft. In the past 1 1/2 years we treated 25 patients who had suffered from herpes disease before keratoplasty for a long time (average 14.3 years), some of them even for over 20 years. They were all resistant both to I.D.U. and T.F.T. the time lapse between grafting and herpes recurrence varied from 1 month to 7 years. This was a group of desperate cases and it was not possible to have a control group because of social consideration. Twelve cases showed an epithelial herpes, 10 cases had stromal damage. We know for experience that an epithelial form can quickly change into a stromal form, especially when the patient does not show up at once and treatment is not started immediately. The time of treatment was long : 8 – 299 days. Sixteen grafts could be saved and cleared. Nine grafts clouded irreversibly while 8 of them had a rejection as well. In 12 of the clear grafts visual acuity became 0.2 or more. Two of the cases with a clear graft had a cataract; cataract extraction will be performed later on. One graft did not reach visual acuity of more than 0.1 because of high astigmatism. We followed the cases at least 1/2 to 2 years after the end of therapy. Two cases showed a second recurrence, had to be treated a second time and healed in the end. No adverse effect was seen on the healing of the epithelium. We saw hardly any side-effects. Only one patient had an allergy with swelling of the eyelids. Of these desperate cases 64 % could be saved. Fig. 3 shows the results.

NUMBER OF GRAFTS

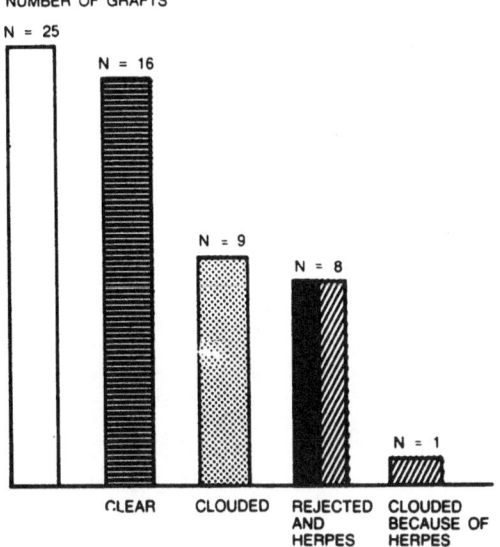

Figure 3.

Conclusion : We concluded that acyclovir is a useful new asset in the treatment of herpes recurrence in the corneal graft.

4. DISCUSSION

In the past ten years we have treated herpes cornea only with perforating keratoplasty, because from our own experience and from the literature (Witmer, 1977) we know that the chances of recurrence in lamellar keratoplasty are higher than in perforating keratoplasty. The numbers of herpes recurrence in grafts mentioned in the literature differ very much. In ten different studies dating between 1977 and 1982 we found a recurrence rate of 8 % – 75 % (Sie, 1980). In our own material we found a ratio of 16.1 %. Sie (1980) treated 18 patients with T.F.T. twice daily and found two recurrences, which is a ratio of 11 1/2. We prefer acyclovir because it is less toxic. When the follow-up was longer we saw a larger number of recurrences. Every virostatic seems useless as a prophylactic when given for a certain time after keratoplasty, because after stopping therapy a recurrence is possible. Since herpes recurrences shortly after grafting have a greater chance of triggering a rejection, prophylaxis for 3 months after operation might be useful, because, in cases of irreversible rejection, the first 3 months are the most dangerous. When treating

corneal grafts with acyclovir we saw no toxicity at all, this in contrast
with T.F.T., which is definitely toxic (Maudgal, 1983).

No literature is available about herpes recurrences in the corneal
graft treated with virostatics. Acyclovir seems to be a useful drug in the
treatment of this condition.

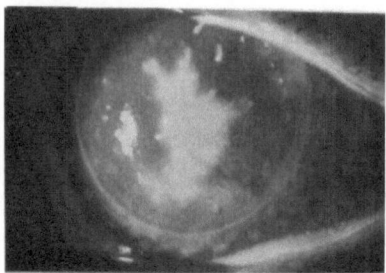 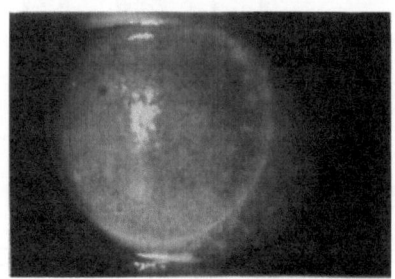

Fig. 4. Herpes recurrences in graft   Fig. 5. Treatment with acyclovir
                                              (after 8 days)

5. ACKNOWLEDGEMENT

The authors wish to thank Wellcome Inc. and particularly Mr. Kuneman
for providing the acyclovir ointment and the placebo, thus making the
study possible.

REFERENCES

1. Maudgal PC, Van Damme B, Missotten L. (1983). Corneal epithelias dysplasia after TFT use. Graefes Arch. Clin. Exp. Ophthalmol.
2. Kok-van Alphen CC, Völker-Dieben HJ, Graniewsky-Wijnands H. (1983).
   Cornea - aesthesiometry after perforating keratoplasty. In press.
3. Peto R, Pike MC, Armitage P, Breslow NE, Cox DR, Howard SV, Mantel
   N, McPherson K, Peto J, Smith PG. (1976). Design and analysis of
   randomized clinical trials requiring prolonged observation of each
   patient. J. Br. J. Cancer 34, 585.
4. Pfister RR, Richards JSF, Dohlman C. (1972). Recurrence of herpetic
   keratitis in corneal grafts. Am. J. Ophthalmol. 73, 192-196.
5. Polack FP, Kaufman HE. (1972). Penetrating keratoplasty in herpetic
   keratitis. Am. J. Ophthalmol. 73, 908-913.
6. Pouliquen J, Goichot EL, Petroutsos G. (1981). Complication des
   kératoplasties sur kératitis herpétiques. J. Fr. Ophthalmol. 4, 12,
   829-832.
7. Rice NSC, Jones BR. (1973). Problems of corneal grafting in herpetic
   keratitis. Ciba Foundation Symposium on Corneal Graft Failure.
   Amsterdam. Associated Scientific Publication, 15, 221-239.
8. Sie SH. (1980). Recidivprophylaxe mit Trifluorothymidin nach Keratoplastik bei Herpes cornea. Ophthalmologica, Basel, 180, 1-8.
9. Skriver K. (1978). Reinnervation of the corneal graft. Acta Ophthalmol. 56, 1013-1015.

10. Völker-Dieben HJ, Kok-van Alphen CC, Lansbergen Q, Persijn GG. (1982). The effect of prospective HLA-A and -B matching on corneal graft survival. Acta Ophthalmol. 60, 203-212.
11. Völker-Dieben HJ, Kok-van Alphen CC, Lansbergen Q, Persijn GG. (1982). Different influences on corneal graft survival in 539 transplants. Acta Ophthalmol. 60, 190-202.
12. Want van der H. (1980). Personal communication.
13. Witmer R. (1972). Resultats des greffes lemellaires et perforantes dans les kerato-uveitis herpétiques. Bull. Mem. Soc. Fr. Ophthalmol. 89, 206.
14. Witmer R. (1981). Results of keratoplasty in meta herpetic keratitis. In: Herpetic Eye Diseases. Sundmacher R. (ed.), Bergmann Verlag, Münich, p. 419.

326

DISCUSSION :

D.L. Easty (Bristol) : In most of our recurrences we have noted
   that they seem to occur at the interface. In one case you
   showed that the recurrence was in the center of the graft,
   do you think that this is unusual or typical ?

C.C. Kok-van Alphen (Leiden) : Well, it's funny. We see a lot
   of recurrences just at the wound edge, but we see them in
   the center too, as in this case. He was a very bad case with
   recurrences for many years.

D.L. Easty (Bristol) : That central ulcer, did it occur long time
   post-op or soon after ?

C.C. Kok-van Alphen (Leiden) : After three years.

G.O. Waring (Atlanta) : I don't know what is in store for
   that ! Could we leave the conference this afternoon with some
   consensus about prophylactic postoperative topical antiviral
   therapy ? You seem to suggest that we should not do it, I
   presume. Is that correct ?

C.C. Kok-van Alphen (Leiden) : I think it does not work. Probably, you have to continue it for very long time, even for
   whole life. So then it would work. But also perhaps, it will
   be toxic and you will have development of virus resistance
   to the drug.

G.O. Waring (Atlanta) : I wonder other people here, who have a
   lot of experience in herpes keratoplasty, might give their
   opinions !

R. Sundmacher (Freiburg) : We don't find it necessary to administer antivirals prophylactically after keratoplasty, except
   in exceptional cases, e.g. persistent deep infiltration at the
   limbus which, presumably, still contains viable herpes viruses.

H.J.M. Völker-Dieben (Leiden) : For how long ?

R. Sundmacher (Freiburg) : As long as the clinical picture indicates viral acitivity in the host cornea. But let me stress
   that you must add antivirals in every situation where an increased dosage of steroids is needed, i.e. mostly in cases of immune reactions against donor endothelium. The one picture
   which you showed with the geographic viral ulcer on the graft

was perhaps triggered by an increased steroid dose without appropriate antiviral cover.

C.C. Kok-van Alphen (Leiden) : We never stop the corticosteroid drops. We continue them in just small doses, because we have always found that if we stop the steroids, you get a rejection.

H.J.M. Völker-Dieben (Leiden) : May I answer on the use of steroids in this patient. As the recurrence of this large central geopgraphic ulcer was three years after grafting, at that moment the patient was not using any steroids at all. There had been epithelial lines at the edge of the graft, but you cann't see them any more. So, it was a kind of dendritic line and in the central part a geographic ulcer. However, I have to admit that his tear production was sub-normal.

H.J. Thiel (Tübingen) : I would like to answer your question too. I agree with Dr. Sundmacher, but even in cases with keratoplasty "à chaud" we never add antivirals with usual therapy. We have never seen the recurrence of herpetic disease in a period of one half or one year.

C.C. Kok-van-Alphen (Leiden) : By virtue of very few recurrences, I think you are a lucky person.

H.J. Thiel (Tübingen) : Thank you very much.

D.L. Easty (Bristol) : We have limited experience in post-op keratoplasty herpes simplex problems. But routinely we use antiviral with good penetration as cover if we use a steroid. We generally use steroids fairly intensively after a penetrating graft. If you just use steroids without antiviral cover, then you run into trouble when you get recurrences. They generally occur at the interface. I regard it as a clinical error not to use antiviral cover post-op.

C.C.Kok-van Alphen (Leiden) : But how long do you use it ?

D.L. Easty (Bristol) : Well, till the eye becomes quiescent, and you can taper down the topical steroids to a low concentration; let us say 0.01% prednisolone. I don't think that concentration will be associated with recurrence of geographic or stromal disease.

C.C.Kok-van Alphen (Leiden) : Our eyes are certainly very quiet after operation, and the trouble comes later.

J. McGill (Southampton) : I agree with David Easty. I use antivirals postoperatively. And on the basis that at least some of your rejections are possibly triggered by viruses, and on the basis of work already published that people have seen virus particles in the rejected grafts, I always increase my antiviral dosage whenever there is a rejection phenomenon. Many of those become quiescent without the added use of steroids. Steroids are kept at the same level, and I add acyclovir, five times a day. Sometimes those grafts can clear, without adding the steroids. This suggests that at least some of the rejection problems are due to viral re-invasion.

F. Lagoutte (Bordeaux) : I think we can do with keratoplasty, as we do with stromal keratitis. What I mean is that as soon as you must use corticosteroids in high dosage, it is necessary to have an antiviral cover. So, again the problem is to know when we consider it as high dosage. It is not really defined.

G.O. Waring (Atlanta) : In your series here, did you use steroids postoperatively, and was the steroid use comparable in both your groups ?

C.C. Kok-van Alphen (Leiden) : Yes, it was just the same; always three drops a day of dexamethasone in both groups.

THE INFLUENCE OF PROSPECTIVE HLA-A AND -B MATCHING IN 288 PENETRATING
KERATOPLASTIES FOR HERPES SIMPLEX KERATITIS

H.J. VÖLKER-DIEBEN, C.C. KOK-VAN ALPHEN, J. D'AMARO and P. DE LANGE

Diaconessenhuis, Leiden, The Netherlands

SUMMARY

A retrospective review of 288 penetrating keratoplasties (PKP) for herpes
simplex keratitis demonstrated a 60.4 % survival rate of clear grafts at
three years. A highly significant difference in corneal graft survival in
severely vascularised corneas (57.1 % at three years) versus non or slightly vascularised corneas (82.8 % at three years) was observed (p = 0.009).
Prospectively HLA-A and -B matched grafts in vascularised corneas revealed
a significantly improved graft survival when compared to unmatched grafts
(p = 0.035 %). Corneal graft survival in eyes grafted "à chaud" was not
significantly below the graft survival of vascularised corneas with a
clinically non-active herpetic corneal disease. Recurrence of herpes simplex in the graft was observed in an earlier post operative period in
HLA-A and -B matched grafts (p = 0.0004).

KEY WORDS : cornea keratoplasty; HLA-typing; herpes keratitis.

1. INTRODUCTION

Recurrent herpes simplex virus (HSV) keratitis leads to corneal scarring and impaired visual acuity. The frequent recurrences of HSV keratitis
and the necessity of frequent visits to the ophthalmologist form a heavy
burden for the social lives of the patients. For many patients a corneal
transplant is the only chance to restore vision and re-establish their
normal social lives.

The main cause of corneal graft failure is immunologic rejection of
the graft. The aim of this study is to determine whether or not prospective HLA-A and -B matching has a beneficial influence on corneal graft
survival.

2. SUBJECTS AND METHODS

In the period from January 1976 to January 1983, 858 penetrating keratoplasties (PKP) were performed, 288 of these were performed because of
recurrent HSV keratitis.

In 250 cases, the diseased corneas were moderately or severely vascularised. 26 Corneas had to be grafted à chaud because of perforation

Maudgal, P.C. and Missotten, L., (eds.) Herpetic Eye Diseases.
© *1985, Dr W. Junk Publishers, Dordrecht/Boston/Lancaster. ISBN 978-94-010-8935-7*

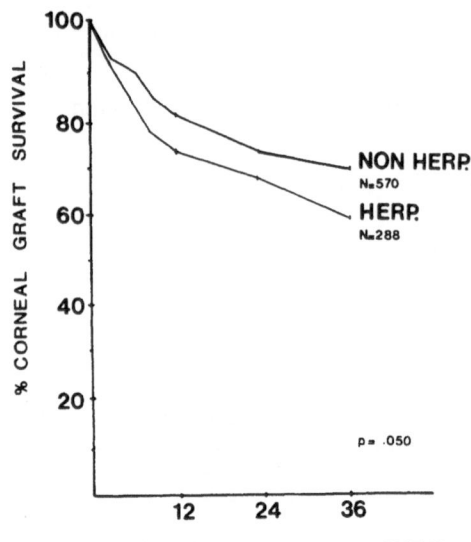

Fig.1: Corneal graft survival
in eyes grafted because of
recurrent herpes simplex virus keratitis versus non
herpetic eye diseases.

or descemetocèle. The remaining grafts were performed in eyes clinically
without active herpes infection at the time of surgery. The visual acuity
of the eyes before grafting was always 0.1 or less. 110 Keratoplasties
were performed with prospectively HLA-A and -B typed donors who were matched as well as possible with the recipients. HLA typings and donor cornea
selection were as previously described (Völker-Dieben et al., 1982).

All grafts were performed by two surgeons (Völker-Dieben and Kok-van
Alphen). Their surgical techniques were identical and conformed to the
method described by Harms and Mackensen (1966). Post operative care was
not changed during the period of this study and was as previously described (Völker-Dieben et al., 1982).

The ages of the 267 patients (288 eyes), 179 men and 88 women, ranged
from 4 to 83 years (mean age 56.3 years). 11 Patients were 15 years of age
or younger. The period of herpetic recurrences before grafting ranged from
2 to 65 years (mean duration 14.5 years). All patients were treated pre-
operatively with antiviral eye drops Idoxuridinum (IDK) 1 mg and trifluorothymidine (TFT) 1 % and corticosteroid eye drops. Antiviral therapy was
not continued post operative.

All patients and graft donors were of Dutch caucasoid origin. All
survival times were calculated using the actuarial life table method. The
significance of the differences between the various classes were tested
with χ^2 statistics derived from the log rank test (Peto et al., 1976).

The numbers to the right of the follow-up curves (Fig. 1-3) indicate the number of patients at the start of the study.

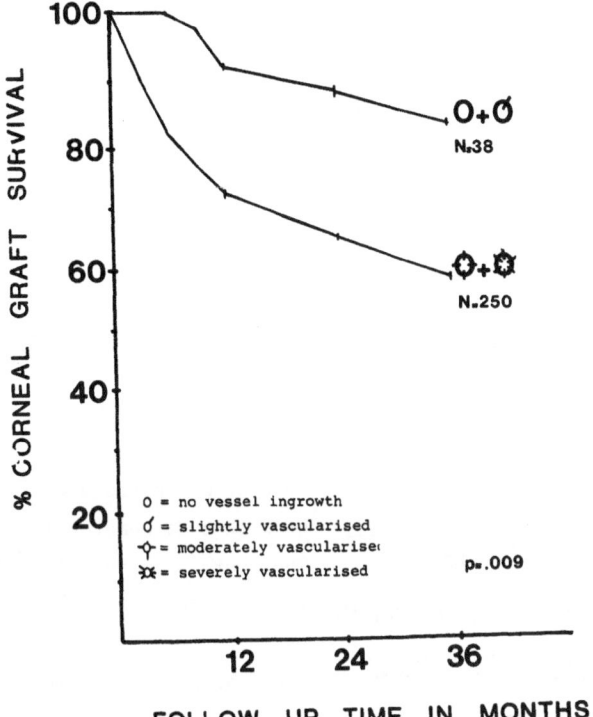

Fig.2: Influence of vas-
cularisation on corneal
graft survival.

3. RESULTS

Corneal graft survival in recurrent HSV keratitis was lower (75.0 %, 68.2 % and 60.4 % at one, two and three years) than in eyes grafted for non herpetic diseases (81.9 %, 73.7 % and 70.9 % at one, two and three years) (overall p = 0.050) (Fig. 1).

250 of the 288 grafts were performed in moderate or severely vascularised corneas and 38 in non or slightly vascularised corneas. The graft survival in vascularised corneas was significantly lower (72.5 %, 65.3 % and 57.1 % at one, two and three years) than in non or slightly vascularised corneas (91.1 %, 87.4 % and 82.8 % at the same time interval) (overall p = 0.009) (Fig. 2).

HLA typed and matched donor corneas were used in the group of vascularised corneas. The matched corneal grafts had a significantly better

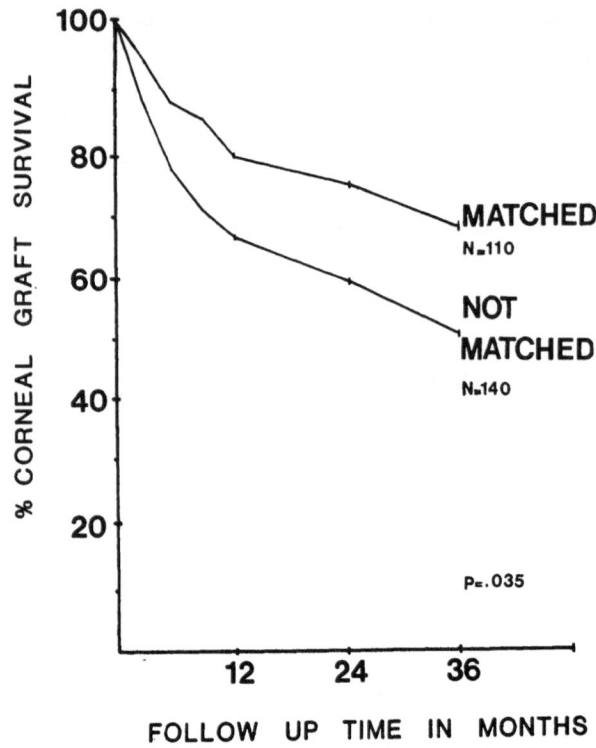

The effect of prospectively HLA-A and -B matching on corneal graft survival in vascularised corneas with recurrent herpes simplex virus keratitis.

survival as compared to the unmatched grafts in vascularised corneas : 80.5 %, 74.1 % and 67.2 % at one, two and three years for the matched grafts, versus 66.7 %, 59.0 % and 50.3 % for the unmatched group in the same time intervals (p = 0.035) (Fig. 3). In 26 cases, it was imperative to perform the corneal graft à chaud. All of those corneas were either perforated or with a descemetocèle. They were all severely vascularised. The corneal grafts in this group of patients demonstrated a lower, but not significantly lower, survival rate when compared to the remaining 224 vascularised corneas; 68.2 %, 58.4 % and 36.7 % versus 73.1 %, 66.1 % and 57.7 % at one, two and three years (Fig. not shown).

Apart from the recurrence of HSV keratitis in the grafts for HSV keratitis, the causes of graft failures (rejection, glaucoma, infection, trauma) are not significantly different when compared to the causes of graft failure in corneal grafts for non herpetic diseases. Since herpetic infection may induce graft rejection it is difficult to determine whether or not grafts became opaque because of HSV infections or because of rejection (Rice et al., 1973). Although not every HSV infection causes a graft rejection, they remain a potential danger. In the 288 corneal grafts for recurrent HSV keratitis, a recurrence of the HSV in the graft was observed in 42 cases. In 15 of them the graft became opaque subsequently. The percentage of herpetic recurrences in the first year after keratoplasty was 9.4 % (17 recurrences of HSV and 181 patients at risk for 12

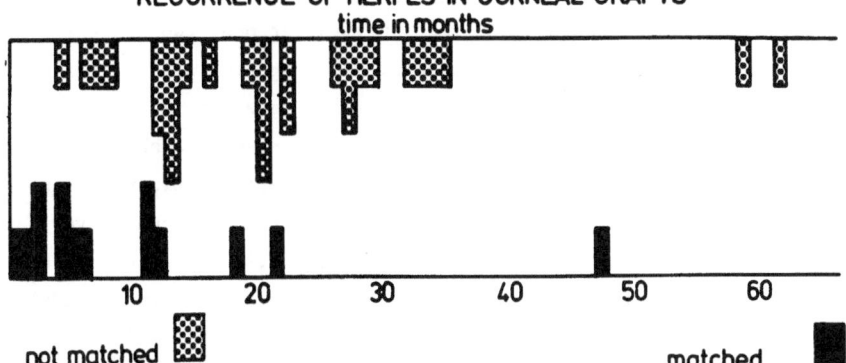

RECURRENCE OF HERPES IN CORNEAL GRAFTS
time in months

not matched ▨   matched ■

Fig. 4. Time interval between penetrating keratoplasty and the recurrence of herpes simplex virus in HLA-A and -B matched grafts as compared with not matched grafts (p = 0.004).

months), in the second year 10.2 % (13 recurrences of HSV and 128 patients at risk for 24 months) and in the third year 11.0 % (9 recurrences of HSV and 82 patients at risk for 36 months).

The time lapse between PKP and the recurrence of HSV in the grafts varied from less than one month to 62 months (Fig. 4). A highly signifi-cant shorter interval between PKP and recurrence of HSV in the graft was observed in HLA-A and -B matched grafts as compared to unmatched grafts : 8.0 months for the matched grafts and 19.4 months for the unmatched grafts (Mann Whitney U test, p = 0.0004).

4. DISCUSSION

The results of the penetrating keratoplasties in herpes simplex virus keratitis are described by several authors (Beekhuis et al., 1983; Cobo et al., 1980, Fine et al., 1977; Foster et al., 1981; Polack et al., 1972).

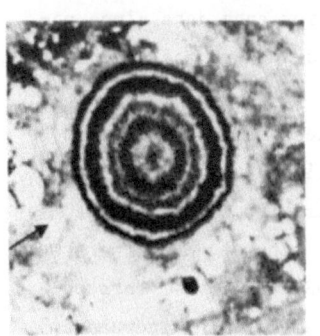

Cobo was the only one who used the actuarial life table method to evaluate the corneal graft survival rates. The number of grafts in this study was 132. A survival rate of clear grafts of 72 % at one year 64 % at two and

Fig. 5. Electron micrographe of herpes simplex virus particle in the corneal stroma of a cor-neal button removed at the time of graft surgery in an eye which was clinically non inflamed during 1.5 years preoperatively.

three years was observed in the entire group. This is comparable to our results of 73.0 %, 68.2 % and 60.4 % graft survival at one, two and three years in the entire group of 288 transplants. Cobo reported also a graft survival rate of 44 % at two years in 33 eyes which were actively inflamed at the time of surgery. This suggests they were transplanted à chaud. His report is comparable to our result of 58.4 % clear grafts at two years in 26 transplants performed à chaud. Cobo's observation that pre-operative vascularisation is the major prognostic factor was previously described by Gibbs et al. (1979), confirmed by us in 1982 and in this study (p = 0.009). Neither in Cobo's study nor in ours was a significant difference in herpetic recurrence found between the group of clinically non-inflamed eyes versus actively inflamed eyes at the time of graft surgery. This observation is not surprising since it was demonstrated by means of electron microscopy that viral particles were present in a corneal button removed at the time of graft surgery in an eye which was clinically non-inflamed during 1.5 years pre-operatively (Fig. 5) (V.d.Want, 1980).

Beekhuis et al. studied 23 patients with active herpetic corneal disease and 23 patients with clinically inactive corneal disease at the time of graft surgery. Although they did not perform the life table analysis to evaluate the percentage of clear grafts, they did follow up all their patients for a minimum of 5 years. Unfortunately both patient groups in their study consisted of lamellar grafts as well as full thickness grafts. The prognosis of lamellar grafts is poorer than for full thickness grafts (Rice et al., 1973). Therefore, we cannot compare their results with ours.

It was not possible to determine if there was any agreement between the results reported by Fine (1977), Foster (1981) and Polack (1972) and ours because the method used to evaluate the percentage of clear grafts was not appropriate to the data. An actuarial life table method as used by Cobo (1980) and in our study is the only valid method for such data since patients are entering the study at different periods and are followed up for different lengths of time (Peto et al., 1976).

The influence of HLA-A and -B matching on corneal graft survival in grafts performed because of recurrent HSV keratitis is to our knowledge not yet described. We observed two influences. Firstly, a significant (p = 0.035) beneficial effect of HLA-A and -B matching on corneal graft survival in vascularised corneas with recurrent HSV keratitis. This observation confirms our previous observation of a significant increased

graft survival with the use of prospectively matched donor corneas in vascularised corneas, independent the initial indication for grafting (Völker-
Dieben et al., 1982). Secondly, there is a significant decrease in time
lapse between PKP and recurrence of HSV in the matched grafts, as compared
to the unmatched graft (p = 0.0004). Since the HSV is a neurotrophical
virus, the reinnervation rate of the denervated donor cornea button may
influence the recurrence of HSV.

Corneal sensibility, as a parameter for corneal nerve ingrowth can be
measured with a corneal aesthesiometer (Skriver, 1978; Draeger, 1979). In
a group of 16 corneas grafted because of recurrent HSV we could not demonstrate corneal sensibility within one year after grafting. However, we
have observed a measurable corneal sensibility in 4 of the 7 HLA-A and -B
matched grafts while only one of the 9 unmatched grafts demonstrated a
measurable corneal sensibility 19 months after keratoplasty (Kok-van
Alphen et al., 1983). Therefore, one may conclude that nerve ingrowth in
an HLA-matched graft is faster than in unmatched grafts. If so, it is not
surprising that recurrences of the HSV are observed in an earlier post
operative period in the well matched group. Although the earlier recurrences of the HSV may induce a rejection episode in a more "dangerous" period
after grafting, it appears that the positive influence of HLA matching
overrules the possible negative influence of early HSV recurrences.

During the past ten years several studies (Cobo, 1980; Foster, 1981;
Colin, 1978; Pouliquen, 1981; Pfister, 1972; Witmer, 1981; Sie, 1980) on
the recurrence of HSV after keratoplasty are reported. The rate of recurrence of HSV reported, varied from 8 % to 75 %. The follow up times varied
from one to 15 years. The HSV recurrence rate seems to increase with time
(Cobo, 1980; Foster, 1981) while Sie (1980) reported in a review of literature that the majority of the HSV recurrences are observed in the first
year after grafting. In our material, we observed almost the same percentage of herpes recurrences in the first, the second and the third year
(9.4 %, 10.2 % and 11.0 %) so we cannot confirm either of the observation
reported by Cobo and Foster nor by Sie. It was difficult to determine
whether or not Cobo and Foster had calculated the percentage of herpes
recurrence by dividing the number of HSV recurrences on the number of patients "at risk" after one, two or three years. In most of the studies
the total number of HSV recurrences is divided on the total number of patients at the start of the study instead of the number of patients that

336

had been followed up for one, two or three years respectively.

5. CONCLUSION

The use of keratoplasty as therapy for herpetic keratitis, is applied, in the vast majority of cases, to corneas with severe vessel ingrowth. The success of penetrating keratoplasties is inversely proportional to the severity of the corneal vascularisation (p = 0.009). We were able to improve our results with the use of HLA-A and -B matched grafts; a significantly better graft survival was observed in matched grafts when compared to unmatched grafts (p = 0.035).

HLA-A and -B matched grafts demonstrated a significantly decreased time lapse between keratoplasty and the recurrence of herpetic simplex in the grafts as compared to unmatched grafts (p = 0.0004). The majority of the herpetic recurrences in the matched grafts was observed in the first post operative year while the unmatched grafts demonstrated the majority of the herpetic recurrences in the second post operative year. Two third of all herpetic recurrences in the graft healed without signs of opcification.

We consider it advisable to use HLA-A and -B matched donor material when grafting vascularised corneas with herpetic keratitis. These patients should be kept under regular ophthalmological control, especially in the first post operative year.

REFERENCES

1. Beekhuis W.H. et al. (1983) Doc. Ophth. 55, 31-35.
2. Cobo L.M. et al. (1980) Arch. Ophth. 98, 1755-1759.
3. Colin J. et al. (1981) J. Fr. Opht. 4, 12, 829-832.
4. Draeger J. et al. (1976) Klin. med. Augenheilk. 169, 407-421.
5. Fine N., Cignetti F.E. (1977) Arch. Ophth. 95, 613-616.
6. Foster C. (1981) In: Herpetic Eye Diseases. Sundmacher R. (ed.), Bergmann Verlag, Münich, p. 425.
7. Harm H., Mackensen H. (1966) Augenoperationen Unter dem Mikroskop. Thieme Verlag, Stutgart, pp. 291.
8. Kok-van Alphen C.C. et al. (1983). Cornea-Aesthesiometry after Perforating Keratoplasty. In press.
9. Peto R. et al. (1976) J. Br. J. Cancer 34, 585.
10. Pfister R.R. et al. (1972). Am. J. Ophth. 73, 192-196.
11. Polack F.P., Kaufman H.E. (1972). Am. J. Ophth. 73, 908-913.
12. Pouliquen J. et al. (1981). J. Fr. Ophth. 4, i2, 829-832.
13. Rice N.S.C. et al. (1973). Ciba Foundation Symposium on Corneal Graft Failure, Amsterdam. Ass. Scienc. Publ., 15, 221-239.
14. Sie S.H. (1980). Ophth., Basel, 180, 1-8.
15. Skriver K. (1978). Acta Opth. 56, 1013-1015.

16. Völker-Dieben H.J. et al. (1982). Acta Ophth. 60, 203-212.
17. Völker-Dieben H.J. et al. (1982). Acta Ophth. 60, 190-202.
18. Want v.d. H. (1980). Personal communication.
19. Witmer R. (1981). In: Herpetic Eye Diseases. Sundmacher R. (ed.), Bermann Verlag, Münich, p. 419.

INTERFERON TREATMENT OF HERPETIC KERATITIS[*]

GILBERT SMOLIN, M.D.

Francis I Proctor Foundation, University of California San Francisco, S-315, San Francisco, California 94143, U.S.A.

Some members of our group have determined the relative activities of natural and biosynthetic interferons in various cell lines; protecting these cell lines from infection with vesicular stomatitis virus. These viruses were normalized for the human WISH cell line. The highlights include : 1) alpha or leukocyte interferon subtypes do have effects across species lines, and 2) the effect will vary depending on the species in which one tests the particular interferon. For example, alpha-A interferon is more effective in the hamster cell line than it is in rabbit. Also, in a given species, we found that a certain subtype may be better than another subtype in vitro. For example, since we are dealing primarily with rabbits in our in vivo work, we found that alpha subtype-D was significantly more effective than alpha subtype-A in protecting rabbit kidney cells from infection with vesicular stomatitis virus. More exactly, it was approximately 40 times more effective.

In our next study we employed four different strains of herpes simplex virus (HSV) type 1 (PH, RA, McKrae and Shealey) and two different type 2 strains (MS and Curtis). We tested alpha-A, -B, -D, and a laboratory synthetic interferon A/D, as well as biosynthetic human gamma interferon in rabbit kidney cells and human corneal cells.

The interferon aliquots were placed on cell monolayers for approximately 18 hours, removed and then the appropriate virus, 50 PFU/mL, were absorbed for about one hour. Virus was then removed, interferon was re-added and incubated. The plates were observed for plaques for approximately 3-4 days, at which time they were stained with 1% crystal violet, fixed with formalin, and read. The tests were performed in triplicate. In each run we had a cell control and a virus control. When we counted the plaques, we averaged the triplicate scores. Our statistician recommended that we explore 50% plaque reduction assay utilising the Cubic Spline technique. For the rabbit kidney cell line the interferon concentration was expressed as units/mL of subtype yielding a

[*]Transcript of the lecture.

Maudgal, P.C. and Missotten, L., (eds.) Herpetic Eye Diseases.
© *1985, Dr W. Junk Publishers, Dordrecht/Boston/Lancaster. ISBN 978-94-010-8935-7*

50% plaque reduction.

The data for the human recombinant gamma interferon was not presented because it was not effective in the rabbit kidney cell line. We have done work in vivo, employing gamma interferon, and found that it was not effective in the rabbit model in protecting against acute herpetic keratitis, apparently it is not effective across species line. The alpha interferon subtype-A was very effective in protecting these cells from HSV infection. The subtype-D was significantly more effective than subtype-A for every HSV strain. In fact, except for one case, it was the most effective alpha subtype tested in protecting these cells from the six strains of HSV. In addition, some strains of HSV are more susceptible to the protecting effects of interferon. For example, the McKrae strain generally tended to be more responsive to treatment with interferon than was the PH strain; the latter strain actually being the one we have been using until we determined these results.

As for as the human corneal cells are concerned, the results are quite interesting in that alpha subtype-A was significantly better than subtype-D. If you recall, it is just reverse in the rabbit kidney cell line. The gamma interferon was moderately effective, as we expected. The laboratory produced or synthetic interferon A/D was the most effective in the human corneal cell line in protecting these cells against HSV. Again, we demonstrated very interestingly that some strains of herpes are more responsive to treatment with interferon, e.g; the Curtis strain was significantly more responsive to treatment than was the McKrae strain.

In conclusion we noted that : 1) Certain virus strains appear to be more susceptible than others to inhibition by interferon. 2) The effect of each interferon subtype is different in the two cell lines that we tested. Anecdotally, other researchers have found that even in the same species, using different cell lines, you may get different results. 3) For a given cell line, the interferon subtypes have different effects on various strains of herpes. We reported in the Current Eye Research, last September, that interferon alpha subtype -D was 20-30 times more effective than subtype-A in vivo. This is what we would have expected from our latest in vitro work. We now infer that in vitro testing of interferon may predict in vivo results. This may have far reaching clinical importance, since we might be able to test a given HSV strain that a patient has against a battery of interferons to find out which subtype may be best suited for that given individual.

Lastly, we tried to determine why one type of interferon was significantly better than another. We thought that it might be related to receptors, i.e; cells of a given species may have more receptors for one type of interferon than another. We treated rabbits with one drop of alpha interferon subtype-A or -D, four times a day for two days, and then collected their tears in micropipettes at 18, 23, and 42 hours after the last topical drop. Significantly more alpha-D interferon was present in tears than alpha-A, consistent with our previous work in rabbits and substantiating our hypothesis. We then radiolabelled interferon and found that for I^{125}-alpha-A interferon there appear to be significant number of receptors in the human corneal cells and much fewer receptors for alpha-A in rabbit corneal cells. It appears that receptors might be responsible for one subtype of interferon being more effective than another in a given species.

DISCUSSION :

T. Doerner (Tel Aviv) : When monitoring the different levels in the tears, do you also monitor the different levels in the serum ? Is there absorption from the eye into the blood ?

G. Smolin (San Francisco) : I have a feeling that there is some interferon in the blood stream, but we did not determine that. In fact, I was surprised to see interferon present to the degree it was, for the length of time it was in the tearfilm. But we only tested the tearfilm.

T. Doerner (Tel Aviv) : We treated patients with interferon beta, and while putting interferon in the tears, we did not find any absorption in the blood. I wonder if alpha interferon behaves differently !

G. Smolin (San Fransisco) : I am afraid I didn't perform that test.

P.A. Asbell (New York) : Have you looked at labeled interferon just on your cell lines in tissue culture ? If so, how much is maintained on different cells after rinsing ?

G. Smolin (San Francisco) : Unfortunately, I guess, I did not explain myself, but that is exactly what we did in the last experiment. We radiolabelled interferon with I^{121} and then counted how much interferon was still present in the cell cultures. We only radiolabelled subtype A. We found that in rabbits almost no A persisted after we washed it off. In the human situation there was significant amounts of A persisting after we washed it off, which implies that there are many more receptors for alpha-A in humans than in rabbits which will be consistent with our previous experiments.

LYMPHOBLAST AND FIBROBLAST - INTERFERON IN A COMBINATION
THERAPY OF KERATITIS DENDRITICA

CHR. FELLINGER, M.E. REICH, H. HOFMANN

INTRODUCTION

The epithelial herpes simplex virus (HSV) keratitis, which
is probably the form of herpes simplex most frequently
occuring on the eye, may differ in its appearance. By
staining with Na-fluorescein keratitis punctata, dendritica,
stellata and geographica can be made visible in the slit
lamp. The herpetic lesions are caused by the viral
reduplication in the corneal epithelium. The clinical
diagnosis is supported by the absence of corneal sensibility
and by isolation of the virus.

Since 1962 , when a virustatic effect could be proved for
IDU , there have been developed many other antiviral drugs
and their effect was tested in clinical studies. Besides
the monotherapy with antiviral drugs the combination
therapies with debridement and virustatics were described.

At the moment interferon treatment is in the centre of
interest. In 1957 Isaacs and Lindenmann discovered
interferon (1). The effectiveness of interferon was proved
in 1962 . From that time placebo controlled clinical trials
on dendritic keratitis were carried out. But it was very
difficult to produce it in large quantities.(2).
At our clinic, we treated the epithelial HSV keratitis
with TFT as a monotherapy or concomitant with iodine
debridement. As, according to our experiences, the healing
progress has not always been satisfactory, we performed a
comparative study with 30 patients suffering from HSV
keratitis applying both TFT as a monotherapy and TFT
combined with interferon. We have been able to obtain human

Maudgal, P.C. and Missotten, L., (eds.) Herpetic Eye Diseases.
© *1985, Dr W. Junk Publishers, Dordrecht/Boston/Lancaster. ISBN 978-94-010-8935-7*

lymphoblast and human fibroblast interferon (HLI and HFI) for the dendritic keratitis treatment. Sundmacher and associates described combined methods with interferon. In clinical trials they tried to find out the most effective concentration of interferon.(4)

MATERIAL AND METHODS

We have treated 30 patients with epithelial HSV keratitis with TFT as a monotherapy and concomitant with human lymphoblast and human fibroblast interferon.

Patients with the clinical diagnosis of superficial H SV keratitis were investigated virologically for the presence of culturable herpes simplex virus in the tear film. Apart from little modification we used the same method as Sundmacher and Neumann-Haefelin.(3)

In group I all patients received 5 drops of TFT 1% daily during the waking hours. In addition they were treated with human serum albumine 2% once in the morning,as a placebo.

In group II all patients received TFT 1% 5 x daily. In addition they were given human fibroblast interferon in a concentration of $1,5 \times 10^7$ U/ml.

In goup III all patients were treated with 5 drops of TFT 1% daily and human lymphoblast interferon in a concentration of $1,5 \times 10^7$ U/ml.

As an additional treatment Mydriaticum Roche was administered. All the groups were studied on a double blind basis.

The ophthalmological examinations were performed daily and included slit lamp controls and viral assays. Slit lamp photographs were taken.

We considered an epithelium healed when it had turned fluorescein-negative, except for some minor punctate epithelial stainings. We defined it as partial healing time.

We applied interferon until the third day of partial healing, the administration of TFT was continued for three more days.

RESULTS

There were 30 patients, who proved positive for herpes
simplex virus by virus isolation. But 7 patients were
excluded from the study because of increasing of the
herpetic lesions after 4 days. Consequently we treated them
with the basic therapy of iodine debridement and TFT. Of
the remaining 23 patients, 9 were treated with HLI and TFT,
8 were treated with HFI and TFT and 6 were treated with
placebo and TFT.

Number of cases   n = 23

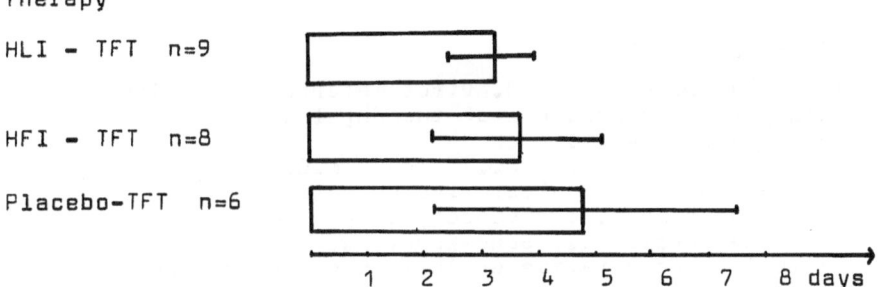

Therapy

HLI - TFT   n=9

HFI - TFT   n=8

Placebo-TFT   n=6

1   2   3   4   5   6   7   8 days

In the figure the average duration of partial healing and
the standard deviations in the treatment of the epithelial
HSV keratitis with TFT as a monotherapy and concomitant with
interferon is shown as a comparative diagram.

In the figure the number of days for partial healing of
dendritic keratitis is given. The average duration of
partial healing of epithelial HSV keratitis with HLI in
a combination therapy with TFT was 3,1 days. The average
duration of healing in the second group, in which all
patients received HFI and TFT was 3,6 days. In the group, in
which all patients received TFT as a monotherapy the
average duration of partial healing was 4,8 days. The
treatment effect is statistically significant. One patient
had a recidive of dendritic keratitis after one year.

346

DISCUSSION

Only those corneal lesions were studied in the trial in
which the virus isolation had been positive. We compared
the effectiveness of TFT as a monotherapy and concomitant
with HFI and HLI. In our former study the average duration
of partial healing with the combined therapy with iodine
debridement and TFT was 5,5 days. In the present double
blind study the average duration of partial healing was
significantly shorter with the interferon groups, namely
3,1 and 3,6 days.

The results obtained in this study correspond on the
whole to the results obtained by other authors as to the
healing duration with TFT as a monotherapy and concomitant
with interferon.

REFERENCES

1. Isaacs A. Lindenmann, J. Virus interference.I The
   Interferon. Proceedings of the Royal society (B),
   1957, 147, 258-267.
2. Jones B.R., Coster, D.J., Falcon, M.G., and Cantell,K.
   Topical Therapy of ulcerative herpetic keratitis with
   human interferon. The Lancet, July 17, 1976, 128.
3. Neumann-Haefelin,D., Sundmacher,R., Skoda,R., and
   Cantell,K. Comparative evaluation of human leukocyte
   and fibroblast interferon in the prevention of herpes
   simplex virus keratitis in a monkey model. Infection
   and immunity, August 1977, 468-470.
4. Sundmacher,R., Neumann-Haefelin, D., Cantell, K.
   Successful treatment of dendritic keratitis with
   human leukocyte interferon. A controlled clinical study.
   Albrecht von Graefes. Arch. Klin. Exp. Ophthalmol.,
   201, 39-45 (1976)

DISCUSSION :

J.O. Oh (San Fransisco) : It has been shown that the combination
of gamma interferon with either alpha or beta interferon has
a synergistic effect. It has been shown in the animal model
as well as the laboratory stage. Have you tried the combination treatment of TFT with combination of your two interferons
to see if they have more effect ?

C. Fellinger (Graz) : We treated with only alpha interferon and
TFT.

J.O. Oh (San Francisco) : My assumption is if you use TFT plus
your both interferons at the same time. You may have more
affect.

C. Fellinger (G raz) : We have not done that.

P.A. Asbell (New York) : How do you control for the size of the
lesions in different groups ? Since, of course, the healing
rate might be related to the initial size of the dendritic lesion
and that might not be equal in all patients.

C. Fellinger (Graz) : We examined all patients on the slitlamp
after fluoresceine instillation. When the lesion was fluoresceine
negative, but only one or two stainings to see, we considered
it as partial healing. Certainly, the healing time would be
longer in large lesions.

T. Doerner (Tel Aviv) : What is rationale of treatment with interferon one drop once daily or one drop five times daily ? There
are several studies which claim that if you apply interferon
several times a day it should be more effective than once a
day. Have you tried in patients treatment with interferon
several times daily ?

C. Fellinger (Graz) : No, we only tried to give our patients interferon in the morning, two drops once daily, and TFT five times.

J. Colin (Brest) : I think that Rainer may answer this question,
may explain this regimen, why only once in the morning.

R. Sundmacher (Freiburg) : We have relied on the results of other
groups. Our own experience has been that application of just
one drop daily gave the satisfactory results which we

published. In your studies, if I understand them correctly, you have used quite low interferon titers, where as we have always used the highest titer available. This is an important difference.

BETA INTERFERON CREAM THERAPY IN PERIOCULAR HERPETIC INFECTIONS.

*   **   ***
ROMANO A., REVEL M., DOERNER T.
*M. AND G. GOLDSCHLEGER EYE INST. TEL AVIV UNIV. - SACKLER SCHOOL OF
MEDICINE CHAIM SHEBA MEDICAL CENTER.
**WEIZMANN INST. REHOVOT. ***INTER-YEDA LTD. NESS ZIONA, ISRAEL

Interferons were used for the local treatment of viral ocular diseases,
in the form of injections, eye drops and cream. Alpha interferon cream
has been used for the treatment of various dermal viral diseases like
labial and genital Herpes, genital warts and other skin manifestations
caused by viruses (verrucas etc..) (1) (2) (3)
Local applications of human interferon for the treatment and prophylaxis
of dendritic keratitis has been used experimentally in animals and
clinical trials in patients.
It was found that a combination of interferon with either mechanical
debridement of the diseased corneal epithelium or with antiviral agents
in the form of eyedrops are more effective than any monotherapy.
Sundmacher, Neumann-Hafelin, Manthey and Muller described the use of
human leucocyte interferon, in combination with thermocautery and
Trifluro thymidine (T.F.T.). It is clear from controlled clinical
trials that Interferon is active in the treatments of established
herpetic eye diseases. It was also shown that interferon has also some
prophylactic effect in preventing recurrent onsets of the disease.
(4) (5) (6).
Usually the dendritic ulcers caused by H.S.V. are treated with various
dosages of alpha interferon,several investigators reported good clinical
results using this treatment. (7) (8) (9).
However, it has been shown in other studies that there are no significant
differences between alpha and beta interferons in the treatment of
Herpetic dendritic Keratitis. (10) Other ocular viral diseases also
responded favourably to beta interferon treatment. (11) (12)
Human beta interferon (FRONE$^{(R)}$, Inter-Yeda Ltd., Israel), developed
at the Weizmann Institute of Science in Rehovot, is produced for clinical
evaluation in lyophilized form for ophthalmic and systemic use (specific

Maudgal, P.C. and Missotten, L., (eds.) Herpetic Eye Diseases.
© *1985, Dr W. Junk Publishers, Dordrecht/Boston/Lancaster. ISBN 978-94-010-8935-7*

activity more than 10^7 I.U./mg protein) and in a cream form for dermal application only (specific activity more than 10^6 I.U./ mg protein). Beta interferon in the form of P.E.G. cream was used in the treatment of periocular H.S.V. infection.

For ethical reasons, we conducted a randomized single blinded trial that was compared to (a)14 similarly treated IDU patients; (b) the natural course of the disease in untreated patients (recorded in our files); published data about acyclovir cream treated patients with recurrent or orofacial herpes simplex infections (13).

14 patients suffering from periocular herpetic lesions and sometimes' from dendritic keratitis were treated by FRONE cream for the periocular herpetic skin lesions and by ARABINOSIDE -A cream, for the corneal lesions, according to the severity of infections.

Among these patients suffering from primary H.S.V. infections and 10 patients suffering from recurred H.S.V. infections.

Table 1

The distributions and the location of the herpetic lesions in 14 interferon cream treated patients.

= Palpebral only

= Palpebral & dendritic keratitis

= Palpebral & facial

Table 2

Age distribution of the interferon cream treated group.

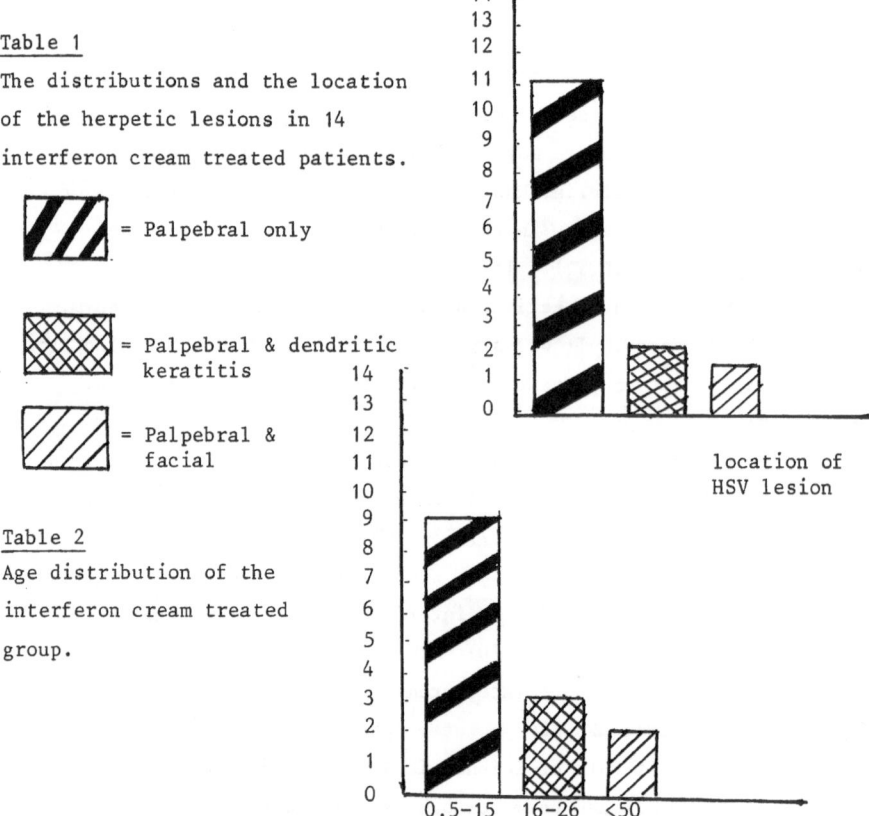

location of HSV lesion

Age (years)

<u>Treatment</u> : Mean duration of FRONE cream application was 6 times daily for 5-7 days by HFIN cream containing : 20,000 I.U./gr daily. Total HFIN used was 100,000 I.U. - 200,000 IU (1-2 tubes) per treatment.

Clinical and Laboratory Results

Patients treated with FRONE (interferon) cream recovered within an average of 6.3 days (3-9 days) comparably to the mean recovery of 7 days for IDU treatments and more than 12 days, which is the natural course of this disease.

Table 3

Mean time until complete healing in patients treated by IDU Acyclovir and FRONE cream.

mean time to complete healing (in days)	FRONE	ACYCLOVIR *	IDU **	NON-TREATED
	6.3	5.6	7.0	>12

* Data taken from published reference (13).

** Our historic group.

It should be noted that the FRONE treated group (14 patients) included 4 primary, local infected patients.

These patients were more sensitive to interferon treatment.
This may require further investigations considering the therapeutic benefits of interferon treatment for patients suffering from primary onsets of the disease.

Table 4

Viral shedding
before and during
the treatment by
interferon cream.

n = No. of
    patients
    with virus
    isolation

n = 12 patients

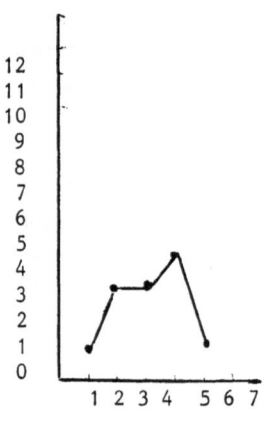

7 days of
viral
shedding.

Positive HSV shedding at time 0 before treatment was found in 12 patients
from periocular area. In two patients 50 years old, though clinically
proven to have palpebralis viruses could not be detected in the
laboratory at time 0 or through the treatment. Six times daily
applications of FRONE of 5-7 days resulted in disappearance of virus
within a mean of 4 days from therapy start. This compared with IDU
treatment where mean viral disappearance time was 4 days.

Side effects :

2 patients out of 14 cases developed allergic reactions : eyelid edema,
erythema and tearing at site of infection after FRONE application.
Both cases were treated by oral antihistamine tablets (INCIDAL) and
FRONE treatment continued till cure.

Antiinflamatory effect :

It should be noted that FRONE cream treatment resulted in an effective
and quick response in reducing the inflamatory reactions, i.e. reducing
the edema within 24 hours of treatment, and the itching, burning and
erythema symptoms. This pronounced antiinflamatory effect somewhat
resembles the steroid activity. This anti-inflamatory effect may be
due to its effect on antibody production and macrophages formation
regulation (15).

SUMMARY AND CONCLUSIONS

Local periocular treatment of HSV by HFIN cream is effective in :
a)   quick disappearance of HSV from infection site.
b)   quick relief response of patients after local administration.
c)   reasonable recovery time as compared to other antiviral agents.
d)   low incidence of side effects.

However considering that 1) antiviral agents are sometimes toxic

2) part of the patients are IDU and Acyclovir resistant (14) and not all patients respond favourably to the other antimetabolic agents.

We believe that treatment with FRONE cream may be beneficial therapy against periocular HSV in ophthalmology, especially in children with periocular lesions and also in other viral skin lesions. The possible synergistic effects between interferon and other antiviral agents as shown in vitro and in vivo and the potential role of HFIN in the prevention of recurrent HSV must still be evaluated.

354

References

1. K., CANTELL, K.& ARMSTRONG, J.A. (1981). Intralesional treatment
   of warts with interferon-a and its long term effect on NK cell
   activity. In The Biology of the Interferon System, ed.E.De Maeyer,
   G. Galasso & H. Schellekens, pp.661-5. London, New York, Amsterdam:
   Elsevier/North-Holland

2. IKIC, D., BOSNIC, N., SMERDEL, S., JUSIC, D., SOOS, E. & DELIMAR,N.
   (1975). Double-blind study with human leukocyte interferon in the
   therapy of condylomata acuminata. In Proceedings of a Symposium
   on Clinical Use of Interferon, ed. D. Ikic, pp.229-33.Zagreb:
   Yugoslav Academy of Sciences and Arts.

3. ISAACS, A. & HITCHCOCK, G. (1980). Role of interferon in recovery
   from virus infections. Lancet, ii, 69-71.

4. SUNDMACHER, R., CANTELL, K. & NEUMANN-HAEFELIN, D.(1978a).
   Combination therapy of dendritic keratitis with trifluorothymidine
   and interferon. Lancet, ii, 687.

5. SUNDMACHER, R., CANTELL, K. & NEUMANN-HAEFELIN, D. (1981).
   Evaluation of interferon in ocular viral diseases. In The Biology
   of the Interferon System, ed.E. De Maeyer, G. Galasso &
   H. Schellekens, pp. 343-50. London, New York,Amsterdam:
   Elsevier/North-Holland.

6. SUNDMACHER, R., NEUMANN-HAEFELIN, D., MANTHERY, K.F. & MULLER, O.
   (1976). Interferon in treatment of dendritic keratitis in humans:
   a preliminary report. Journal of Infectious Diseases, 133,
   A160-A164.

7. SUNDMACHER, R., NEUMANN-HAEFELIN, D. & CANTELL, K.(1976).
   Successful treatment of dendritic keratitis with human leucocyte
   interferon - a controlled clinical study. Graefes Archiv fur
   Klinische und Experimentelle Ophthalmologie, 201, 39-45.

8. KAUFMAN, H.E., MEYER, R.F., LAIBSON, P.R., WALTMAN, S.R.,
   NESBURN, A.B. & SHUSTER, J.J.(1976).Human leukocyte interferon
   for the prevention of recurrences of herpetic keratitis. Journal
   of Infectious Diseases, 133, A165-A168.

9. MERIGAN, T.C.,REED, S.E., HALL, T.S.& TYRRELL, D.A.J.(1973).
   Inhibition of respiratory virus infection by locally applied
   interferon. Lancet i, 563-7.

10. LINDENMANN, J., BURKE, D.C. & ISAACS, A.(1957). Studies on the production, mode of action and properties of interferon. British Journal of Experimental Pathology, 38, 551-62.

11. ROMANO, A., REVEL,M., GUARARI-ROTMAN, D., BLUMENTHAL, M.& STEIN, R. (1980). Use of human fibroblast derived (Beta) interferon in the treatment of epidemic adenovirus keratoconjunctivitis. Journal of Interferon Research, 1, 95-100.

12. SACKS, S.L., SCULLARD, G.H., POLLARD, R.B., GREGORY, P.G., ROBINSON, W.S. & MERIGAN, T.C. (1982). Antiviral treatment of chronic hepatitis B virus infection IV. Pharmacokinetics and side effects of interferon and adenine arabinoside alone and in combination. Antimicrobial Agents and Chemotherapy, 21, 95-100.

13. WILLIAM, A., VAN VLOTEN, ROBERT N.J.,STEWART AND FRANS PUB. (1983) Topical acyclovir therapy in patients with recurrent orofacial herpes simplex infections. Journal of Antimicrobial chemother. 12. Suppl. B 89-93.

14. DEKKER, C., ELLIS, M.N., McLAREN, C., HUNTER, G., ROGERS, J., BARRY, D.W.
(1983) Virus resistance in clinical practice. Journal of Antimicrobial chemotherapy, 12, Suppl. B., 137-152.

15. HOOKS, J.J., DETMICK-HOOKS, B.,
Immunoregulatory actions of interferon. Molecular aspects Med. Vol. 5, p. 183-196., 1982.

Address reprint requests to :

Dr. AMALIA ROMANO

HEAD OF LAB. FOR OPHTHALMIC MICROBIOLOGY AND EYE INFECTION

MAURICE AND GABRIELA GOLDSCHLEGER EYE INSTITUTE

RESEARCH DEPARTMENT

TEL AVIV UNIVERSITY - SACKLER SCHOOL OF MEDICINE

CHAIM SHEBA MEDICAL CENTER

TEL HASHOMER 52621, ISRAEL

356

DISCUSSION :

B. Juel-Jensen (Oxford) : I am slightly worried by some of the
things you said. First of all you say that your method of
treatment is particulary useful in primary herpes. It is likely
that the skin infection you are dealing with was primary herpes because you said it lasted 21 days. In recurrent herpes
the average duration in untreated patients is about 8 days.
But you did not produce any proof that your patients had a
primary infection. That is to say you did not tell us anything
about antibodies. Whether you started with no antibodies and
there was a rise. Second, some twenty years ago, Burnett and
Katz[1] and we in Oxford [2], and seven years later Kibrich and
Katz[3] showed that IDU in cream does not cross the skin. In
other words it is inactive. I wonder what magic you had in
your base to make it cross the skin. One wonders whether, in
fact, there was any effect other than placebo effect from your
interferon. The last point is that the first slide you showed of
zoster, was not ophthalmic zoster. It was the zoster of the
maxillary division of the nerve.

1. Burnett, J.W. and Katz, S.L. : A study of 5-iodo-2'-deoxy-
   uridine in cutaneous herpes simplex. J.Invest-Dermatol. 40 :
   7,1963

2. Juel-Jensen, B.E. and Mac Callum, F.O. : Treatment of herpes
   simplex lesions of the face with idoxuridine : results of a
   double-blind controlled trial. Brit. Med. J., II, 987-988, 1974.

3. Kibrick, S. and Katz, A.S. : Topical idoxuridine in recurrent
   herpes simplex. Ann. N.Y. Acad. Sci; 173, 83-89, 1970.

A. Romano (Tel Hashomer) : Viral isolation from dermal lesions
were obtained only during the acute phase of the disease. In
our experience, in dermal recurrent H.S.V. infections, the
average duration of periocular skin lesions in untreated patients is usually 12-14 days. Only in mild cases is the
duration of infection about 8 days. However, in the primary
infections the duration of the disease is about 21 days. As for
the other part of your question, we perform virological and
serological tests in all new patients and we follow the titers of

antibodies at the beginning of the disease (before starting the treatment), during the testing, and at the end of the acute phase. We then also follow-up the patients during the latent periods. In these tests we search for specific antibodies against H.S.V. and for IgG, IgA, IgM in serum and tears. Presence of IgM is a marker for primary infection. Interferon titration in tears and serum was also performed and we also looked for specific antibodies for beta-interferon. Please note that our interferon treatment in patients suffering from severe recurrent infections with periocular vesicles and their reaction to the antiviral agents were known. Regarding the last part of the question, IDU cream may well penetrate the skin as during the acute phase of the infection, the skin is not intact.

Also at the time of the study this IDU cream was our only dermal agent for H.S.V. skin infections. Unlike ophthalmic infections, dermal infections were open wounds, vesicles and ulcers of the skin ; there is a close contact between the antiviral agent and the viruses. To conclude, the clinical and laboratory results of interferon treatment showed reduction of acute phase of the disease and the reduction of the time to viral negative shedding. This was especially noted in those patients who were previously treated by other antiviral agents.

We can therefore conclude that the interferon treatment is effective in the acute phase of the disease.

B. Juel-Jensen (Oxford) : Yes. You still have not answered my question. You made the assumption that your results would appear to bear out that IDU cream is active. You gave examples of patients most of whom may have had primary infection of the skin, as you said virus was isolated for three weeks. I find it surprising that you did not specify that all your patients in your series had primary infections. Because if you compare recurrent with primary, you are not comparing like with like. And you still haven't answered my question. What base do you have your IDU in, since you claim that it is active. This is very strange since three independent groups have shown in the past that it doesn't work.

T. Doerner (Tel Aviv) : IDU cream is registered in Israel, I suppose also in other countries, for treatment of herpes labialis
and herpes genitalis. We don't have data on this cream
because we are not the manufacturer of this cream. We can
have the same assumptions about the acyclovir cream which is
new dermal 5% cream. Again you can ask how does it penetrate into the skin ? The IDU cream is our control, we suppose
as it is registered and it has been proven for the treatment of
skin herpes. It is the only agent available anyway. Regarding
the duration, I don't agree to the mean duration of recurrent
herpes, type 1 and type 2. There are many patients whose
recurrent herpes simplex virus infection took about 21 to 24
days even with treatment.

B. Juel-Jensen (Oxford) : My dear, read the literature.

HUMAN LEUKOCYTE INTERFERON PLUS TRIFLUOROTHYMIDIN VERSUS
RECOMBINANT ALPHA 2 ARG INTERFERON PLUS TRIFLUOROTHYMIDIN
FOR THERAPY OF DENDRITIC KERATITIS. A CONTROLLED CLINICAL
STUDY

R.Sundmacher[1], D.Neumann-Haefelin[2], A.Mattes[1], W.Merk[3],
G.Adolf[4], and K.Cantell[5]

[1]University Eye Clinic, D7800 Freiburg, West-Germany
[2]Institute of Virology of the University, D-7800 Freiburg
[3]Dr.Karl Thomae GmbH, D-7950 Biberach 1, West-Germany
[4]Ernst-Boehringer-Institut für Arzneimittelforschung,
                              A-1121 Wien, Austria
[5]National Public Health Institute, SF-00280 Helsinki,
                                            Finland

1. SUMMARY

Thirty-two patients with virologically proven dendritic keratitis received trifluorothymidine eye drops as a basic
therapy. In addition, they were treated at random with either huIFN alpha (Le)($30x10^6$ IU/ml, 1 drop daily), or with
rhuIFN alpha 2 arg ($23x10^6$ IU/ml, 1 drop daily). The natural
interferon preparation from human leukocytes proved to be
more effective than the E.coli derived alpha 2 interferon.
The average healing times were 2.6 days and 3.6 days respectively.

2. INTRODUCTION

Healing of dendritic keratitis is considerably accelerated
if interferon is topically applied in addition to a potent
synthetic antiherpetic agent. This has not only been shown
for the combination trifluorothymidine-interferon (Sundmacher et al, 1978; de Koning et al, 1982) but also for the
combination acyclovir-interferon (Colin et al, 1983; de Koning et al, 1983). The enhancing effect of interferon is

Maudgal, P.C. and Missotten, L., (eds.) Herpetic Eye Diseases.
© *1985, Dr W. Junk Publishers, Dordrecht/Boston/Lancaster. ISBN 978-94-010-8935-7*

titer-dependant. The best results have up till now been obtained with interferon titers ranging from 30 to 100×10^6 IU/ml (Sundmacher, 1982, 1984; Sundmacher et al, 1981, 1984). All published studies were performed with human leukocyte interferon, of which the subtype alpha 2 is a major constituent. The aim of the present study was to investigate whether a highly purified E.coli derived alpha 2 subtype has the same enhancing effects as natural leukocyte interferon.

3. PATIENTS, MATERIALS AND METHODS

Selection of patients, virological controls, randomization, and the procedures for evaluating the results were the same as in our previous studies (Sundmacher et al, 1978, 1981, 1984). Patients with a clinical diagnosis of dendritic or geographic keratitis were randomly allocated to groups 1 or 2. First corneoconjunctival washings were performed with Eagle's minimal essential medium. They were later processed for virus culture on human foreskin fibroblasts. Then, the patients received one drop of interferon preparation 1 or 2 respectively into the cul de sac, and remained in a reclined position for 10 minutes to ensure sufficient contact time for the interferon preparation with the ocular surface. Preparation 1 contained rhuIFN alpha 2 arg (23×10^6 IU/ml), and preparation 2 consisted of huIFN alpha (Le)(30×10^6 IU/ml).The leukocyte interferon was the same as used by us in previous clinical studies.The specific activity was $\leq 1.25 \times 10^7$ IU/mg of protein (Cantell and al, 1981). The E.coli derived interferon was provided by Boehringer, Ingelheim. Human IFN alpha 2 arg mRNA derived from Sendai virus-induced Namalwa cells was cloned in E.coli (Dworkin-Rastl et al, 1982). The amino acid sequence of this IFN is identical with that of IFN alpha 2 described by Streuli et al (1980) except for amino acid 34 which is arginine instead of histidine. The protein was expressed in E.coli (Dworkin-Rastl et al, 1983) and purified to homogeneity (purity $\geq 98\%$). The preparation was stabilized by addition of human serum albumin (20mg/ml). The specific activity of the rhuIFN alpha 2 arg preparation was 2×10^8 IU/mg protein. Contaminating proteins larger than 70.000 daltons could not be found, nor were there detectable amounts of foreign antigens. The endotoxin content was less than 0.5 nanogram/ml.

The patients were instructed to apply 5 drops of trifluorothymidine 1% (TFT)(Dr.Mann,Berlin) during the course of the day. Every morning, they received their coded interferon preparation after virus isolation. Interferon was given for the last time when the corneal epithelium had healed fluorescein-negative (except for minor punctate stainings). The time required to achieve this criterion was termed healing time, and evaluated statistically (Chi-square tests with Yates correction). TFT was given for three more days after healing time, and then also withdrawn. Usually, artificial tears were additionally administered for some weeks as a prophylactic measure against postherpetic (metaherpetic) healing disorders. Only those patients were accepted for final evaluation in whom at least one virus culture was positive for herpes simplex virus. Thus the viral etiology of the disease treated was proven, and it was assured that no protracted aviral (metaherpetic) cases complicated evaluation of the results.

4. RESULTS

Of 42 patients who entered the study, 32 fulfilled the criteria of the protocol and could thus be evaluated. Seventeen received leukocyte interferon, and 15 were treated with recombinant alpha 2 arg interferon. Virus shedding was equal in both groups (fig.1).

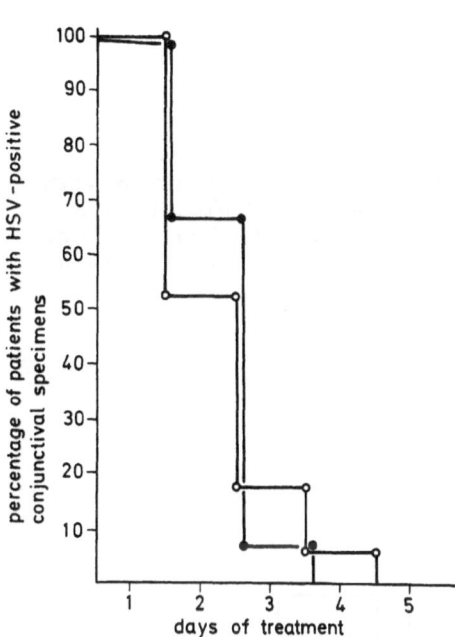

fig.1   Virus shedding curves after treatment with TFT plus huIFN alpha (Le)(●——●, average shedding time 1.73 days), and with TFT plus rhu-IFN alpha 2 arg (o——o, average shedding time 1.76 days).

However, the time course of healing was clearly different (fig.2). The average healing times were 3.6 days with alpha 2 arg interferon, but only 2.6 days with leukocyte interferon (fig.3). The difference was significant on the third day of therapy (X^2=8.58; p=0.003)

5. DISCUSSION

Since alpha 2 interferon is a major constituent of natural human leukocyte interferon, we expected to find similar results when combining leukocyte interferon or a recombinant alpha 2 interferon respectively with TFT for treatment of dendritic keratitis. This assumption turned out to be only partly correct.

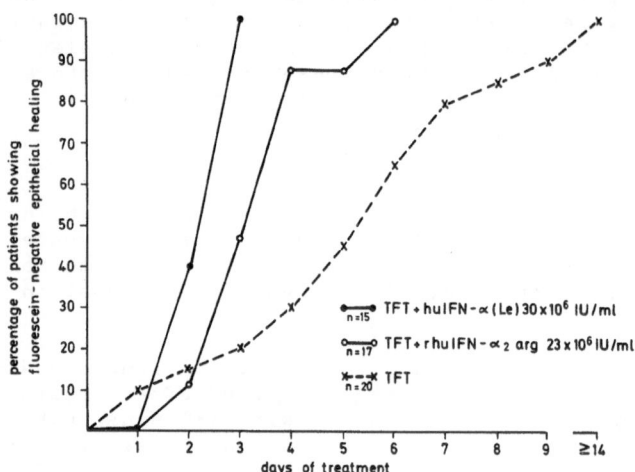

fig.2   Healing curves of dendritic keratitis treated with
either TFT plus huIFN alpha (Le) or with TFT plus rhuIFN
alpha 2 arg respectively. For comparison, the healing curve
after therapy with TFT alone is included. This curve stems from
a former study (Sundmacher et al, 1981).

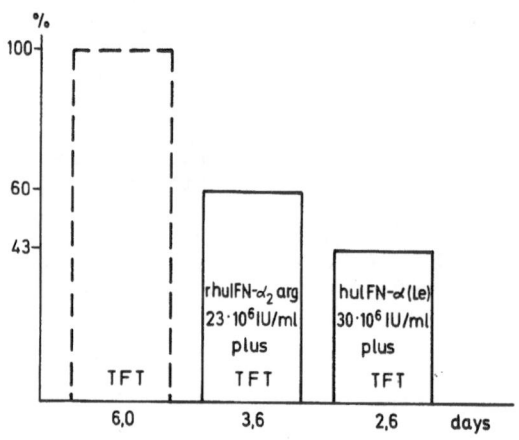

fig.3   Average healing times of dendritic keratitis (same
groups as in fig.2)

Although we did not test rhuIFN alpha 2 arg plus TFT directly against TFT plus placebo, a comparison with the data of a pure TFT group shows that the recombinant interferon was effective (fig.2).The TFT data stem from a previous study of our group and were collected in a randomized, placebo-controlled procedure following the same criteria as in the study here presented. Though strictly speaking not allowed, it is possible to illustrate the effectiveness of the rhuIFN alpha 2 arg - TFT combination therapy by calculating the probabilities of error according to the Chi-square test with Yates correction. During the first three days of therapy there is is no difference between both types of treatment. Then the difference becomes highly significant: day four $p=0.001$, day five $p=0.01$, day six $p=0.02$.

So far, our assumption was correct that a recombinant alpha 2 interferon should be effective in a combination therapy with TFT of dendritic keratitis. This is in accordance with the results of other studies, which demonstrated effectiveness of alpha 2 interferon preparations for prophylaxis of respiratory diseases (Hayden and Gwaltney, 1983; Herzog et al, 1983; Scott et al, 1982) or simian varicella virus infections in monkeys (Soike et al, 1983).

However, the natural human leukocyte interferon was still more effective then the recombinant alpha 2 interferon with a significant difference on the third day ($p=0.003$). This difference is larger than could be attributed to the relatively small difference in interferon titers ($\Delta \log=0.12$). Thus we have to look for some other reasons which may explain the difference. Firstly, it may be that the recombinant interferon preparation had some toxic effect which could have hindered epithelial resurfacing. Biomicroscopically, however, there were no signs of epithelial toxicity in either group. Secondly, the minor variation of the alpha 2 interferon used (arginine instead of histidine in position 34) may have been operative. This is unlikely, at least in terms of antiviral activity. We did not only test both interferons in the standard assay with vesicular stomatitis virus, but also in multiple assays with herpes simplex virus type 1. In both types of interferon assay we found only the same slight difference of about Δ 0.12 log units/ml, which does not explain the observed clinical differences. Third, natural human leukocyte interferon is composed not only of alpha 2 interferon but also of other different interferon species and other plasma proteins, the biological activity of which is not well defined at present. It may be thatthe combination of different interferons and the presence of these plasma proteins has advantages over the application of pure interferon species. To clarify the latter possibility, more experimental and clinical studies with different types of interferons as well as with different interferon combinations are needed.

REFERENCES

Cantell K, Hirvonen S, Koistinen V (1981) Partial purification of human leukocyte interferon on a large scale. Meth.Enzymol. 78, 499-505

Colin J, Chastel C, Renard G and Cantell K (1983) Combination therapy for dendritic keratitis with human leukocyte interferon and acyclovir. Amer.J.Ophthal. 95, 346-348

Dworkin-Rastl E, Swetly P and Dworkin MB (1983) Construction of expression plasmids producing high levels of human leukocyte-type interferon in E.coli. Gene 21, 237-248

Dworkin-Rastl E, Dworkin MB and Swetly P (1982) Molecular cloning of human alpha and beta interferon genes from Namalwa cells. J.Interferon Res.2, 575-585

Hayden FG and Gwaltney JM jr (1983) Intranasal interferon alpha 2 for prevention of rhinovirus infection and illness. J.Infect.Dis. 148, 543-550

Herzog CH, Just M, Berger R, Havas L and Fernex M (1983) Intranasal interferon for contact prophylaxis against common cold in families. Lancet II, 962

De Koning EWJ, van Bijsterveld OP and Cantell K (1982) Combination therapy for dendritic keratitis with human leukocyte interferon and trifluorothymidine. Br.J.Ophthalmol. 66, 509-512

De Koning EWJ, van Bijsterveld OP and Cantell K (1983) Combination therapy for dendritic keratitis with acyclovir and alpha-interferon. Arch.Ophthalmol. 101, 1866-1868

Scott GM, Wallace J, Greiner J, Phillpotts RJ, Gauci CL and Tyrell DAJ (1982) Prevention of rhinovirus colds by human interferon alpha-2 from E.coli. Lancet II, 186-188

365

Soike KF, Kramer MJ and Gerone PJ (1983) In vivo antiviral activity of recombinant type alpha interferon A in monkeys with infections due to simian varicella virus. J.Infect.Dis. 147, 933-938

Streuli M, Nagata S and Weissmann C (1980) At least three human type alpha interferons: structure of alpha 2. Science 209, 1343-1347

Sundmacher R (1982) Interferon in ocular viral diseases. In: Interferon 4 (I Gresser, ed.) pp 177-200, London - New York, Academic Press

Sundmacher R (1984) The role of interferon in prophylaxis and treatment of dendritic keratitis. In: Herpes Simplex Infections of the Eye (FC Blodi, ed.) in press, Contemporary Issues in Ophthalmology, Churchill Livingstone

Sundmacher R, Cantell K and Mattes A (1984) Combination therapy for dendritic keratitis with high-titer alpha-interferon and trifluorothymidine. Arch.Ophthalmol. 102, 554-555

Sundmacher R, Cantell K and Neumann-Haefelin D (1978) Combination therapy of dendritic keratitis with trifluorothymidine and interferon. Lancet II, 687

Sundmacher R, Neumann-Haefelin D and Cantell K (1981) Therapy and prophylaxis of dendritic keratitis with topical human interferon. In: Herpetic Eye Diseases (R Sundmacher, ed.) pp 401-407, Munich, Bergmann

DISCUSSION :

C. Claoué (Southampton) : I go back to your slide where you combined the data from this study with the pure TFT study. In your first day both interferon groups showed no healing where as in your TFT only trial 20% of your patients had completely healed. Do you think that is just the chance observation ?

R. Sundmacher (Freiburg) : Yes, That's a chance observation.

J. Colin (Brest) : Are you sure that the difference in titer could not explain the difference in healing ?

R. Sundmacher (Freiburg) : I must admit that I was really annoyed when I learnt that the titers of both interferons had not been adjusted to exactly the same level. However, in all test systems which we tried; vesicular stomatitis virus as well as herpes simplex virus tests, we consistently found only the small titer difference of log 0,1. From my experience that is too little to account for the highly significant clinical difference.

J. Colin (Brest) : Have you treated with interferon the patients who have ever been treated with interferon in previous studies ? If so, what were the results ?

R. Sundmacher (Freiburg) : Yes, I have. There were no differences in the results.

G. Smolin (San Fransisco) : I wanted to ask you whether or not you know if there is any difference in recurrence rate between the patients that were just given an antiviral, like trifluorthymidine, and those who were treated with interferon and antiviral.
Have you had opportunity to follow these patients ?

R. Sundmacher (Freiburg) : Yes. We have about thousand herpes patients on file. I did not look them up with this special question in mind. From my clinical judgment, however, the recurrence rate does not depend on the type of previous therapy. In making this statement, I speak only of true recurrences and not of flaring up of an insufficiently treated chronic process.

ACYCLOVIR AND RECOMBINANT HUMAN ALPHA 2 ARG INTERFERON TREATMENT FOR
DENDRITIC KERATITIS

P.J. MEURS AND O.P. VAN BIJSTERVELD (KONINKLIJK NEDERLANDS GASTHUIS
VOOR OOGLIJDERS,UNIVERSITY OF UTRECHT,UTRECHT,HOLLAND)

1. INTRODUCTION

Since the clinical introduction of anti-herpes virus agents there has
been progressive improvement in the treatment of herpetic epithelial
keratitis.It was Kaufman in 1962 who introduced idoxuridine(IDU) in the
treatment of dendritic keratitis.In many studies the efficacy of IDU was
confirmed but it had many toxic side-effects,especially when used over
a long period of time,as demonstated by Jones in 1967.In 1972 Wellings
found trifluorothymidine(TFT) to be more effective than IDU.At the
same time Pavan-Langston and Dohlman concluded arabinoside(ara-A) to be
more effective than IDU.Van Bijsterveld and Post compared TFT and ara-A
and found no difference in antiviral activity between these two drugs.
In 1979 Jones published for the first time the positive results of the
treatment of dendritic keratitis with acycloguanosine(Acyclovir,ACV,
Zovirax^R).
Kaufman and Jones used Interferon(IFN) in epithelial herpetic keratitis
as antiviral agent.If given alone this drug did not appear to be very
effective,but Interferon in combination with TFT was found to be more
effective than TFT alone by Sundmacher et al. and de Koning et al.
Similar results were found for the combination of ACV and Interferon by
de Koning et al.In all these cases human leucocyte alpha-Interferon was
used.
As a result of the development of gen-technology,recombinant human
alpha 2 arg Interferon(rHu alpha 2 arg IFN)became available.In a double
masked randomised trial we compared the results of the combination of ACV
and rHu alpha 2 arg IFN with ACV and human serum placebo.In all thirty-
six eyes we treated,all patients had dendritic keratitis or one of its
superficial variants.Patients with metaherpes or stromal forms of herpes
keratitis were excluded from the trial.

Maudgal, P.C. and Missotten, L., (eds.) Herpetic Eye Diseases.
© *1985, Dr W. Junk Publishers, Dordrecht/Boston/Lancaster. ISBN 978-94-010-8935-7*

2. MATERIALS AND METHODS

Of the thirty-six patients 28 were male and 8 were female.They all had
a recent history of herpes dendritic keratitis or other superficial
forms or with a recurrence which occured six weeks after healing of the
preceeding attack of illness at the earliest.These patients were
included in a double blind placebo controlled trial to compare the
results of the combination of ACV and rHu alpha 2 arg IFN with ACV and
Placebo on the healing time of acute dendritic keratitis.All patients
received ACV ointment every 2 hours.In addition they received every
morning at the same time after careful eye examination one drop of
rHu alpha 2 arg IFN or Placebo in a recumbent position.After a ten
minutes interval each patient received a second drop,the patient
remained in a reclined position for another ten minutes to insure that
the recombinant IFN or Placebo kept in contact with the epithelial
lesion in the cornea.Treatment with rHu alpha 2 arg IFN or Placebo was
done in a double blind way.The trial medication is embodied in a plastic
tube of about 12 cm length -a both side welded 'drop-cannula'- which is
enclosed in an applicator (Fig. 1).

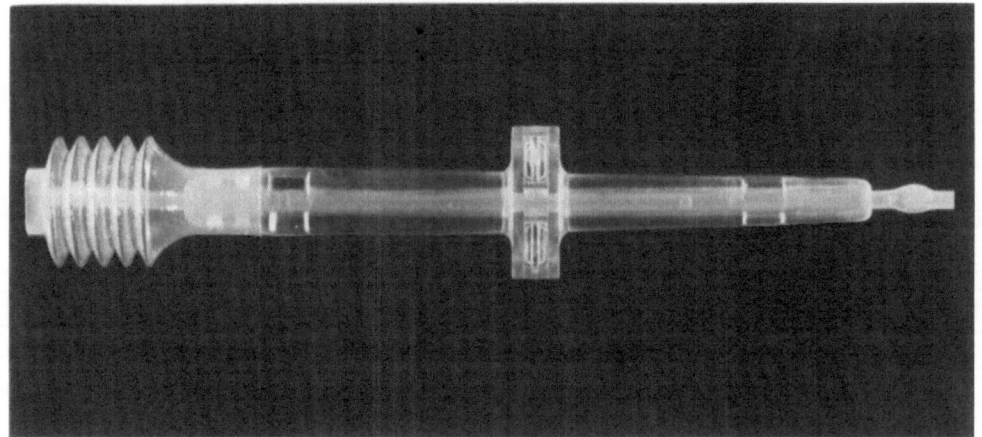

FIGURE 1. A both side welded 'drop-cannula',which contains 0.05 ml
rHu alpha 2 arg IFN or 0.05 ml human serum albumin(Placebo).

These tubes are numbered 1 to 36 and stored at -20° C or colder.The
thawing and warming to the approximate room temperature takes about
twenty minutes.Each verum tubulus containes 0.05 ml Interferon solution

$\triangleq 1.5 \times 10^6$ IU rHu alpha 2 arg IFN.Each Placebo tubulus containes 0.05
ml human serum albumin solution 3 %.

Before treatment we isolated herpes simplex virus from the corneal lesion
by minimal whiping and also from the conjunctiva,which was carried out
with two cotton wool sticks.These sticks were brought into a Gly medium.
Virus isolation and identification was done at the National Institute
of Public Health in Bilthoven,the Netherlands.Two criteria for healing,
as used by van Bijsterveld,Post and de Koning,were used,i.e.:
partial healing,a condition whereby no staining of the epithelium of the
cornea with fluorescein is found and complete healing,the situation
whereby in addition there is absence of the epithelial oedema and
microcystic changes.We gave the rHu alpha 2 arg IFN or Placebo untill
complete healing was reached.ACV was continued six days after complete
healing had occured.

3. RESULTS

Treatment did not fail in any of the patients probably due to the
carefully selection criteria we used,because only patients with a fresh
epithelial herpetic keratitis were admitted to the trial.Of the 36
patients(28 male and 8 female),17(15 male and 2 female) were treated
with the ACV and Placebo combination and 19(13 male and 6 female) with
the ACV and rHu alpha 2 arg IFN combination.

Table 1. Characteristics of the two treatment groups.

	PLACEBO GROUP(N=17)	INTERFERON GROUP(N=19)
SEX,FEMALE	N = 2 PATIENTS	N = 6 PATIENTS
MALE	N = 15 PATIENTS	N = 13 PATIENTS
MEAN AGE(YEARS ± S.D.)	36.8 ± 15.8	46.3 ± 20.7
AFFECTED EYE,OD	N = 7 PATIENTS	N = 8 PATIENTS
OS	N = 10 PATIENTS	N = 11 PATIENTS
RECURRENCE,YES	N = 8 PATIENTS	N = 9 PATIENTS
NO	N = 9 PATIENTS	N = 10 PATIENTS

S.D = Standard Deviation

370

The age of the patients varied from 11 to 86 years,with an average of
42 years.Two patients had herpetic keratitis on both eyes;17 patients
had a large dendritic ulcer,15 a small dendritic lesion and 4 patients
had a geographic (ameboid) ulcer.9 patients had a concomitant cutaneous
herpes when treated.During the trial 2 patients had a recurrence in the
study period.Table 1 shows the patient characteristics in the two
treatment groups.In Fig. 2 the cumulative frequency distribution of the
partial healing time is given in patients treated with rHu alpha 2 arg
IFN and ACV and those treated with Placebo and ACV.

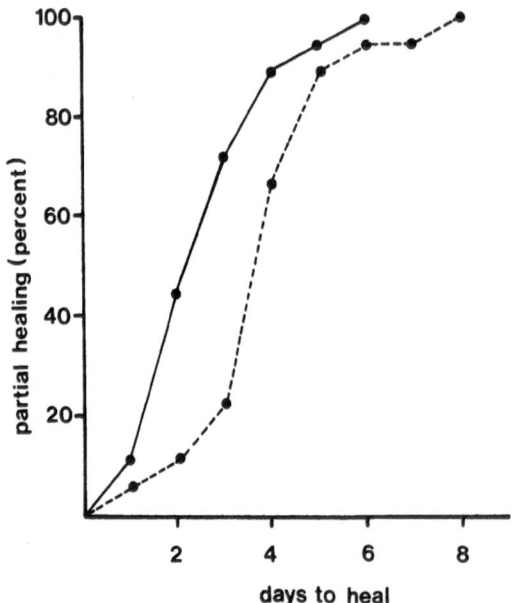

FIGURE 2. Cumulative frequency distribution of the partial healing
time.The black line represents the rHu alpha 2 arg IFN-ACV combination
and the dotted line the Placebo-ACV group.

The partial healing time of the group treated with ACV and rHu alpha 2
arg IFN was on the average 2.95 days and for the Placebo-ACV group 4.06
days.Table 2 shows the statistical data of partial healing.Table 3 is
the table of analysis of variance for these data.The difference of the
two groups is significant,P smaller than 0.05.

Table 2. Statistical data of partial healing.

	PLACEBO–ACYCLOVIR COMBINATION	RHU ALPHA 2 ARG IFN–ACYCLOVIR COMBINATION
NUMBER OF OBSERVATIONS (N)	17	19
AVERAGE DAYS TO HEAL	4.06	2.95
S.D. (N)	1.59	1.28
S.D. (N–1)	1.64	1.31

Table 3. Analysis of variance.Data of partial healing.Placebo-Acyclovir combination (N=17) versus rHu alpha 2 arg IFN-Acyclovir combination (N=19)

SOURCE	SUM OF SQUARES	DF	MEAN SUM OF SQUARES
TREATMENT	11.0837	1	11.0837
RESIDUAL	73.8885	34	2.1732
TOTAL	84.9722	35	

DF = Degrees of freedom.Treatment F^1_{34} = 5.1002   P smaller than 0.05

In Fig. 3 the number of days of complete healing in both treatment groups is given in a cumulative frequency graph.

The time for complete healing in the group treated with ACV and rHu alpha 2 arg IFN is on the average 5.58 days and in the Placebo-ACV group 7.47 days.Table 4 shows the statistical data of complete healing.

Table 4. Statistical data of complete healing.

	PLACEBO–ACYCLOVIR COMBINATION	RHU ALPHA 2 ARG IFN–ACYCLOVIR COMBINATION
NUMBER OF OBSERVATIONS (N)	17	19
AVERAGE DAYS TO HEAL	7.47	5.58
S.D. (N)	2.23	2.14
S.D. (N–1)	2.29	2.19

S.D. = Standard Deviation

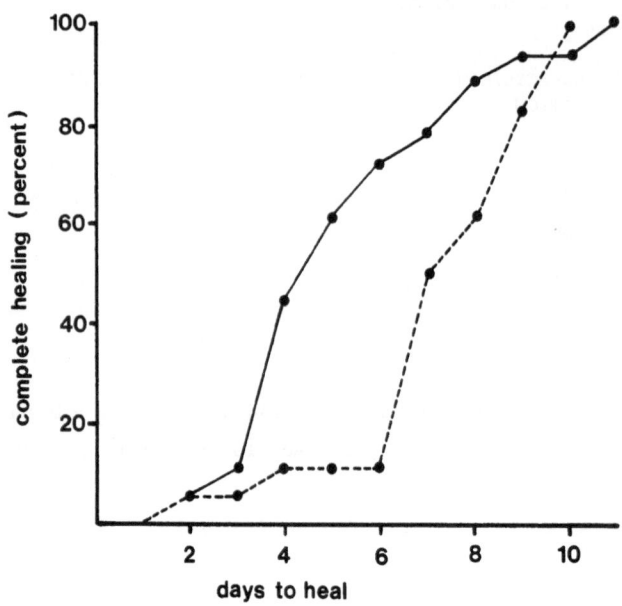

FIGURE 3. Cumulative frequency distribution of the complete healing
time.The black line represents the rHu alpha 2 arg IFN-ACV combination
and the dotted line the Placebo-ACV group.

Table 5 is the table of analysis of variance for the data of complete
healing.The difference between the two groups is significant,P smaller
than 0.025.

Table 5. Analysis of variance.Data of complete healing.Placebo-Acyclovir
combination(N=17) versus rHu alpha 2 arg IFN-ACV combination(N=19).

SOURCE	SUM OF SQUARES	DF	MEAN SUM OF SQUARES
TREATMENT	32.1053	1	82.1053
RESIDUAL	170.8669	34	5.0255
TOTAL	202.9722	35	

DF = Degrees of freedom.Treatment F^1_{34} = 6.4   P smaller than 0.025

4. DISCUSSION

In this study ACV was effective in the treatment of dendritic keratitis
but the lesions healed significantly more rapidly when rHu alpha 2 arg
IFN was combined with the virostatic therapy.

At the present time the best known treatment for herpetic epithelial
keratitis appears to be ACV or TFT in combination with potent
Interferon,either buffy coat leucocyte Interferon or rHu alpha 2 arg
IFN.

REFERENCES

1. Van Bijsterveld OP,Post H. 1980. Trifluorothymidine versus adenine
   arabinoside in the treatment of herpes simplex keratitis. Br. J.
   Ophthalmol. 64,33-36.
2. Jones BR. 1967. Prospects in treating viral disease of the eye.
   Transactions of the Ophthalmological Socities of the United
   Kingdom. 87,537-579.
3. Jones BR. 1981. Human Interferon in topical therapy of herpetic
   keratitis. In:Sundmacher R. ed. Herpetic eye diseases. Munich
   395-400.
4. Kaufman HE, Mantola EL, Dohlman C. 1962. Use of 5-iodo-2'-deoxy
   uridine (IDU) in treatment of herpes simplex keratitis. Arch.
   Ophthalmol. 68,235-239.
5. Kaufman HE, Meyer RF, Laibson PR, Waltmann SR, Nesburn AB, Shuster
   JJ. 1976. Human leucocyte Interferon for prevention of recurrences
   of herpetic keratitis. J. Infect. Dis. 133,165-168.
6. De Koning EWJ, van Bijsterveld OP, Cantell K. 1982. Combination
   therapy for dendritic keratitis with human leucocyte Interferon and
   trifluorothymidine. Br. J. Ophthalmol. 66,505-512.
7. De Koning EWJ,van Bijsterveld OP, Cantell K. 1983. Combination
   therapy for dendritic keratitis with Acyclovir and human alpha
   Interferon. Arch. Ophthalmol. 101,1866-1869.
8. Pavan-Langston D, Dohlman C. 1972. A double-blind clinical study
   of viral keratoconjunctivitis. Am. J. Ophthalmol. 74,81-88.
9. Sundmacher R,Cantell K, Neuman-Haefelin D. 1978. Combination therapy
   for dendritic keratitis with trifluorothymidine and Interferon.
   Lancet. ii:687.
10.Wellings PC, Awdry PN, Bors FH, Jones BR, Brown DC,Kaufman HE. 1972.
   Clinical evaluation of trifluorothymidine in the treatment of herpes
   simplex corneal ulcers. Am. J. Ophthalmol. 73,932-942.

ACKNOWLEDGEMENT

We are very indepted to the firms Bender,Thomae and Boehringer
Ingelheim for supplying us with recombinant human alpha 2 arg Interferon.

374

DISCUSSION

G. Smolin (San Francisco) : I would like to make the comment
that in some animal experiments we performed, despite what
has been stated in the literature, we found there is an optimal
dose of interferon. In the model we used, it wasn't one drop
a day, it was two drops twice a day. I also believe that it
is true, once you reach the optimal dose increasing the amount
of interferon you give, doesn't significantly alter the course
of disease. The question I have is, how do we know that the
dosage you have used was the optimal dose of interferon ?

P.J. Meurs (Utrecht) : It was the only dose we could get from
the firm. So, I could not experiment with the concentration
of interferon drops I get.

G. Smolin (San Francisco) : In the regimen you used, do you give
interferon just once a day or twice a day ?

P.J. Meurs (Utrecht) : I gave every morning when I see the patient in the Department, at 9 o'clock sharp. They get one drop,
in reclining position, and another drop 10 minutes later, and
then wait another 10 minutes. And that's it.

R. Sundmacher (Freiburg) : Perhaps I can provide some more information on Dr. Smolin's question. In our earliest studies with
low titer interferon we started with 6 drops of interferon daily.
We then reduced it to 4 drops daily with high titer interferon.
Currently, we administer only one drop of high titer interferon
daily, and we have not observed any loss of clinical efficacy.

A. Patterson (Liverpool) : Just three little questions. First is,
you did not present it here, but it will be interesting, do you
have in your clinic a group where you just treat the patients
with interferon alone to compare with other groups ? This will
appear to give a better base line, if you can. Second is, what
was the distribution between the two groups of the four patients
who had geographic ulcers ? I presume these were steroid induced geographic ulcers. Thirdly, could you explain why you
have designed a trial combining acyclovir and interferon versus

acyclovir alone ? In the acyclovir interferon group which drug to you think is more effective, is there any evidence of a synergistic effect between the two ?

P.J.Meurs (Utrecht) : To start with the last question, others have shown that interferon alone is not effective in the treatment of dendritic herpetic keratitis. At least not as effective as you might expect.

A. Patterson (Liverpool) : We did a trial which we reported in the literature in 1962. I quite agree with you, we compared patients with simple dendritic ulcers who received human interferon supplied by Isaac's from Covendale versus those who received water drops. Just over 50% of the patients with interferon healed in the usual time compared with 33% of patients who received water. So, for our clinic this provided the baseline that we expected with the interferon available to us then, to heal about 50% of patients. In your data here, 50% of the patients are healing with interferon. The rest are healing with acyclovir or what permutation do you think you are getting, or is there some chemical interaction between an antiviral agent and interferon which boosts the one or the other ?

P.J. Meurs (Utrecht) : I don't know the mechanism how acyclovir is working together with interferon or may be against it. Our results show that the placebo controlled group has definitely a longer healing time than the combination with interferon.

R. Sundmacher (Freiburg) : First of all, what you got from Sir Isaacs nobody can tell in terms of interferon units. There were certainly some molecules in it, but most of it was water and non-interferon molecules. So I don't know what your base line realy expressed. Secondly, there is good agreement now that even high titer interferon is not effective if it is applied as the only therapeutic agent in a true thereapeutic situation. Thirdly, the rationale for today's combination therapy of dendritic keratitis with high titer interferon plus antivirals has been the attempt to exploit the prophylactic potencies of interferon in a therapeutic situation. That sounds difficult, but it is not. Presumably, herpes simplex virus is not only shed once

from the terminal nerve endings in the cornea, but for a prolonged period of time, or repeatedly over a period of days.
The proposed role for interferon has been to inhibit this prolonged or repeated virus shedding, whereas the role for the
antivirals has been to eliminate virus from the cornea. I must
admit that I don't know whether this concept is true from the
pathophysiological point of view or whether other modes of action
are involved, e.g. the activity of interferon as immunomodulator.
This remains an open question. It is a fact, however, that
the combinations work excellently.

A. Romano (Tel Hashomer) : I have some experience about effectiveness of interferon in herpetic keratitis. Interferon does not
inhibit the re-epithelialization of the lesion. That is the reason,
I think, that high doses of interferon after two to four days
of treatment heal the dendritic lesion. The virus diseappears
after two days interferon application. Perhaps, it is good to
take the first day a high dose of interferon externally, and
in the 2nd, 3rd and 4th day a low dosage. A combination of
external interferon and inducer of interferon is perhaps a good
combination.

E. De Clercq (Leuven) : I would like to return to the question
of combination therapy of interferon with any of the other antiviral drugs, or combination of the antiviral drugs themselves.
There are some indications from in vitro experiments, that if
you have right compounds at the right concentrations at the
right time, you may have a synergistic effect; for instance,
between interferon and acyclovir. You have to remember that
the results depend on both the doses and the time of administration. In the optimal conditions you may have a benefit by
combining these antiviral drugs. Likewise, the effect of combination therapy on herpetic keratitis may depend on the timing
and the concentration of the drugs. If you want to establish
all the parameters that are required for an optimal synergistic effect, you may be busy for another 20 years.

THE ACUTE RETINAL NECROSIS SYNDROME AND RETINAL NECROSIS ASSOCIATED WITH ENCEPHALITIS

A. LEYS, B. DE CNODDER, AND L. MISSOTTEN*

The acute retinal necrosis syndrome (ARNS) is a well-established unilateral or bilateral condition of possibly herpetic origin in otherwise healthy patients (1,9-11,15,17,18, 33,36,38,39,41). Similar retinal necrosis can be the terminal stage of the chronic spreading retinitis of cytomegalovirus (CMV) inclusion disease or may result from a herpes simplex or herpes zoster infection (2-8,12,14,16,20-26,28-32, 34,35,37,40). Necrotic retinitis is rare disease relative to the incidence of localizations of CMV, herpes simplex, and herpes zoster elsewhere in the body and in the eye (8,13,19, 22,28,29). In the last five years, we have had one case of ARNS and observed two immunosuppressed patients who developed necrotic retinitis and encephalitis.

CASE 1

A 53-year old woman had had from childhood a bilateral optic atrophy with a stable visual restriction to light perception in her right eye and 1/15 in her left eye.

Three days after a slight contusion on her left temple, she developed misty vision in her left eye that progressed to blindness in a few days. The eye became red and tender due to hypertensive uveitis. One week after the contusion, she was referred to us by her ophthalmologist.

We observed a fresh necrotic retinitis complicated with hemorrhages spread out over the entire retina except for for the papillomacular region (Fig. 1a,b). The vitreous cleared

*Department of Ophthalmology, Katholieke Universiteit Leuven, U.Z. St. Rafäel, Kapucijnenvoer 7, B-3000 Leuven, Belgium.

Maudgal, P.C. and Missotten, L., (eds.) Herpetic Eye Diseases.
© *1985, Dr W. Junk Publishers, Dordrecht/Boston/Lancaster. ISBN 978-94-010-8935-7*

under local corticotherapy, and, three days later, when we compared the lesions with their previous condition, we saw that
they had become a denser yellow but that there was also partial
resorption of the necrotic tissue along the retinal vessels.
During the following weeks, further resorption of the blood
and the necrotic material was observed, along with an increase
of retinal atrophy. The optic disc appeared particularly pale,
and all the arterial vessels appeared to be occluded. Fluoro-
graphically, we saw thread-like filling of the major arterial
vessels, and extinction of the fluorographic arterial picture
during the venous filling phase.

The vitreous became progressively more cloudy and more
organized. A central retinal detachment was observed three
months after the first signs of necrosis, which we attempted
to repair by means of a vitrectomy. After the vitreous
cleared, reapposition of the retina was not possible. No
tears were observed, but there was a central, flat detachment
due to tension from a circumferential fibrotic band. The
optic disc had a peculiar pigmentation (Fig. 1c,d). Fluoro-
graphically, we noted deep, peripheral atrophy with sharp
demarcation from the central retinal detachment (Fig. 1e,f).
The large retinal vessels manifested irregular segments and
occlusions, and the retinal capillary bed was virtually absent.
Leakage of fluorescein was the most striking on the fibrous
membranes.

The culture of the rinse water used during the vitrectomy
was virus negative, as was electron microscopic examination of
the filtered remnants. The clinical course was that of the
ARNS, and there were no arguments for an immune deficiency.
The titres for herpes and CMV remained low for the entire
observation period.

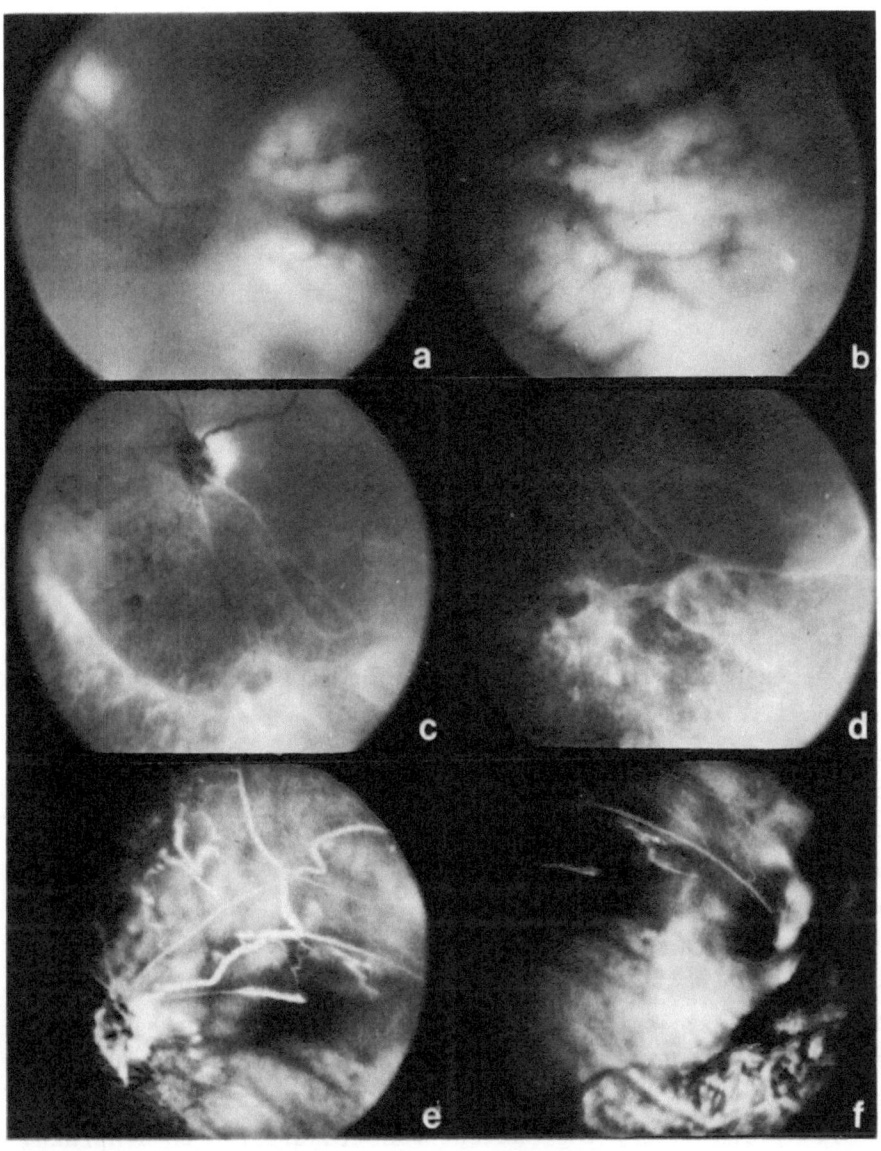

FIGURE 1: (Case 1) Fresh necrotic lesions in the papillomacular area (a) and temporally (b). Atrophic retina and retinal
detachment after the vitrectomy in the nasal (c) and lower
temporal regions (d). Fluorography AV filling stage (e,f),
same fields and on the same date as (c) and (d).

CASE 2

This case of retinal necrosis occurred in a 26-year old immunosuppressed woman three months after a kidney transplant. Fresh peripheral retinal lesions were discovered in her right eye during an examination for hypertensive uveitis (Fig. 2a). One month after the onset of the eye disease, hemiplegia and homonymous hemianopia developed. Moniliasis of the mouth was also observed, and systemic fungistatic treatment was commenced. Complement fixing antibody titers for herpes and CMV remained low initially, and no viruses could be isolated in the lumbal fluid, so no virostatic treatment was administered.

It was only four months after the onset of the eye symptoms that the serum titers for CMV rose progressively from 1/32 to 1/256. The lumbal fluid was not examined in this period. It was supposed that the immunosuppression was responsible for the absence of antibody formation in the acute phase since the total picture was very compatible with CMV infection (12). Arguments for CMV retinitis are seen when we examine the lesions closely: initially, the necrotic lesions are white with a slight transparency and are crumbly around the edges (Fig. 2a). In a photo taken three days later, we see, in the same sector, a constriction of the arterial caliber and denser and more yellow necrotic tissue, but the necrotic material is also beginning to resorp, particularly along the retinal veins (Fig. 2b). Atrophied tissue remains. Seven days later, there was further cicatrization (Fig. 2c), and we observed a few retinal hemorrhages in these lesions. Temporal and nasal lesions developed somewhat later. They were still white and bloody while the initial lesions in the lower sector had already cicatrized.

Two years later, the patient was transferred to a nursing home because of serious psychomotoric sequels of encephalitis. At that time, the necrotic scars were still limited to the retinal periphery of one eye, the vitreous was organized, but the retina was attached.

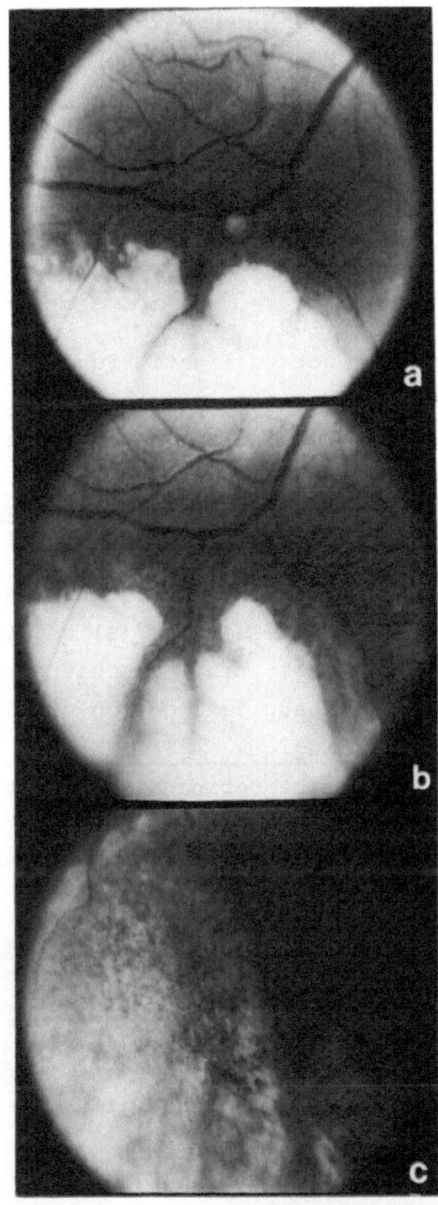

FIGURE 2: (Case 2) Fresh necrotic lesions (a), partial resorption of necrotic tissue three days later (b), and almost total cicatrization seven days later (c).

382

CASE 3

Bilateral necrotic retinitis was observed in another 58-year old woman, who had been immunosuppressed because of a proliferative glomerulonephritis. Her symptoms began with a sore throat, labial herpes, and recurring gastriculcer bleeding and progressed to bilateral deafness, blindness, and encephalitis.

In her serum, the titers rose both for herpes simplex (1/32 to 1/512) and for CMV (1/256 to 1/1024); in her lumbal fluid, there was a titer increase for CMV (1/8 to 1/32), and CMV was isolated in her urine.

Her pupils did not react to light. Fundoscopy initially showed some cottonwool exsudates. Twelve days later, two necrotic retinal plaques were noted in her right eye, and more striking lesions with papiloedema, retinal vasculitis, and retinitis with bleeding and exsudates were observed in her left eye.

During the subsequent months, the retinal necrosis spread. Figure 3 shows necrotic tissue nasally (a) and in the lower part of the retina (b). The retinal vascular occlusions, the cloudy vitreous, and the sharp demarcation of the necrotic retinal tissue were striking.

In two months, the entire retina of her left eye had become necrotic; the necrosis in her right eye remained limited. Because of the serious incapacities of the patient, no virostatics were administered.

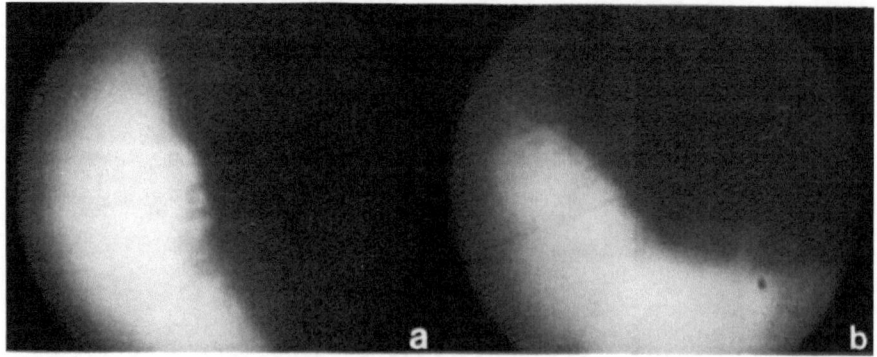

FIGURE 3: (Case 3) Extensive necrotic tissue nasally (a) and in the lower part of the retina (b).

DISCUSSION

Herpes virus can be responsible for necrotic retinitis, which has a well-defined clinical picture.

Necrotic retinitis can be part of a generalized cytomegalovirus or CMV infection congenitally in children (8,28) and in immune-suppressed patients (24,29,32), particularly those with kidney transplants (2,4,19,21,23,26,28-32), Hodgkin's disease (12,37), or the auto-immune deficiency syndrome (16,34).

Generally, there is a positive serology with an increase of CMV complement fixing antibodies, and, in many cases, the diagnosis was confirmed by histopathology.

Necrotic retinitis can also occur during the course of herpes simplex encephalitis (3,20,25) or during the course of opthalmic zoster (10).

Similar but more rapidly evolving lesions occur in the acute retinal necrotic syndrome or ARNS in the form of an isolated unilateral or bilateral eye disease in otherwise healthy people with a negative serology for herpes and CMV. Culbertson demonstrated the herpetic nature of this syndrome in two patients with ARNS enucleated during the active phase (9-11,15). On the basis of the histopathology, electron microscopy, and positive cultures, he concluded that at least some cases of ARNS are secondary to retinal infection by a herpes virus. He recommends the use of acyclovir and anticoagulants during the early stages and periocular or systemic corticosteroids in the later stages. Nevertheless, papillitis and difficult to repair retinal detachments are common complications contributing to the pessimistic prognosis that is associated with retinal necrosis.

Our purpose here has been primarily to present the pathognomonic clinical picture of herpetic retinitis and of the acute retinal necrosis syndrome. This picture can orient diagnostic procedures and therapeutic practice.

REFERENCES

1. Ando, F., M. Kato, S. Goto, K. Kobayashi, H. Ichikawa & T. Kamiya. Platelet function in bilateral acute retinal necrosis. Am. J. Ophthal. 96: 27-32 (1983).
2. Astle, J.N. & P.P. Ellis. Ocular complications in renal transplant patients. Ann. Ophthal. 6: 1269-1274 (1974).
3. Bloom, J.N., J.I. Katz & M.E. Kaufman. Herpes simplex retinitis and encephalitis in an adult. Arch. Ophthal. 95: 1798-1799 (1977).
4. Carson, S & S.N. Chatterjee. Cytomegalovirus retinitis: Two cases occurring after renal transplatation. Ann. Ophthal. 10: 265-279 (1978).
5. Chawla, H.B., M.J. Ford, J.F. Munro, R.E. Scorgie & A.R. Watson. Ocular involvement in cytomegalovirus infection in a previously healthy adult. Br. Med. J. 2: 281-282 (1976).
6. Chumbley, L.C., D.M. Robertson, T.F. Smith & R.J. Campbell. Adult cytomegalovirus inclusion retino-uveitis. Am. J. Ophthal. 80: 807-816 (1975).
7. Cogan, D.G. Immunosuppression and eye disease. Am. J. Ophthal. 83: 777-788 (1977).
8. Cox, F., D. Meyer & W.T. Hughes. Cytomegalovirus in tears from patients with normal eyes and with acute cytomegalovirus chorioretinitis. Am. J. Ophthal. 80: 817-824 (1975).
9. Culbertson, W.W., J.G. Clarkson, M. Blumenkranz & M.L. Lewis. Acute retinal necrosis. Am. J. Ophthal. 96: 683-685 (1983).
10. Culbertson, W.W., M.S. Blumenkranz, H. Haines, J.D.M. Gass, K.B. Mitchell & E.W.D. Norton. The acute retinal necrosis syndrome. Part 2: Histopathology and etiology. Ophthalmology 89: 1317-1325 (1982).
11. Culbertson, W.W., J.G. Clarkson, M. Blumenkranz, M.L. Lewis. Reply. Am. J. Ophthal 97: 662 (1984).
12. Diddie, K.R. D.J. Schanzlin & F.A. Mausolf. Necrotizing retinitis caused by opportunistic virus infection in a patient with Hodgkin's disease. Am. J. Ophthal. 88: 668-673 (1979).
13. Fiala, M., J.E. Payne, T.V. Berne, T.C. Moore, W. Henle, J.Z. Montgomerie, S.N. Chatterjee & L.B. Guze. Epidemiology of cytomegalovirus infection after transplantation and immunosuppression. J. Infect. Dis. 132: 421-433 (1975).
14. Fiala, M., S.N. Chatterjee, S. Carson, S. Poolsawat, D.C. Heiner, A. Saxon & L.B. Guze. Cytomegalovirus retinitis secondary to chronic viremia in phagocytic leukocytes. Am. J. Ophthal. 84: 567-573 (1977).
15. Fisher, J.P., M.L. Lewis, M. Blumenkranz, W.W. Culbertson, H.W. Flynn, J.G. Clarkson, J.D.M. Gass, E.W.D. Norton. The acute retinal necrosis syndrome. Ophthalmology 89: 1309-1316 (1982).
16. Friedman, A.H., J. Orellana, W.R. Freeman, M.H. Luntz, M.B. Starr, M.L. Tapper, I. Spigland, H. Rotterdam, R.M. Tejada, S. Braunhut, D. Mildvan & U. Mathur. Cytomegalovirus retinitis: a manifestaition of the acquired

immune deficiency syndrome (AIDS). Br. J. Ophthal. 67: 372-380 (1983).

17. Hayasaka, S., T. Asano, K. Yabata & A. Ide. Acute retinal necrosis. Br. J. Ophthal. 67: 455-460 (1983).

18. Hayreh, S. Correspondence. Acute retinal necrosis. Am. J. Ophthal. 97: 661-662 (1984).

19. Ho, M., S. Suwansirikel, J.N. Dowling, L.A. Youngblood & J.A. Armstrong. The transpanted kidney as a source of cytomegalovirus infection. N. Engl. J. Med. 293: 1109-1112 (1975).

20. Johnson, B.L. & H.W. Wisotzkey. Neuroretinitis associated with herpes simplex encephalitis in an adult. Am. J. Ophthal. 83: 481-489 (1977).

21. Madge, G.E. Cytomegalovirus infection of the eye in a case of renal homotransplantation. MCV Quarterly 8: 251-253 (1972).

22. Masuyama, Y., M. Fukuzaki, Y. Baba, A. Sawada, A. Sumiyoshi. Histopathological study of adult cytomegalic inclusion retino-uveitis. In: R. Sundmacher (ed.), Herpetische Augenerkrankungen-- Herpetic Eye Diseases. J.F. Bergmann Verlag, Munich, pp. 495-500 (1981).

23. Merritt, J.C. & C.O. Callender. Adult cytomegalic inclusion retinitis. Ann. Ophthalmol. 10: 1059-1063 (1978).

24. Michelson, J.B., R.F. Stephens & J.A. Shields. Clinical conditions mistaken for metastic cancer to the choroid. Ann. Ophthalmol. 11: 149-153 (1979).

25. Minckler, D.S., E.B. McLean, C.M. Shaw, A. Hendrickson. Herpesvirus hominis encephalitis and retinitis. Arch. Ophtahlmol. 94: 89-95 (1976).

26. Murray, H.W., D.L. Knox, W.R. Green & R.M. Sussel. Cytomegalovirus retinitis in adults: a manifestation of disseminated viral infection. Am. J. Med. 63: 574-584 (1977).

27. Nahmias, N.G., R.J. Whitley, A.N. Visintine, Y. Takel, Y. & C.A. Alford, Jr. Herpes simplex virus encephalitis: Laboratory evaluations and their diagnostic significance. J. Infect. Dis. 145: 829-836 (1982).

28. Polak, B.C.P. Ophthalmological complications of haemodialysis and kidney transplantation. Dr. W. Junk, B.V., The Hague, pp. 5, 43, (1980).

29. Pollard, R.B., P.R. Egbert, J.G. Gallagher & T.C. Merigan. Cytomegalovirus retinitis in immunosuppressed hosts. I. Natural history and effects of treatment with adenine aribinoside. II. Ocular manifestations. Ann. Intern. Med. 93: 655-670 (1980).

30. Pollard, R.B., P.R. Egbert, J.G. Gallagher & T.C. Merigan. Infections with cytomegalovirus in adult and the natural history and treatment of cytomegalovirus retinitis. In: R. Sundmacher (ed.), Herpetische Augenerkrankungen--Herpetic Eye Diseases. J.F. Bergmann Verlag, Munich, pp. 495-500 (1981).

31. Porter, R., A.L. Crombie, P.S. Gardner & R.P. Uldall. Incidence of ocular complications in patients undergoing renal transplantation. Br. Med. J. 3: 133-136 (1972).

32. Porter, R. Acute necrotizing retinitis in a patient receiving immunosuppressive therapy. Br. J. Ophthal. 56: 555-558 (1972).

33. Price, F.W. & T.F. Schlaegel, Jr. Bilateral acute retinal necrosis. Am. J. Ophthal. 89: 419-424 (1980).

34. Rodrigues, M.M., A. Palestine, R. Nussenblatt, H. Masur & A.M. Macher. Unilateral cytomegalovirus retinochoroiditis and bilateral cytoid bodies in a bisexual man with the acquired immunodeficiency syndrome. Ophthalmology 90: 1577-1582 (1983).

35. Russell, A.S. & A. Saertre. Antibodies to herpes-simplex virus in "normal" cerebrospinal fluid. Lancet, Vol. 1, 64-65 (1976).

36. Topilow, H.W., J.J. Nussbaum, H. Mackenzie Freeman, G.R. Dickersin, W. Szyfelbein. Bilateral acute retinal necrosis. Arch. Ophthalmol. 100: 1901-1908 (1982).

37. Toy, J.L. & R.P. Knowlder. Cytomegalovirus retinitis misdiagnosed as Hodgkin's lymphoma deposits. Br. Med. J. 2: 1398-1399 (1978).

38. Verhoeven, D.C., S.H. Oei & J.E. Winkelman. Acute retinale necrose. Ned. Tijdschr. Geneeskd. 127: 2442 (1983).

39. Willerson, D., T.M. Aaberg & F.H. Reeser. Necrotizing vaso-occlusive retinitis. Am. J. Ophthal. 84: 209-219 (1977).

40. Wyhinny, J., D.J. Apple, F.R. Guastella & C.M. Vygantes. Adult cytomegalic inclusion retinitis. Am. J. Ophthal. 76: 773-781 (1973).

41. Young, N.J.A. & A.C. Bird. Bilateral acute retinal necrosis. Br. J. Ophthal. 62: 581-590 (1978).

DISCUSSION :

D.L. Easty (Bristol) : We have seen two patients both of whom
   were immunosuppressed, who had this very typical appearance.

A. Leys (Leuven) : Slowly spreading necrosis ?

D.L. Easty (Bristol) : I did not see them through that phase,
   but we have photographic evidence of it, and they survived.
   However, I think the prognosis is bad.

A. Leys (Leuven) : Only children die.

D.L. Easty (Bristol) : Is that so ? Eventually they had a sector atrophy, very classical appearance. The other case, just
   as you showed, eventually expired. She had a second transplant.

R. Sundmacher (Freiburg) : Even after this excellent presentation,
   I feel uncomfortable regarding the differential diagnosis between certain types of CMV retinitis and the acute retinal necrosis syndrome. In the literature I found that all kinds of
   herpes viruses have been incriminated to cause acute retinal
   necrosis. Isn't it only a very severe type of herpes retinitis ?

A. Leys (Leuven) : Yes.

R. Sundmacher (Freiburg) : What would then be the practical value of separating this type of presumed herpes retinitis from
   the other ones ?

A. Leys (Leuven) : The necrosis syndrome is a problem for the
   ophthalmologist. The CMV retinitis is only a small part of
   generalised disease. So the responsibility of treatment is in
   medicine for CMV retinitis and with the neurologist for herpes
   encephalitis. The acute retinal necrosis syndrome is a problem
   that needs to be resolved by the ophthalmologist.

R. Sundmacher (Freiburg) : That is generally true; but I am
   aware of papers describing CMV retinitis without general disease, just as in the retinal necrosis syndrome. So, what
   is the difference then ?

A. Leys (Leuven) : Usually you need to have immuno-suppression or congenitally acquired disease to be able to use the term CMV retinitis.

B. Juel-Jensen (Oxford) : In your first patient, did you say that the herpes simplex virus titer was negative ?

A. Leys (Leuven) : It was negative.

B. Juel-Jensen (Oxford) : In the CSF ?

A. Leys (Leuven) : Yes, also during the acute phase.

B. Juel-Jensen (Oxford) : But, may I consider the CSF ? One thing one can say with absolute certainty, is that the patient did not have herpes simplex virus encephalitis because there is always antibody in the CSF.

A. Leys (Leuven) : In literature it has been described that titers don't rise if the patient is severly immuno-suppressed. So, I agree for our first patient we only have clinical arguments.

B. Juel-Jensen (Oxford) : This is true. But your patient was not immuno-suppressed, because your patient was perfectly capable of producing herpes simplex virus antibody in the circulation. Therefore that patient did not have herpes encephalitis, because if she had had herpes encephalitis she would have produced antibody in the CSF.

A. Leys (Leuven) : Several months after the acute phase serum titers rose for CMV. We have no data on titers in the CSF because lumbal puncture was not done in that stage. During the active phase of the eye disease and encephalitis titers were negative, both in serum and in spinal fluid.

CLINICAL COMPARISON BETWEEN HERPES SIMPLEX AND HERPES ZOSTER OCULAR
INFECTIONS
R. AHONEN AND A. VANNAS (Helsinki University Eye Clinic, Helsinki,
Finland)

1. INTRODUCTION

Both herpes simplex virus (HSV) and varicella zoster virus (VZV)
are known to penetrate the cornea and cause endothelitis, anterior
uveitis, trabeculitis and focal iritis (Sundmacher and
Neumann-Haefelin, 1979; Sundmacher and Muller, 1982; Vannas et al.,
1983; Ahonen et al., 1983). However, the incidence and nature of
tissue damage in the anterior chamber during herpetic kerato-uveitis
are not clear. In the present paper special attention has been paid to
the occurrence and type of acute anterior segment disease during HSV
and VZV infections.

2. MATERIAL AND METHODS

2.1 HSV group

Fifty-seven patients with primary HSV keratitis were monitored
with slit-lamp and specular microscopy for two years on average.
Twenty-two of the cases were female and 35 were male. Their age ranged
from 4 to 82 (mean 43) years. Trifluridine 1% eye drops were used
routinely as treatment. In addition topical corticosteroids were used
in 16 cases when the epithelium was infact. Ten patients suffering
from HSV kerato-uveitis were studied for endothelial cell alterations
with both non-contact and wide-field specular microscopes.

Maudgal, P.C. and Missotten, L., (eds.) Herpetic Eye Diseases.
© *1985, Dr W. Junk Publishers, Dordrecht/Boston/Lancaster. ISBN 978-94-010-8935-7*

2.2 VZV group

Thirty patients, 17 female and 13 male, with unilateral VZV ocular infection were examined with biomicroscopy and specular microscopy. They ranged in age from 27 to 82 (mean 67) years. The patients were admitted to the Helsinki University Eye Clinic with early kerato-uveitis in 1981 and were monitored for two years period on average. Scopolamin 2.5mg/ml was used routinely for mydriasis. Topical corticosteroids were included in the treatment in 18 patients when the epithelium was infact. No antiviral drugs were used. Fourteen cases were studied for endothelial cell alterations using specular microscopy.

2.3 Specular microscopy

The endothelial mosaic was examined and photographed with both non-contact and wide-field specular microscopes. After stromal edema and uveitis had subsided photographs were taken for analysis of endothelial cell density. Endothelial cell density was determined with variable frame analysis using a digitizer. Healthy contralateral eyes served as controls.

3. RESULTS

3.1 HSV group

During early keratitis 52 corneas presented a dendritic epithelial ulcer and five a geographic ulcer. Twenty-five eyes (44%) developed anterior uveitis. Transient endothelial changes, as a sign of endothelitis, followed by severe anterior uveitis were observed in 11 cases (19%) from two to five weeks from the onset of the disease.

Involvement of the trabecular meshwork or trabeculitis was detected in two eyes (4%). There were 2 cases (4%) of elevated IOP.

Time for complete healing ranged from 7 to 77 (mean 20) days. During the follow-up herpetic keratitis recurred in 19 patients (33%). The latency period varied from 1 to 21 months, average 9.9 months. Nine corneas (16%) developed chronic herpetic keratitis.

Specular microscopy showed a 12% lower endothelial cell density on average in the eyes with endothelitis and severe anterior uveitis. Endothelial cell density remained unchanged in the eyes without endothelitis.

3.2 VZV group

All cases with VZV ocular infection showed a punctate epithelial keratitis and anterior uveitis whilst a dendritic ulcer developed in five eyes. During the early stages, 13 cases (43%) developed endothelitis, trabeculitis was seen in five eyes (17%) and focal iritis in four (13%). Eight eyes (27%) had elevated IOP.

Complete healing time ranged from 13 to 294 (mean 61) days. A new episode of corneal edema and anterior uveitis as a sign of recurrent infection was seen in four eyes (13%) from 1 to 11 (mean 5.7) months later. Chronic keratitis was seen in two eyes.

Endothelial cell density was reduced on average 15% in the eyes with endothelitis. Patients with endothelitis and an episode of elevated IOP had a 20% lower cell count. The endothelial cell density remained unchanged in the eyes without endothelitis.

392

4.DISCUSSION

Though clinically very different, both HSV and VZV effect the anterior segment of the eye similarly. In the present study there was a high incidence of endothelitis and a decrease in endothelial cell density in these eyes. After endothelitis, trabecilitis and focal iritis were further signs of viral penetration into the anterior chamber.

The present findings are in agreement with other observations suggesting a productive type of HSV and VZV infection in the endothelial cells resulting in endothelitis, endothelial cell death and liberation of living viruses into the anterior chamber (Sundmacher, 1981; Ahonen et al., 1984). Recent papers have reported on the efficacy of acyclovir and bromovinyldeoxyuridine in HSV and VZV infections. During next years we can determine their value in preventing virus penetration into the anterior chamber.

REFERENCES
1. Ahonen R, Vannas A, Mäkitie J. 1983. Endothelial cell loss in herpes zoster keratouveitis. Br. J. Ophthalmol. 67:751-754
2. Ahonen R, Vannas A, Mäkitie J. 1984. Virus particles and leucocytes in herpes simplex keratitis. Cornea, in print.
3. Sundmacher R, Neumann-Haefelin D. 1979. Herpes simplex virus-positive and -negative keratouveitis, in Silverstein AM and O'Connor GR (eds): Immunology and Immunopathology of the Eye. New York, Masson Publishing, pp. 225-229.
4. Sundmacher R. 1981. A clinico-virologic classification of herpetic anterior segment diseases with special reference to intraocular herpes, in Sundmacher R (ed): Herpetische Augenkrankungen. Munich, JF Bergman Verlag, pp. 203-210
5. Sundmacher R, Muller O. 1982. Das Hornhautendothel bei zoster ophthalmicus. Klin. Monatsbl. Augenheilkd. 180:271-274.
6. Vannas A, Ahonen R, Mäkitie J. 1983. Corneal endothelium in herpetic keratouveitis. Arch. Ophthalmol. 101:913-915.

DISCUSSION :

C. Claoué (Southampton) : Would you please explain to us exactly
how you diagnose the patients as having endothelitis or trabeculitis ?   Secondly, is there histopathological evidence of acute
inflammatory response in the endothelium or trabecular meshwork at that time ?

R. Ahonen (Helsinki) : Firstly, when we diagnose endothelitis it
is easily seen with the slitlamp and we also take specular
micrographs from the endothelium. It was not seen in all cases of herpetic ocular infection, it was only in the percentage
I described. Endothelitis was mostly present in the central
endothelium and the keratic precipitates appeared later. It
is possible to diagnose trabeculitis by gonioscopy when the
corneal edema does not hinder the view of trabeculum. In most
cases it was not possible. When we saw keratitic precipitates
all over the corneal endothelium and there was high intraocular pressure, like in those cases we could see with a gonios-
cope, we decided that it was a trabecular infection. What
was your third question ?

C. Clauoé (Southampton) : I was asking if there was any histopathological evidence of an acute inflammatory infiltrate in
the endothelium or trabecular meshwork. Could I just get back
to your previous answer : you have still not told me how I
can recognise endothelitis. Do you mean swollen cells seen
on specular microscopy, or cellular atypy, or do you think
that the presence of keratitic precipitates means that endothelitis is present ?

R. Ahonen (Helsinki) : There are transient endothelial changes.
You can see black holes in the endothelial mosaic during endothelitis. First they are small and afterwards they coalesce
and become larger.

R. Sundmacher (Freiburg) : I think we better come back to this
question in the General Discussion later on.

B. Juel-Jensen (Oxford) : A simple question. You talk about recurrences in varicella-zoster infection. Was there any evidence
of recurrence in the skin ? Because, I presume these patients

had V^I or ophthalmic zoster at the same time. Recurrences are very uncommon in non-immunosuppressed people in ordinary segmental zoster.

R. Ahonen (Helsinki) : We diagnosed a recurrence of varicella-zoster infection when cornea was edematous and associated with anterior uveitis.

R. Sundmacher (Freiburg) : The unsolved question with "recurrences" in zoster is that we do not know whether it is only flaring-up of subclinical peripheral disease, i.e. persistence of varicella zoster e.g. in endothelial cells, or whether we deal with true neuronal recurrences. Both pathways may be operative. It has been my view that in most clinical situations we deal with virus persistence.

D.L. Easty (Bristol) : Could I ask you a simple question too ? It is actually not clear in my mind why you are comparing these two diseases. I am not sure what your philosophy is in comparing herpes zoster with herpes simplex.

R. Ahonen (Helsinki) : As I said earlier, we were interested in the corneal endothelium, and started comparing the endothelium involvement in the two diseases. These findings are a sort of side results from this study. Since we had no knowledge of the incidence of the anterior segment pathology in herpetic ocular infection, primarily this study was meant for our own information.

J. I. McGill (Southampton) : Can I come back to Dr. Juel-Jensen's question about what is a recurrence and why it begins; we really don't know. I agree with Rainer that probably it is persistent infection. Nobody has actually produced the histopathology on this. We have seen one recurrent ulcer eight months after the initial attack from which we isolated the virus. But it is the only time we have ever done it. It could well be a complex situation where viral reactivation starts with an immune mechanism which we don't know.

CORNEAL COMPLICATIONS OF HERPES ZOSTER OPHTHALMICUS

T. J. LIESEGANG, M.D.

The chronological order and pathogenesis of the diverse corneal
lesions in herpes zoster ophthalmicus (HZO) have not been adequately
documented. The role of viral infection, vasculitis, immune reaction,
and tissue damage remains unclear. The morphology of the corneal
lesions was reviewed in a series of consecutive patients followed after
an attack of acute HZO. Based on this study and a review of the literature, the current concepts of the pathogenesis involved in the corneal
disease is summarized. More effective therapy may be directed with a
better understanding of these mechanisms.

MATERIAL AND METHODS
    The records of all patients seen in the Department of Ophthalmology
at the Mayo Clinic with HZO between January, 1978 and January, 1984 were
reviewed to select only those patients seen acutely and followed for at
least four months after the onset of the illness. Demographic data,
history of systemic disease, and the course of their ocular disease was
reviewed. The morphology of the corneal lesions was obtained from
descriptions and drawings in the chart and supported in most situations
with stereo-slit lamp photographs.

RESULTS
    Of the 213 patients seen with HZO over the six-year period, 94 had
adequate follow-up after acute HZO. The remainder were seen for chronic
HZO. Sixty-one of the 94 patients (64.2%) developed some form of
corneal involvement. In this group of 61 patients with corneal disease,
85.2% had dermatological evidence of involvement of the nasociliary
division of the ophthalmic nerve, although none had isolated nasociliary
nerve involvement. In 14.7% there was extension to some of the branches
of the maxillary division, and the disease progressed to cutaneous or
visceral dissemination in 6.5%. Prior medical disease was present in

Maudgal, P.C. and Missotten, L., (eds.) Herpetic Eye Diseases.
© *1985, Dr W. Junk Publishers, Dordrecht/Boston/Lancaster. ISBN 978-94-010-8935-7*

several: lymphoma or leukemia in four, cancer in four, collagen or immune disease in five, and orbital injury in three. During the follow-up period, none of the patients developed new significant medical diseases, although four patients had later symptoms and signs compatible with central nervous system zoster vasculitis.

The incidence, morphology, chronology, and pathogenesis of the corneal lesions in these patients is described below.

Punctate Epithelial Keratitis (51%). The earliest corneal manifestation (at one to ten days) was a coarse, punctate epithelial keratitis (PEK) with blotchy, swollen epithelial cells. The lesions were peripheral, multiple, small, and focal. They were transient or coalesced to a pseudodendrite (in 55%) and were followed by anterior stromal infiltrates (in 33%). One of six patients grew the varicella zoster virus (VZV) in culture from a corneal debridement.

Early Pseudodendrites (51%). Multiple, small, fine dendrites or stellate lesions of swollen, raised epithelial cells occurred at 2-15 days. They were peripheral and were frequently a coalescence of previous PEK. They were slightly broader and more plaque-like than the dendrites of HSV with an absence of the central ulcer trough (1). VZV was cultured from four of seven corneal lesions. Other authors have identified zoster viral antigen with immunofluorescence (2). Corneal scrapings revealed multinucleated giant cells and intranuclear inclusions within epithelial cells, as reported by others (1). They were self-limited (3).

Anterior Stromal Infiltrates (41%). Single or multiple patches of dry granular infiltration developed in the anterior stroma beneath Bowman's layer at 6-21 days. They were subsequent to one of the previous epithelial lesions (in 92%) and probably represent soluble antigen eliciting an immune response. They respond to steroids but may relapse.

Sclerokeratitis (1%). Localized stromal infiltration with or without an epithelial defect may develop in the periphery of the cornea adjacent to an episcleral or scleral nodule. These occur early or later in the course. This probably results from a vasculitis of the scleral vessels with ischemia and immune complex deposition (4). It may progress to vascularization, lipid deposition, or scarring.

Keratouveitis/Endotheliitis (35%). Striate keratitis with epithelial and stromal edema may occur suddenly at 1-21 days. It may be diffuse or localized and associated with underlying large, smudgy KP, anterior chamber reaction, and elevated IOP (in 33%). The uveitis is caused by an ischemia of the pars plicata (5) and may manifest with hypopyon, hyphema, and anterior segment ischemia. It led to phthisis or pre-phthisis in two patients. Endothelial cell loss is a frequent feature relating to the severity of the uveitis, although the mechanism may be a specific endothelial attack by virus or immunological mechanisms (6,7).

The keratouveitis may smolder secondary to a vasculitis and nutritive ischemia to the cornea. The end stage corneal picture is an interstitial keratitis with scarring, lipid deposition, and deep active vessels. The histopathologic counterpart is a granulomatous inflammatory reaction and giant cells around Descemet's membrane (8).

Serpiginous Ulceration (7%). Acute stromal edema, cellular infiltration, and a crescent-shaped ulcer with a grey-white base may develop in the corneal periphery at 2-20 weeks. Perforation occurred in one, as reported by other (9). This may be related to a vasculitis and responds to anti-inflammatory measures.

Delayed Corneal Mucous Plaques (13%). Elevated, coarse, opaque, grey-white lesions on the surface of swollen epithelial cells may occur with a sudden onset at 1-16 weeks. They can form complex pseudodendritic patterns with sharp margins but lack the terminal branches and delicate features of HSV. They are culture negative and cytology showed ballooned epithelial cells with overlying mucous plaques. The morphology and course suggest that the mechanism may be similar to the abnormal epithelial receptor sites seen in keratitis sicca (10).

Disciform Keratitis (10%). A deep central or peripheral disc of corneal edema with minimal stromal infiltration and an intact epithelium occurs at 1-9 months. The time, the course, the presence of immune rings, the rapid response to steroids, the documentation of prior corneal exposure to viral antigen, and the histopathology confirmed that it is a cell-mediated, delayed hypersensitivity response.

Neurotropic Keratitis (25%). The corneal sensation is usually depressed at 3-21 days but returns in most. Additionally, in some patients it develops at 2-6 months and causes a neurotropic keratitis from the nerve degeneration following ganglion necrosis. Early there is a lack of corneal luster, an irregular corneal surface, and mild punctate epithelial erosions. Later, fine intraepithelial vesicles or exfoliation occurs. Horizontal oval epithelial defects and boggy stromal ulcers may

develop in the lower cornea. Keratouveitis, exposure keratitis, and tear
dysfunction enhance the risk of scarring, thinning, or perforation.
Therapy with tears, mucolytic agents, and soft contact lenses are
temporary measures; tarsorrhaphy is required in recalcitrant cases.
Exposure Keratitis (11%). Cicatricial retraction of the upper lid or
ectropion of the lower lid from dermal scarring may produce an ineffective blink or a frozen lid as early as 11 days and as late as 3 years
after the acute attack. Lid thickening, meibomian gland and lash
follicle damage, and neurotropic keratitis again enhance the potential
for corneal erosion and perforation (11). Drying skin preparation used
early in the course may enhance these contractures; moist wet compresses
are preferable. Once scarring is established, plastic surgical repair
may be required.

DISCUSSION

Permanent corneal scarring may result from the multiple mechanisms
mentioned above. It may assume the pattern of nummular scar, a diffuse
severe deep interstitial keratitis, or a peripheral stromal scar with a
vascular leash and lipid deposition. The inflammation may proceed slowly
and silently, inspite of topical corticosteroids. Corneal perforation or
permanent endothelial decompensation with phthisis may result.

The elucidation of the exact mechanisms awaits further exquisite
immunologic testing and viral detection. Tissue has generally been
available for pathological examination only in advanced cases (8).
Better knowledge of the mechanism will allow more direct therapy as newer
and less toxic topical and systemic antiviral agents become available
(12,13).

Topical corticosteroids are beneficial but definitely prolongs some
of the corneal components of the disease. Patients with corneal complications must be seen frequently to detect silent progression of the
corneal disease, to monitor for complications of steroid therapy, and to
detect conditions requiring discontinuance of topical steroids (for
example, neurotropic and exposure keratitis). Damage to the lids and
interference with tear function requires therapy directed toward maintaining surface lubrication. Surgical procedures on the lids and cornea
may be required to protect or to restore the corneal integrity.

REFERENCES
1. Marsh RJ, Fraunfelder FT, and McGill JI (1976) Herpetic corneal
    epithelial disease. Arch Ophthalmol 94, 1899-1902.
2. Hayashi S (1975) Study of herpes zoster keratitis, demonstration of
    virus particles in corneal scrapings. ACTA Soc Ophthalmol Japan
    79, 1542-1549.
3. Pavan-Langston D, and McCulley JP (1973) Herpes zoster dendritic
    keratitis. Arch Ophthalmol 89, 25-29.
4. Marsh RJ (1973) Herpes zoster keratitis. Trans Ophthalmol Soc UK
    93, 181-192.
5. Crock G (1967) Clinical syndrome of anterior segment ischemia.
    Trans Ophthalmol Soc U.K. 87, 513-533.
6. Reijo A, Antti V, and Jukka M (1983) Endothelial cell loss in
    herpes zoster keratouveitis. Brit Jour Ophthalmol 67, 751-754.
7. Maudgal PC, Missotten L, DeClercq E, and Descamps J (1980)
    Varicella-zoster virus in the human corneal endothelium: a case
    report. Bull Soc belge Ophthalmol 190, 71-86.
8. Hedges TR and Albert DM (1982) The progression of the ocular
    abnormalities of herpes zoster: histopathologic observations of
    nine cases. Ophthalmol 89, 165-176.
9. Mondino BJ, Brown SI, and Mondzelewski JP (1978) Peripheral cor-
    neal ulcers with herpes zoster ophthalmicus. Amer Jour Ophthalmol
    86, 611-614.
10. Fraunfelder FT, Wright P, and Tripathi RC (1977) Corneal mucous
    plaques. Amer Jour Ophthalmol 83, 191-197.
11. Waring GO and Ekins MB (1981) Corneal perforation in herpes
    zoster ophthalmicus caused by eyelid scarring with exposure kera-
    titis. Sundmacher, R (ed). Herpetic eye diseases. J. F. Bergman
    Verlag Freeburg, 469-478.
12. Balfour HH Jr, Bean B, and Laskin OL, et al (1983) Acyclovir halts
    progression of herpes zoster in immunocompromised hosts. New
    England Jour Medicine 308, 1448-1453.
13. McGill J, Chapman C, and Mahakasingam M (1983) Acyclovir therapy
    in herpes zoster infection: a practical guide. Trans Ophthalmol
    Soc U.K. 103, 111-114.

DISCUSSION :

C.R. Dawson (San Francisco) : That is a very nice study. Does this represent the natural history of herpes zoster ophthalmicus ?

T.J. Liesegang (Rochester) : No antiviral therapy was used.

C.R. Dawson (San Francisco) : I was referring to the natural history of herpes zoster under steroid treatment.

T.J. Liesegang (Rochester) : I think 11 received systemic steroids. Some of them received topical steroids.

C.R. Dawson (San Francisco) : What percentage of these patients had steroids by neither route ?

T.J. Liesegang (Rochester) : I could get you the exact figures. The study is a relatively natural course, because topical steroids were not used until the patients developed a complication. This study can be used to compare with future antiviral studies. As some of you may be aware, ophthalmic acyclovir ointment is not available to the clinician in the United States. Intravenous acyclovir has recently become available.

Y. Centifanto (New Orleans) : Your presentation was excellent, but I have a few questions, and I hope you will forgive me as I don't know very much about varicella. If epithelial lesions followed by stromal involvement constitute the natural course of the disease, then I suppose there is viral replication first and then later some sort of persistence, but we don't know if it is still actively multiplying virus, slow virus, or the presence of viral antigens. Is this correct, or do we know what the picture is in terms of the virus ?

T.J. Liesegang   : I think there are several mechanisms acting here. Certainly, I think the virus is present in the early epithelial lesions. Doctor Maudgal has shown by viral antigens that the virus is perhaps present in the endothelium, although virus has never been seen within the eye. More of the damage may result from a vasculitis. The virus probably gets into blood vessels and causes a giant cell reaction in either large or small blood vessels and occludes the blood vessels. Thrombosis and ischemia are very important mechanisms in zoster as opposed to simplex. Five of the patients in this series developed central nervous system zoster. The reason that I make this point is that it was never diagnosed by the neurologist. These patients came in with stroke symptoms. In these five patients, in addition to the zoster going down the nerve and showing up in the skin, it went up to the carotid system and the patients developed a giant cell arteritis in the cranial vessels, causing stroke symptoms and even death. I think it is also very important for the ophthalmologist to know that in follow-up of the patients in this series, no other significant medical diseases appeared. All the diseases with immune incompetence were therefore known before the zoster occured.

O.P. van Bijsterveld (Utrecht) : If you put these patients on steroids, will you ever be able to get them off steroid treatment ?

T.J Liesegang (Rochester) : I try not to put them on topical steroids. Once on topical steroids, I have gotten many of them off but it is with difficulty, titrating the dose very carefully and slowly over a long period of time.

C.R. Dawson (San Francisco) : With the numerous difficulties in managing the cornea in patients with ophthalmic zoster, do you think that early penetrating keratoplasty is a useful modality in the management of this problem ?

T.J. Liesegang (Rochester) : I am not sure you can predict who is going to do well or poorly with regard to the cornea. The disease may smolder for years. You will see patients and they will look healed and are off steroids. Some may return 6 months later without any specific complaints, but they may have developed a tremendous interstitial keratitis with deep vessels. So I have patients with corneal herpes zoster return frequently because they have a tendency to develop smoldering keratitis and may not be aware of it. I do not have a specific therapy. Although I have tried steroids on some patients with deep interstitial keratitis and it may respond. The one lady demonstrated in the photographs who progressed over the two year period of time was from the Bahamas and was not followed closely. She was treated with topical steroids and progressed nonetheless.

ORAL BROMOVINYLDEOXYURIDINE TREATMENT OF HERPES ZOSTER OPHTHALMICUS

P.C. MAUDGAL[1], M. DIELTIENS[1], E. DE CLERCQ[2] and L. MISSOTTEN[1]
[1]Eye Research Laboratory of the Ophthalmology Clinic, and [2]Rega Institute for Medical Research, Katholieke Universiteit Leuven, B-3000 Leuven, Belgium.

1. INTRODUCTION

Bromovinyldeoxyuridine $\big[$(E)-5-(2-bromovinyl)-2'-deoxyuridine, BVDU$\big]$ is a highly potent and selective antiherpes agent that inhibits the replication of herpes simplex virus type 1 (HSV-1) (1-3) and varicella-zoster virus (VZV) (4,5) at a very low concentration (0.002 - 0.01 µg/ml), while 5,000 to 10,000-fold higher concentrations are needed to affect normal cell metabolism.

When applied to rabbit eyes as either eye ointment or eyedrops, BVDU is superior to 5-iodo-2'-deoxyuridine (IDU) in suppressing the development of HSV-1 keratitis, and in promoting the healing of established epithelium disease (6,7). BVDU is also superior to 1 % TFT eyedrops in the treatment of stromal keratitis produced by intrastromal inoculation of HSV-1 (8), and keratouveitis caused by inoculation of HSV-1 into the anterior chamber (9). Oral administration of BVDU to rabbits at 10 mg/kg/day or 100 mg/kg/day also promotes healing of keratouveitis (9). BVDU eyedrops have been found efficacious in the treatment of corneal dendritic or geographic ulcers and stromal keratitis (10-12).

Efficacy of oral BVDU therapy has been demonstrated in the treatment of severe herpes zoster in cancer patients, and herpes zoster ophthalmicus with or without involvement of the ocular tissue (13-15). In this paper we report on the results obtained in 15 herpes zoster ophthalmicus patients who were treated with oral BVDU combined with topical 0.1 % BVDU eyedrops.

2. SUBJECTS AND METHODS

Seven male and eight female patients who presented with typical symptoms of herpes zoster ophthalmicus were admitted to the study. Except for one young patient (age : 31 years), other patients were either elderly (12 patients) or middle-aged (2 patients). Skin eruption consisted of papules,

Maudgal, P.C. and Missotten, L., (eds.) Herpetic Eye Diseases.
© *1985, Dr W. Junk Publishers, Dordrecht/Boston/Lancaster. ISBN 978-94-010-8935-7*

vesicles, bullae with or without hemorrhage, necrotic lesions, and sometimes crusts on the scalp, forehead, temporal region, nose, cheek and
periorbital skin. One patient had disseminated skin lesions. All subjects
had experienced prodromal symptoms in the involved dermatome before skin
lesions appeared. The lesions themselves had been present for an average
time of 5.6 days when the patients presented to us. All patients complained
of severe neuralgic pain in the involved dermatome. Various associated
systemic disorders were present in 11 patients, i.e. hyperthyroidism, hypo-
thyroidism after partial thyroidectomy, angina pectoris, old myocardial
infarction, liver cirrhosis, gallstones, rheumatism, Reiters disease, dia-
betes mellitus, asthma and recurrent epididymitis.

Lesions of periorbital skin or ulcerative blepharitis were noted in
13 patients. Ptosis of the upper eyelid was present in 2 patients, one of
them having total ophthalmoplegia. Two patients had mild conjunctivitis
whereas all others had marked conjunctivitis and chemosis. Two patients
had corneal ulcers. Dendritic keratitis was observed in 2 other cases,
and 5 patients had diffuse punctate keratitis. Stromal edema or infiltrates were noted in 3 patients. Aqueous flare was present in 7 eyes, two of
these also having keratic precipitates. Associated ocular diseases were
lid lag of the other eye (hyperthyroidism), absent eye movements and pu-
pillary reaction (total ophthalmoplegia), limited elevation (superior
rectus palsy), vitreous hemorrhage in the fellow eye, diabetic cataract
and retinitis pigmentosa.

All patients were hospitalized and informed consent was obtained for
BVDU treatment. BVDU 125 mg capsules were administered orally at 8 hour
intervals (375 mg/day) for 5 days. Hospitalized patients were examined
daily and at regular intervals thereafter. Routine blood and urine tests
as well as urea, creatinine, platelets, electrolytes and liver enzymes
(SGPT, SGOT, γGT) measurements were done before, during and after BVDU
therapy. Drug levels in blood and urine were determined by a bio-assay
based on the inhibition of HSV-1 cytopathogenicity in cell cultures. All
patients also received topical 0.1 % BVDU eyedrops administered hourly
during the day only. Patients who developed corneal edema due to endothelium damage were also given topical corticosteroids.

3. RESULTS

Within 24 hours after the start of BVDU treatment all patients felt
markedly better. New skin lesion formation ceased within 1-2 days (Table
1). Existing lesions started to scab from 1-3 days onwards and the skin
eruption healed in an average time of 9 days (from 6 to 12 days). Neuralgic pain subsided within 2-3 days if the treatment was started at an early
stage of skin eruption. Treatment did not influence neuralgic pain in two
patients and it took 3 - 4 weeks to subside in the other three cases. Postherpetic neuralgia reappeared later in one patient. Almost all patients
complained of severe itching in the involved skin dermatome during the
follow-up period; this itching subsided gradually over several weeks.

Keratitis healed within 6 - 12 days (Table 1). Conjunctivitis subsided
in the same period; however, slight redness of the conjunctiva persisted
for up to one more week in two patients. Aqueous flare generally resolved
within 1 week; however, in one case it persisted for 3 weeks. With the
resolution of eye disease, visual acuity improved markedly (10/10 in 7 patients, 9/10 in one patient, 8/10 in 2 patients, 7/10 in 2 patients, 5/10
and 4/10 in one patient each, and unrecorded in one patient). Complications observed in these patients were lower canaliculitis (2 patients),
dry eye (1 patient), and exposure keratopathy between treatment day 3 to
5 (1 patient). Associated senile disciform degeneration of the macula was
observed in one patient, when her fundus could be examined properly following BVDU treatment. Most likely this macular pathology was already present before the VZV infection or BVDU treatment.

Apparent VZV eye disease recurred in one patient 20 days after BVDU
treatment. It presented as stromal keratitis and internal rectus palsy.

Table 1. Oral BVDU treatment of patients with ophthalmic zoster

Treatment regimen : oral BVDU at 375 mg/day for 5 days, combined with BVDU
   0.1 % eyedrops.
Number of patients : 15.
Average duration of symptoms before BVDU treatment : 5.6 days.
Average healing time on BVDU therapy :
   - cessation of new lesion formation : within 1-2 days
   - crust formation of skin lesions : within 2-3 days
   - complete healing of skin lesions : within 6-12 days
   - resolution of keratitis : within 6-12 days
   - resolution of conjunctivitis : within 8-20 days
Duration of neuralgia on BVDU therapy : variable (2 days - 4 weeks).

Complete resolution occurred in one month upon topical 0.5 % BVDU and topical corticosteroid administration.

Routine urine and blood tests, and measurements of urea, creatinine, blood platelets, electrolytes and liver enzymes (SGPT, SGOT, γGT) did not reveal any toxicity of BVDU.

4. COMMENT

This study demonstrates that BVDU is an effective and safe drug when administered orally at 375 mg/day and topically as 0.1 % eyedrops to patients with herpes zoster ophthalmicus. The formation of new skin lesions was arrested within 2 days of BVDU therapy and the skin eruption healed within at maximum 12 days. Similarly, the eye disease responded quickly to BVDU therapy, although topical corticosteroids were needed in some patients to suppress corneal edema resulting from endothelium involvement. Apparent VZV eye disease recurred in one patient 20 days after BVDU therapy was stopped. This recurrence resolved upon treatment with topical 0.5 % BVDU eyedrops and topical corticosteroids.

One might argue whether 5 days of oral BVDU are sufficient for the treatment of ophthalmic zoster. A 5-day duration of therapy was chosen based on our experience in cancer patients (14,15), where 5 days of oral BVDU treatment sufficed to effectively treat localized or disseminated herpes zoster skin eruption. No recurrences were noted during the follow-up period (14, 15 and the present study), except for one recurrence of ocular disease.

A number of patients in our series had associated systemic disorders, i.e. thyroid dysfunction, heart disease, liver cirrhosis, gallstones, or asthma. BVDU treatment did not adversely affect these systemic disorders. Furthermore, no toxic effects of BVDU therapy were revealed by whole blood cell counts, blood platelets, urea, creatinine, electrolytes and liver enzymes (SGPT, SGOT and γGT) measurements.

REFERENCES

1. De Clercq E, Descamps J, Barr PJ, Jones AS, Serafinowski P, Walker RT, Huang GF, Torrence PF, Schmidt CL, Mertes MP, Kulikowski T, Shugar D. 1979. Comparative study of the potency and selectivity of anti-herpes compounds. In: Antimetabolites in Biochemistry, Biology and Medicine. Skoda J, Langen P (eds.), Pergamon Press, Oxford, pp. 275-285.
2. De Clercq E, Descamps J, De Somer P, Barr PJ, Jones AS, Walker RT. 1979. (E)-5-(2-Bromovinyl)-2'-deoxyuridine : a potent and selective anti-herpes agent. Proc. Natl. Acad. Sci. USA 76, 2947-2951.

3. De Clercq E, Descamps J, Maudgal PC, Missotten L, Leyten R, Verhelst G, Jones AS, Walker RT, Busson R, Vanderhaeghe H, De Somer P. 1980. Selective anti-herpes activity of 5-(2-halogenovinyl)-2'-deoxyuridines and -2'-deoxycytidines. In: Developments in Antiviral Therapy. Collier LH, Oxford J (eds.), Academic Press, London, pp. 21-42.
4. De Clercq E, Descamps J, Ogata M, Shigeta S. 1982. In vitro suscepti-bility of varicella-zoster to E-5-(2-bromovinyl)-2'-deoxyuridine and related compounds. Antimicrob. Agents Chemother. 21, 33-38.
5. Shigeta S, Yokota T, Iwabuchi T, Baba M, Konno K, Ogata M, De Clercq E. 1983. Comparative efficacy of antiherpes drugs against various strains of varicella-zoster virus. J. Infect. Dis. 147, 576-584.
6. Maudgal PC, De Clercq E, Descamps J, Missotten L, De Somer P, Busson R, Vanderhaeghe H, Verhelst G, Walker RT, Jones AS. 1980. (E)-5-(2-Bromovinyl)-2'-deoxyuridine in the treatment of experimental herpes simplex keratitis. Antimicrob. Agents Chemother. 17, 8-12.
7. Maudgal PC, De Clercq E, Descamps J, Missotten L. 1979. Comparative evaluation of BVDU (E)-5-(2-bromovinyl)-2'-deoxyuridine) and IDU (5-iodo-2'-deoxyuridine) in the treatment of experimental herpes sim-plex keratitis in rabbits. Bull. Soc. belge Ophtalmol. 186, 109-118.
8. Maudgal PC, De Clercq E, Descamps J, Missotten L, Wijnhoven J. 1982. Experimental stromal herpes simplex keratitis. Influence of treatment with topical bromovinyldeoxyuridine and trifluridine. Arch. Ophthal-mol. 100, 653-656.
9. Maudgal PC, Uyttebroeck W, De Clercq E, Missotten L. 1982. Oral and topical treatment of experimental herpes simplex iritis with bromo-vinyldeoxyuridine. Arch. Ophthalmol. 100, 1337-1340.
10. Maudgal PC, Missotten L, De Clercq E, Descamps J, De Meuter E. 1981. Efficacy of (E)-5-(2-bromovinyl)-2'-deoxyuridine in the topical treat-ment of herpes simplex keratitis. Albrecht von Graefes Arch. Klin. Ophthalmol. 216, 261-268.
11. Maudgal PC, De Clercq E, Descamps J, Missotten L. 1981. Efficacy of E-5-(2-bromovinyl)-2'-deoxyuridine in the topical treatment of herpe-tic keratitis in rabbits and man. In: Herpetische Augenerkrankungen. Sundmacher R (ed.), J.F. Bergmann Verlag, München, pp. 339-341.
12. Maudgal PC, De Clercq E, Missotten L. 1984. Efficacy of bromovinyl-deoxyuridine in the treatment of herpes simplex virus and varicella-zoster virus eye infections. Antiviral Res. 4, 281-291.
13. Maudgal PC, Dralands L, Lamberts L, De Clercq E, Descamps J, Missot-ten L. 1981. Preliminary results of oral BVDU treatment of herpes zoster ophthalmicus. Bull. Soc. belge Ophthalmol. 193, 49-56.
14. De Clercq E, De Greef H, Wildiers J, De Jonge G, Drochmans A, Des-camps J, De Somer P. 1980. Oral (E)-5-(2-bromovinyl)-2'-deoxyuridine in severe herpes zoster. Brit. Med. J. 281, 1178.
15. Wildiers J, De Clercq E. 1984. Oral (E)-(2-bromovinyl)-2'-deoxyuridine treatment of severe herpes zoster in cancer patients. Eur. J. Cancer Clin. Oncol. 20, 471-476.

DISCUSSION :

L.M.T Collum (Dublin) : It is not criticism, but could I perhaps
talk in the nicest possible way. I accept entirely what you
say that BVDU may do what you have shown. Taking the cases
that have been minor attacks with just a little rash, get better fairly quickly on their own. The rash disappears quickly
and their symptoms will tend to regress reasonably well. What
you say may be correct, but unless you can compare it with
a control group it is very difficult to prove the beneficial
effect of BVDU. In the more severe cases you seem to get good
results. I think this is a slight point to make. Perhaps
you have any comment to make about that ?

P.C. Maudgal (Leuven) : In this series only one patient had mild
skin eruption, but all other patients had very severe skin
disease. However, you are right in raising that point. We
have seen some other patients with ophthalmic herpes zoster
who had only a mild rash, or just a few skin vesicles, which
disappeared without any treatment.

C.C. Kok-van Alphen (Leiden) : I think the management of pain
was very impressive; because it is very painful disease. I
think it is very important, when you can do anything about
this. Then I should like to ask : do you know anything about
the tear production in those patients ? Has therapy anything
to do with it ? Was it better afterwards ? We see patients
with bad tear production later, I should say.

P.C. Maudgal (Leuven) : Some of the patients had dry eyes.
Most of the patients were elderly people, and you have yourself
said that you see such cases. We don't believe it is due to
BVDU treatment. The dry eye condition is managed by artificial tear substitutes, hydroxypropylmethyl cellulose inserts
etc.

B. Juel-Jensen (Oxford) : May I say how much I enjoyed listening
to this series of clinical cases, because we all start that way
with a new drug, we have to. But I would make a plea, not
least to myself, that when we are dealing in controlled trials
with agents with a possible action on zoster, that we record

two things, one, at least, we in Oxford have often failed to run. One is, how long after the onset of the first clinical observable signs was the drug given and second, how long after the first clinical symptoms ? I think this is important, for the incubation period (so colled) of zoster can vary from one day to 21 days. And God only knows what is going on in the nerves during the 21 days. It happened to Fred Mac-Callum, my partner. We did not make the correct diagnosis for three weeks. Some of the patients you showed have had zoster perhaps for several weeks. I think it may be doubted whether you are doing your antiviral drug justice when you give it that late.

P.C. Maudgal (Leuven) : I agree with you in general. But I don't know how to start treating a patient during the incubation period.

B. Juel-Jensen (Oxford) : I don't either. But I think it is important in the assessment of the double blind trials that we take this into account. It could just be that the patients with a long incubation period respond less favourably than those with a short. It could be, and it may be too simplistic, that the virus in those with a short incubation period have managed to do less harm to various structures in which the virus is present. That's my point.

P.C. Maudgal (Leuven) : I agree with you again that this might be a possibility. But concerning your second point that whether we are doing justice by administering the compound to these patients, if you compare the natural course of zoster infection, it takes much longer time before the skin lesions are healed, especially if the disease is severe. I think we have enough specialists in the audience who whill agree to that.

B. Juel-Jensen (Oxford) : It is a mutual admiration society.

P.C. Maudgal (Leuven) : Thank you.

R. Sundmacher (Freiburg) : May I ask you a last question : what was the rationale for the treatment period of five days ? In our experience with Zovirax, five days have not been suffi-

cient. We currently treat 10 or more days; and the important
observation even with two weeks of systemic treatment is that
the severe neuralgic pain, which usually is relieved promptly
by systemic Zovirax, may recur. In some instances patients
complain that the pain may even be worse. Our interpretation
of these observation has been that zoster is some kind of
"slow" virus disease which must be treated on a prolonged
basis.

P.C. Maudgal (Leuven) : Professor De Clercq suggested that we
should treat the patient only for five days; perhaps he would
like to explain this ?

E. De Clercq (Leuven) : You should see this in context with the
cancer patients with herpes zoster that we treated with BVDU.
In our Oncology Clinic, we have additional experience in the
treatment of localised or disseminated herpes zoster in cancer
patients. The majority of the patients, i.e. about 60 % responded after one day of BVDU treatment. This means that at least
in these patients, the treatment period could be limited to two
or three days.

R. Sundmacher (Freiburg) : No, our expierence has been completely
different, with ACV. When you withdraw the drug the disease
recurs. If your statement is correct, then BVDU must be terribly more potent that ACV, or your cases belonged to the ones
which spontaneously heal within a couple of days, such cases,
of course, exist.

E. De Clercq (Leuven) : We have not seen any recurrence after
BVDU treatment. You should not forget that BVDU is about
1000-fold more potent in its activity against varicella-zoster
virus than acyclovir.

R. Sundmacher (Freiburg) : I know, you have been telling this,
but one should note that you refer to in vitro differences of
which nobody knows what they mean in the clinical situation.

E. De Clercq (Leuven) : There are several compounds which are
effective in vitro, but ineffective in either experimental models
or in a clinical situation. Soike has tested BVDU and ACV in
the simian varicella virus model in monkeys and found that

BVDU is far more effective than ACV. (Soike et al. : Antimicrob. Agents Chem. 20 : 291-297, 1981 and Soike et al : Antiviral Res. 1 : 325-337, 1981). Our results further demonstrate
the efficacy of BVDU in the treatment of herpes zoster infections. But, we could indeed discuss whether five days therapy is sufficient for the treatment of ophthalmic zoster. Five
days was chosen on an arbitrary basis and for the treatment of
ophthalmic zoster it may be too short; but for those patients
that we treated in the Cancer Clinic, we found that the five
day treatment regimen was effective and we have not changed
this protocol so far.

C.C. Kok-van Alphen (Leiden) : Did you see side effects of the
therapy ? Because I think when you didn't, perhaps we can
extend the therapy.

P.C. Maudgal (Leuven) : We didn't observe any side effects.
Prof. De Clercq objected to prolonging of therapy, because you
should not treat the patient for longer period than required.
In fact, till now we have not felt any need of prolonging therapy.

R. Sundmacher (Freiburg) : Didn't you see any recurrences in
the cornea which arose from presumed virus persistence ? If
so, my clue would be that the treatment was not totally effective.

P.C. Maudgal (Leuven) : There was recurrence of stromal disease
in one patient several weeks later, and I am not sure whether it was a viral or immunological problem. In this patient
stromal disease recurred when topical corticosteroids were stopped.

R. Sundmacher (Freiburg) : I think there is no immunological
problem without an underlying viral background.

P.C.Maudgal (Leuven) : I agree to that, but it does not necessarily mean the reactivation of VZV in the cornea, especially when
the corneal edema suddenly re-appears when you have just
stopped the topical corticosteroids; and it subsided quickly
when you re-institute corticosteroid therapy.

HERPES ZOSTER TREATMENT

J.I. McGILL, Southampton

SUMMARY

A retrospective study was carried out at Southampton Eye Hospital on the
files of 144 patients with ocular herpes zoster seen over the last four
years.   Treatment duration and recurrence rates were significantly lower
in the Acyclovir group compared to the steroid treated group, and the
Acyclovir with steroid treated group.   Progression of the disease was
more evident in the steroid treated group as new parts of the eyes that
were not involved in the initial attack were affected when recurrences
had occurred.

INTRODUCTION

Herpes zoster is a common affliction affecting both the skin and the eye.
There is an estimated incidence of 0.2% of herpes zoster in the general
population, of whom 7% to 20% will develop ocular involvement.   Ocular
involvement can be lengthy, particularly if treated with topical steroids,
often resulting in ocular damage and visual loss.   The currently accepted
theory of the aetiology of herpes zoster infection is that after an initial
attack of chicken-pox the virus remains latent in the dorsal root ganglion
of the trigeminal nerve.   Trigger factors reactivate the virus.   It was
first suggested by von Bokay (1909) that varicella and zoster were the
same viral agent, and Weller et al. (1958) isolated the virus from patients
either with varicella or zoster infection and found that the isolates
were indistinguishable.

Previous work (McGill, 1981; McGill and Chapman, 1983) has shown that
topical Acyclovir has a role to play in the treatment of herpes zoster
ocular involvement, and that it is superior to steroids in terms both of
treatment duration and of recurrence rates.   However, in this work no

Maudgal, P.C. and Missotten, L., (eds.) Herpetic Eye Diseases.
© *1985, Dr W. Junk Publishers, Dordrecht/Boston/Lancaster. ISBN 978-94-010-8935-7*

control or placebo treated patients were included, as it was found
ethically difficult to justify treating with placebo patients with painful
red inflamed eyes.   There are two ways out of this dilemma.   Firstly,
the prophylactic role of Acyclovir can be tested in patients who develop
a skin rash, who have not yet developed ocular involvement, and clinical
trials are at present under way to determine this.   The second way out
of the dilemma is to review retrospectively all patients treated by many
different doctors in a set period with either form of treatment.
Obviously such a retrospective analysis has many pitfalls.   By considering
the treatment of many different doctors, different regimes were used, but
the main point is that such a retrospective analysis, because it covers
many doctors, will overcome any observer bias shortfall.   With prolonged
follow-up, too, it will determine how individual groups fare, and whether
any one treatment is associated with unacceptable side effects.

MATERIAL

Files for all 144 immuno-competent patients attending Southampton Eye
Hospital with herpes zoster ophthalmicus between 1977 and 1983 were surveyed.
The name, age, sex and entry date to the Eye Hospital of each patient was
recorded.   Details of the onset of the rash, initial crusting, termination
of the rash, duration of progermal symptoms, presence of post-herpetic
neuralgia and eye signs prior to the start of treatment were noted.
Recorded also were the presence or absence, and duration, of conjunctival
injection, corneal epithelial disease, and stromal disease, be it disciform
or numular keratitis, episcleritis, scleritis and uveitis.   Any details
of iris involvement, rise in intraocular pressure, change in lens clarity,
fundal appearance or extraocular muscle balance were recorded, as was the
visual acuity on the Snellen chart.   Patients were seen every two to three
days during the acute phase of the disease, and thereafter two-weekly,
two-monthly, and subsequently once every six months, depending on the
course of the disease.

RESULTS

The age range of the patients varied from 20 to 93 years.   The average
age was 63 years with 51 patients in the 7th, 8th and 9th decade of life.
65 patients were female, 56 male.   Overall there was no difference in the
change in visual acuity in the three groups, namely the steroid treated

TABLE I

Change in visual acuity of patients with herpes zoster ophthalmicus
from the onset of treatment on different treatment regimes

	Steroids	Acyclovir	Steroids & Acyclovir
% improved by two lines	35%	36%	29%
% declined by two lines	30%	15%	43%
% with no significant change	35%	49%	28%

TABLE II

Acyclovir treated patients

Number	Controlled by Acyclovir	Steroids added
56	51	5

51 of the 56 patients initially treated with Acyclovir responded
favourably, but in 5 cases the clinical signs failed to subside
in 4 weeks, and steroids were added.

TABLE III

Summary of treatment duration and recurrence rates of the different
treatment regimes

	Acyclovir	Steroids	Acyclovir & Steroids
Number of patients	56	74	14
Average duration of treatment	62.3	200	197
Total Recurrence rate	6% (2)	50% (37)	57% (8)
% Recurrences after one year	6% (2)	5.4% (4)	7.1% (1)

TABLE IV

To show the average duration of interval after cessation of treatment
and before the first recurrence

	Acyclovir	Steroids	Acyclovir & Steroids
Average duration in weeks	67	19	18

TABLE V

A summary of recurrences occurring on and off treatment on the different treatment regimes

	Acyclovir	Steroids	Acyclovir & Steroids
Recurrences on treatment	0	5 (2) *	2 (1)
Recurrences on treatment being withdrawn	0	15 (8)	3 (3)
Recurrences after treatment was stopped	2	27	7

* Numbers in brackets denote patients who had recurrences after treatment was stopped as well as recurrences on treatment

TABLE VI

To show treatment duration and number of recurrences demonstrating that duration of treatment has no effect on incidence of recurrences

	Steroids	Steroids & Acyclovir
50 - 100 (days)	12	2
101 - 200 (days)	11	2
201 and over (days)	14	4

patients, the Acyclovir treated patients, or the steroid and Acyclovir treated patients (Table I). The average duration of treatment for Acyclovir treated patients was significantly shorter than that for steroid treated patients, with only two out of 56 patients having a recurrence, and this occurring after 18 months in the Acyclovir treated patients, whereas 50% of the steroid treated patients recurred in the first year and 5% after one year (Table III). The average duration of the interval from the cessation of treatment to the first recurrence was shortest for the steroid treated patients (Table IV). A significant proportion of patients treated with topical steroids had a recurrence or exacerbation of their disease whilst still on treatment (Table V). It is apparent that there is a difference in outcome of the patients treated with the different treatment regimes. The addition of steroids appears to lead to prolonged treatment, but the duration of treatment with steroids had no effect on the incidence of recurrence (Table VI).

CONCLUSIONS

This retrospective study of patients treated at the Southampton Eye Hospital and using Acyclovir alone or in combination with steroids, or steroids alone, has shown that Acyclovir treated patients fare much better than steroid or steroid plus Acyclovir treated patients. The addition of steroids leads to prolonged treatment, frequent recurrences occurring either as treatment is being withdrawn or after it had been withdrawn. In addition, steroid treated patients often showed a progression of their disease in the recurrence to parts not initially affected.

Not all patients treated with topical Acyclovir responded favourably, and my policy is that if stromal involvement or uveitis persists for more than three weeks after the onset of the Acyclovir treatment, then steroids topically should be added. Prolonged stromal involvement or uveitis lead to marked endothelial loss and can result in endothelial decompensation.

From the practical point of view, patients presenting initially with herpes zoster kerato-uveitis, not initially treated with steroids, should be treated with topical Acyclovir 3.3% ointment five times a day until the disease resolves, and thereafter twice a day for two weeks before stopping treatment.

ACKNOWLEDGEMENTS

I am most grateful to Mr M.J. Absolon, Mr I.H. Chisholm, Mr A.R. Elkington
and Mr C.B. Walker for allowing the case notes of their patients to be
studied.

Thanks are also due to my wife for typing the paper.

REFERENCES

1. von Bokay J. 1909 Uber den aetiologischen Zusammenhang der
    Narizellen mit gewissen Faellen von Herpes Zoster. Wien, Klin
    Wschr 22: 1323-1326.
2. Weller TH, Witton HM, Bell JE. 1958 Etiological agents of
    varicella and herpes zoster: Isolation, propagation and cultural
    characteristics in vitro. J Exp Med 108: 843-868.
3. McGill J. 1981 Topical acyclovir in herpes zoster ocular
    involvement. Br J Ophthalmol, 65: 542-545.
4. McGill J, Chapman C. 1983 A comparison of topical acyclovir
    with steroids in the treatment of herpes zoster keratouveitis.
    Br J Ophthalmol, 67: 746-750.

DISCUSSION :

R. Sundmacher (Freiburg) : You did not try systemic therapy yourself ?

J. McGill (Southampton) : Yes, we have done a placebo controlled
study of intravenous acyclovir on the acute stage rash (McGill
et al. J. Infection 1984). There was even distribution of patients with ocular involvement in the intravenous study. The
five days course of intravenous therapy was not enough to affect the eye. All patients with eye involvement treated with
intravenous acyclovir for five days required subsequent topical
acyclovir. So, that rather confirms what you were saying before.

J. Colin (Brest) : We have treated 18 patients with systemic acyclovir during five days and then by tablets during 10 more
days. We have seen after the end of treatment two recurrences with skin vesicles in another skin area. Have you any
idea of this mechanism ?

J. McGill (Southampton) : No. I suppose it must be recurrence
of a slow virus. I agree, it can happen. It will fit in the
eye picture, wouldn't it, if you get recurrences later. But
was the eye involvement treated with five or 12 days treatment ? Does that successfully treat the eye involvement ?

J. Colin (Brest) : Yes.

J. McGill (Southampton) : It did ! It is interesting.

B. Juel-Jensen (Oxord) : Mr McGill, first thank you for a most elegant paper. Just to ask again about this magic five days, I
don't know where the medical profession collected it, although
as my neighbour suggested it may originate from the five-day
working week. You may remember the work by Bean and colleau-
gues in Minneapolis : their placebo group all grew varicella-
zoster virus for five days. It makes one wonder whether in
fact we are treating for long enough. You don't know, even
though it disappears in what you can swab locally, that the
virus is not still active in the nerve, we have now started in
severe zoster to treat the patient for at least a week and sometimes for 10 days.

J.McGill (Southampton) : Thank you, you have got a very good
    point here. Certainly we are now treating for seven days.
    We are doing an oral trial again on seven days. The only
    guidelines we have got is that we cultured the skin lesions
    after five days, they were crusted which meant that they proba-
    bly started to heal, we assume they were healing and we could
    not isolate virus from these lesions. It may be that there
    is still live virus deep down in the nerve or under the skin.
    There was certainly no virus or virus particles in those lesions
    after five days. But it is totally empirical as far as I am
    concerned. As for the working week, I don't think that is
    right because the law is that all zoster patients come in on
    Friday evening just as you are getting off for the week - end !

M. Shield (High Wycombe) : I would like to raise the possibility
    that we are in fact confusing two separate issues here. The
    first is that you have got persistant virus and the other is
    the persistance of virus antigens. And a lot of the features
    that you see in varicella-zoster virus infections would fit in
    very well with soluble antigen progressing through anatomical
    sites and being taken up by the lymphatic drainage. As is
    characteristic for certain infections in which there is a cell-
    mediated response you may well get persisting antigen, perhaps
    there for many many years. One can think of conditions where
    you get antigens deposited in the skin (such as tuberculin)
    and when they (meaning people) are re-challenged with the
    same antigen in the form of infective particles, either orally
    or by inhalation, then you actually get a response also in
    the skin around where the antigen is fixed. So, if you have
    a re-challenge say in the nasal area or orally with herpes
    virus, you may well provoke an immunological response to an-
    tigen which is present elsewhere, in this case in the eye.
    I also suggest that with things like acyclovir, perhaps BVDU
    and other antiviral agents, that you may get an effect of these
    compounds actually on immunologically functioning units such
    as lymphocytes.These drugs may alter the immunological func-
    tions that you see in these diseases.

J.McGill (Southampton) : It is a good point there. But if it is just viral antigen why does it always flare up in the eye, firstly. And secondly if it is just viral antigen, parts of the eye not initially treated become affected in recurrences. If they had antigen there initially, you would have thought that they had shown the disease process in the initial attack. But sometimes they don't.

M. Shield (High Wycombe) : These are interesting things for which to have to provide answers. I imagine that you can get infiltration and distribution of the antigen over a period of time as a consequence of handling by phagocytic cells.

T.J. Liesegang (Rochester) : If you ask the patients carefully enough, you will find that about 10% to 15% will have vesicles in other areas of their body. They may not tell you about them and you need to ask them. Many of them experience a viremia that has been proven by cultures. About 10% in a recent zoster series that I was evaluating for other reasons had dissemination of a very mild degree, and this is particularly true if they are immunologically suppressed. These patients can go on with skin dissemination for months. Virus has been cultured from a few of those, although by the time you see them they are usually crusted and nothing is there to culture. It depends on how often you see the patients.

I do not necessarily think that the severity of the eye disease relates to the severity of the skin disease. Obviously the nasociliary nerve is the most important nerve relating to eye involvement. The most common nerves to be involved, however, are the supraorbital and the supratrocheal nerves on the forehead, and this does not usually lead to eye involvement. They may have a heavy involvement of the nasociliary nerve and can get eye involvement without getting any skin disease. In fact, I am sure that we see patients with pseudodendrites, or with disciform keratitis, or with interstitial keratitis without a history or evidence of any skin disease. But if you were astute enought to do serological studies, you might pick up an increase in the zoster titer. As I mentioned before, the virus can go up the central nervous system, down the nerve, or just into the eye. So it does not necessarily have to have skin involvement.

We are involved in a placebo controlled study of 10 days of oral acyclovir. We have over 85 patients in a collaborative multi-center study. I am not free to give you all the information, because it is still preliminary. It was not startling enough to break the study, but our patients with oral acyclovir are doing better as far as the acute symptoms and as far as the early ocular disease. We hope that this holds up over the length of the study.

J.McGill (Southampton) : What about the postherpetic neuralgia?

T.J.Liesegang (Rochester) : It is too early to tell, and I do not have any information.

J.McGill (Southampton) : Have any one of your treated patient had a segmental arteritis or the stroke ?

T.J. Liesegang (Rochester) : One of my patients died, and I do not know whether he got the placebo or whether he got acyclovir.

J.McGill (Southampton) : Because we have seen that patients die in the first six weeks. What the percentage is, I don't know. But our number of patients is small.

T.J. Liesegang (Rochester) : The treatment of central nervous system zoster is still debatable. Some neurologists feel that they should be given antivirals. Some of them have been given antivirals and have died inspite of the treatment. Others feel steroids are indicated or anticoagulants. I do not know how to treat this aspect of the disease at the present time.

B. Juel-Jensen (Oxford) : Just one comment. This business of outlying lesions is a well known fact. Those of you who read the paper by Tomlinson and MacCallum[1] about 15 years ago will know why. They demonstrated quite clearly that in people over 45 to 50, there is no detectable compliment fixing antibody to varicella-zoster. Peripheral lesions only stop if you produce these antibodies. That probably is the main function of the humoral element of the immunity in the patient.

[1]Tomlinson, A.H. and MacCallum, F.O. (1970) : The incidence of complement fixing antibodies to varicella-zoster virus in hospital patients and blood donors. J. Hyg. (Camb.) 68, 411

GENERAL DISCUSSION ON THE MANAGEMENT OF HERPETIC EYE DISEASES

P.C. MAUDGAL(Leuven)

During this meeting we have heard some
very elegant papers on the current problems in herpes virus eye
infections. However, every clinician has his or her own approach
to deal with specific conditions. I thought that before we depart,
perhaps we should exchange views and discuss different approaches
available to us. I have requested Dr. Sundmacher to continue to
chair this session. I have also brought with me some slides of
herpetic ocular lesions, and I shall point out what difficulties we
face in diagnosis and management of the herpetic eye diseases.
Please feel free to ask questions or to make comments at any
moment. I shall appreciate if you will tell us how you manage a
particular case. It will be a "general discussion" in the real
sense of the word, if questions are asked from the floor and the
answers are also provided from the floor.
So, in the management of herpetic eye diseases we have several
problems. We have heard during this meeting that herpes virus
infection may present with conjunctivitis. When there are associated skin lesions, it is easy to diagnose the condition. But if
there are no skin lesions in a patient who has a red eye, we
are confronted with the problem of diagnosis. This particular
patient had a combined infection by adenovirus and herpes simplex
virus. I would like to know the opinion of other sepcialists here,
what should be done in such a case to make the diagnosis and to
institute appropriate therapy ? How should we proceed ?
C.R. Dawson (San Francisco) : In our patients who have previously had ocular herpes and then present with conjunctivitis,
   I start all of them on prophylactic antivirals. In this case,
   trifluoridine twice daily. Dr. Field will object, but we feel
   this prevents the recurrence of corneal disease. We have not
   observed significant epithelial keratitis with this twice daily
   dosage, even with the more toxic antivirals such as idoxuridine. It is a problem to identify those cases of acute follicular
   conjunctivitis due to herpes simplex in patients who do not

Maudgal, P.C. and Missotten, L., (eds.) Herpetic Eye Diseases.
© *1985, Dr W. Junk Publishers, Dordrecht/Boston/Lancaster. ISBN 978-94-010-8935-7*

have a previous history of herpetic eye disease. Acute follicular conjunctivitis is a relatively common condition and herpetic infections make up less than 10% of cases. While rapid viral diagnosis may be ideal, it may not be cost-effective. In every case of acute follicular conjunctivitis, however, we examine the lids very carefully, especially at the base of the cilia, for small, discrete ulcers which may be hidden on a more superficial examination. We also actively discourage the use of corticosteroids during the acute phase of any follicular conjunctivitis; there is no rationale for their use and the consequences can be devastating if the conjunctivitis is caused by herpes simplex.

P.C. Maudgal (Leuven) : Well, you have as well pointed out the problem. Are there any further comments ?

P. Wright (London) : I think I am known as a therapeutic nihilist throughout the world, but it is my philosophy, that on the whole these are toxic compounds which will produce confusing epithelial changes very readily. One thing I do not want somebody to do is to present to me this case three days later when there is spotty epithelial keratitis that may be due to the co-existent adenovirus or may be due to an antiviral. So my rule is that if you have no clinical grounds including this careful search for small vesicles to believe that this is a recurrence of herpetic disease or primary herpetic disease, you treat it only with topical antibiotics until you have some evidence to alter that. We have 48-hour isolation for virus and we have rapid micro IF antibody titers. So my instruction is that you send up isolates, you do daily blood and tears, and unless you have good laboratory support you continue without antiviral therapy.

R. Sundmacher (Freiburg) : If I see no corneal or anterior segment involvement, I tend to give no antivirals - and above all no steroids. However, a proper control for a couple of days is advisable. The other problem is that "experienced people", who have had a number of corneal recurrences, will feel very uneasy without antiviral cover - even if it is not

absolutely necessary. In these cases antiviral therapy may
be justified for these more general reasons.

P.C. Maudgal (Leuven) : We make smears of conjunctival scrapings in such patients and stain them by Gram stain and Giemsa stain. We also use immunofluorescence staining technique
using fluorescein tagged antiherpes antibodies. Immunofluorescence technique may not be a 100% reliable method, but it
can give a correct diagnosis in about 80% cases. Combined
with the cytological results by Gram or Giemsa stain, you can
nearly be sure of the diagnosis. However, to do this one
needs suitable equipment. Diagnostic problem also arises in
cases of punctate herpetic keratitis. Our policy is again to
proceed in the way as we do for follicular conjunctivitis. Are
there any further suggestions or comments ?
Let us go to the next slide. These are typical dendritic ulcers
caused by herpes simplex virus infection. If we see that picture, I am sure we all agree that we can manage them in different ways. We know that one may just scrape the lesions
mechanically or apply cauteries using different types of chemicals, or cryotherapy. One may also use antivirals or may com-
bine antivirals with interferon. Are there people in this audience who routinely use debridement instead of antivirals ?

C.R.Dawson (San Francisco) : I agree that I am in this minority
but there is clear evidence that gentle, wiping debridement
with a dry, cotton-tipped applicator removes 99,9% of the virus
present on the surface of the cornea. This is done after the
application of topical anesthesia. The loose epithelium is removed at the slitlamp with a dry, cotton-tipped applicator up
to the edge where it is firmly attached. The debridement does
not involve the use of toxic antiseptic compounds such as carbolic acid or iodine. Following debridement, we place a relatively long-acting dilating medication in the eye (e.g. homatropine), one application of an antiviral compound and an antibiotic drop. The patient is then patched firmly for 24-48 hours.
Debridement is contra-indicated if there is a herpetic lesion of
the lid or a follicular conjunctivitis, both of which can act as

sources of reinfection for the corneal epithelium. It has recently been shown that there may be a localized conjunctivitis
of the tarsal plate directly overlying the corneal epithelial lesions, which can also be a source of infection; thus the tarsal
conjunctiva must be examined carefully with the slitlamp before
debridement is done. This treatment clearly shortens the duration of the corneal ulceration and reduces patients morbidity
(Whitcher et al., Arch. Ophthalmology 94 : 589, 1976). When
the patch is removed at 24-48 hours full antiviral therapy is
instituted. With the antiviral therapy alone, without debridement, however, the course is more prolonged.

P.C.Maudgal (Leuven) : Although very potent antivirals are becoming available, personally I would still prefer debridement,
if the dendritic lesion is present in the prepupillary region;
because the patient may develop stromal disease despite antiviral treatment. If it happens in the prepupillary area, the
vision will mostly remain affected after the keratitis is healed.

M.G. Falcon (London) : I certainly support those views too. At
Moorfields we did a study in which we have shown that debridement combined with an antiviral lead to more rapid healing
than antiviral alone.

P.C. Maudgal (Leuven) : I would like to comment on that point.
Of course you can use antivirals after debridement, and I understand the rationale behind it. Replica histology has shown
us that only a limited number of epithelial cells are involved
in a dendritic ulcer. If you debride this lesion, the focus
of infection is removed, as Dr. Dawson has already pointed
out. If you then administer antivirals you are using them as
prophylaxis. In terms of healing time by this approach, you
are in fact observing the regeneration time of the epithelium
in the presence of the antiviral drug. I am unable to understand how any antiviral drug can make the epithelium wound
heal quickly after debridement.

C.R. Dawson (San Francisco) : I feel that a single dose of antiviral, even a relatively toxic one such as idoxuridine, has

only a slight effect on retarding epithelialization in 48 hours.
If acyclovir is available for this purpose, however, the effect
would be very small indeed, if present at all.

P.C. Maudgal (Leuven) : I agree, but I made that point because
I don't understand why the healing should be quicker if you
use antivirals after debridement than the debridement alone.
I accept that the recurrence rates would be higher after debridement if you don't use antivirals with it; but I don't think
that the use of antivirals leads to quicker healing. I might
be wrong, but I feel it is slight misinterpretation of the studies in the literature, whether these studies relate to antivirals or interferon. The credit for a rapid healing should be
given to debridement and not to the antivirals or interferon.

P. Wright (London) : I don't believe you have any evidence
though that those cells which you show have got beautiful epi-
theliolysis. You know, they are very sick cells indeed. Is
there any evidence that these can get their act together again
and stick down and be of any use to you ? Most certainly,
I believe that removing cells which have little potential for
replication improves the chances of those viable cells around
the edge to replicate and spread across that patch.

P.C. Maudgal (Leuven) : Yes, that is true. These cells are very
sick cells and are not going to regain their normal function.
However, if there is associated epithelium edema, corneal replica studies indicate the presence of virus in the distant
cells. In those cases I would not choose to scrape the epithelial lesion. If it is a localized dendrite like this one, although this is a large one, you can scrape it without fearing
any problems afterwards.

G.O. Waring (Atlanta) : Is there any role at all of cautery or
anything like that at this stage of treatment ?

P.C. Maudgal (Leuven) : Personally, I have no experience.
have never used cautery. Perhaps you can tell something.

G.O. Waring (Atlanta) : No, it would seem to me inappropriate
at this point. Given the evidence that simple wiping debridement is effective, that we have antiviral back up, that we

know that applying toxic chemicals to the eye can cause increased scarring, it seems to be an inappropriate thing to do.

P.C. Maudgal (Leuven) : I thought so too.

R. Sundmacher (Freiburg) : I think everybody agrees, at least in the room here.

P.C. Maudgal (Leuven) : Since we are short of time I shall skip the slides relating to the points we have already discussed during this meeting. In these slides we just see a dendritic ulcer developing into a geographic ulcer. I think if there is marked necrosis of the epithelium cells only then you get a geographic ulcer. You can have initially a dendritic ulcer which can enlarge to become a geographic ulcer. It is possible that the shape and size of the ulcers depends on the strain of the virus. Dr. Centifanto has already showed us that different strains of herpes viruses produce different pathology. Would you like to comment further on this point, Dr. Centifanto ?

Y. Centifanto (New Orleans) : Yes, we did show that the morphology of the ulcer depends on the genome of the infecting virus strain. Some strains produced short, stubby dendrites, some produced long, thin lesions, and some produced only punctate keratitis. There is a definite basis in virus genetics for the shape of the ulcers and how they progress from day one to day seven.

P.C. Maudgal (Leuven) : Thank you, Dr. Centifanto. These slides show other examples of geographic ulcers. I think, we skip the treatment part unless somebody wants to make a comment.

C.R. Dawson (San Francisco) : Would you give us your treatment of geographic ulcers ?

P.C. Maudgal (Leuven) : Well, I don't make replicas in these cases because when the epithelium is more or less intact, amyl acetate penetrates into the superficial stromal layers. I have not done any studies by making replicas of a denuded cornea.

D.L. Easty (Bristol) : A case of geographic ulcer you are going to treat with antivirals immediately. But I am never quite sure, when you have a steroid treated patient like this with

a geographic ulcer, whether you should cut your steroid just
at that time completely, or whether you should wean it off.
It sounds a bit strange to ask this question, but I have seen
cases that have been treated with antiviral and they got a
steroid rebound. Have you any experience with this ?

P.C. Maudgal (Leuven) : What we do when we see such a case, we
stop steroids and we treat with antivirals. If the ulcer heals
and there is no stromal edema, we don't prescribe steroids.
Yesterday I talked about the residual epithelium defects, or
aseptic defects, or metaherpetic keratitis-whatever you call it,
in those cases we start steroids again, but under antiviral
cover.

C.R. Dawson (San Francisco) : I feel a bit like the surgeon in
George Bernard Shaw's play "The Doctor's Dilemma", who has
only one procedure for all conditions, but here again I use
gentle, wiping debridement. The patching is continued, however, until the epithelial defect has healed. In some cases
a soft contact lens may be substituted for the patch. In these
large ulcers I find it difficult on clinical grounds alone to
differentiate those due to indolent epithelial defects and those
associated with viral replication. It is with these cases that
I find laboratory diagnosis most helpful. In an early series,
our group recovered virus from only 20% of these larger epithelial defects ,Coleman et al., Arch. Ophthalmol. 81 : 22, 1969).
Clearly, with the idoxuridine and other antiviral treatment,
I think we contribute to the persistence of these longstanding
epithelial defects. With these lesions we, again, carry out
gentle, wiping debridement and patching. There is no question
that they heal slowly, but re-epithelialization occurs much
sooner with debridement and patching than with antiviral treatment alone. For those patients who have been on topical corticosteroids for some period of time, they must continue to
receive this medication. Once the patch is removed the dosage
of the corticosteroid should be governed by the response of
the stromal disease or uveitis because there is little evidence
that the epithelial disease responds to the steroid therapy.

P.C. Maudgal (Leuven) : That is a justified approach. Regarding
your question of differention between the postherpetic indolent
ulcers and herpetic geographic ulcers, we look carefully at
the ulcer margin. If you have an undermined edge of the
ulcer, perhaps only in a small part, then you can be sure that
this ulcer will develop into an indolent ulcer. At this stage
viral replication may still be going on in other parts of the
ulcer. So our approach to treatment in these cases would be
either debridement or topical antivirals. If the ulcer edge is
undermined all around, you are dealing with an indolent ulcer,
and in this case antivirals will have no effect. Are there any
further comments on that point ?

Then let us move to the next slides. In one slide we have
epithelial and stromal disease, accompanied by corneal neovascularisation. It is a longstanding recurrent infection. In the
other slide we see only some stromal haze. Now, I wanted to
come to the problem of terminology used to describe different
types of stromal keratitis; because we hear different terms like
interstitial, disciform, or necrotising keratitis, or stromal infiltrates and endothelitis. I think it is very important, especially to conduct studies, that we understand each other precisely
what we are talking about. Personally I feel confused. Yesterday we saw some slides showing disciform keratitis, which I do
not diagnose as disciform keratitis. I believe there are other
people in this audience who describe these conditions using
different terms.

Someone from audience : Appoint a committee.

R. Sundmacher (Freiburg) : No, that is no matter for a committee.
If you give me some time, I will try to define "endothelitis".

P.C. Maudgal (Leuven) : You are most wellcome.

R. Sundmacher (Freiburg) : Let me start with the term "disciform"
keratitis, which is a historical expression for a mostly round
shaped corneal haze in an inflamed herpes eye. Herb Kaufman
has always called this "disciform edema", which is a very

good expression from the pathophysiological point of view, because the disciform edema is caused by an underlying endothelial disease, which makes the endothelium leaky and brings
about corneal swelling. In the beginning, pure disciform edema is not associated with any stromal infiltration. If stromal
infiltration is a prominent feature of the disease, then we call
it interstitial herpetic keratitis. However, what makes the
clinical pictures sometimes confusing is the fact that with long-
standing corneal edema as well as with repeated attacks of
"disciform edema" one usually gets secondary stromal infiltration with subsequent scarring; and some patients experience,
of course, both - interstitial and endothelial herpetic disease
either concomitantly or subsequently.   This calls for clinical
signs which enable us to diagnose endothelitis and separate
herpetic endothelitis from other types of disease.

Let me first stress that it is impossible to make or reject the
diagnosis of endothelitis purely on the basis of specular microscopy. What you see with specular microscopy is blebs, dark
areas etc. which indicate nothing but sick endothelial cells,
i.e. endothelial edema (intra- and intercellular). There are
two classes of diseases which lead to acute endothelial edema.
The first group we call endotheliopahty, and the second group
endothelitis. What is the difference ? Endotheliopathy compri-
ses a rather heterogenous group of diseases with endothelial
trauma of any kind, e.g. surgical trauma, toxic influences,
severe iridocyclitis, etc. The trauma is not specifically directed against the endothelial cells; they suffer more or less because they are exposed to traumatizing events in their neigh-
bourhood. With endothelitis it is totally different. In this
case the endothelial cells are directly attacked by inflammatory cells. It is logical that these inflammatory cells must be
immune cells which are primed to attack a target in the cell
membrane of the endothelial cells. In the case of herpetic
endothelitis it is presumably herpes antigens located in the
cell membranes.

434

This type of "immune-endothelitis" has special features which
allow for a clinical diagnosis : normally the process is focal
and does not involve the entire endothelium. From the strict
correlation between (immune-) precipitates on the endothelium
and overlying "disciform edema" the diagnosis of endothelitis
is made. Of course, one doesn't necessarily need a disciform
edema for the diagnosis. If localized precipitates are correlated with endothelial edema visible by specular microscopy,
and all other areas of the endothelium do not show involvement, then it is also a slight form of endothelitis.
Coming back to the group of endotheliopathies. With these
you may, of course, also have edema and precipitates; however, you never have the strict local correlation between the
two of them.
Nomenclature is never agreed upon unanimously. Everybody
may use his nomenclature as long as he himself and others
know of what he is speaking. For us, disciform keratitis and
endothelitis have come to be interchangeable terms.
G.O. Waring (Atlanta) : Would you then define allograft rejection
in the penetrating keratoplasty as a focal endothelitis ?
R. Sundmacher (Freiburg) : Excellent brain ! Exactly that !
G.O. Waring (Atlanta) : That's what you asked me to ask, wasn't
it ?
R. Sundmacher (Freiburg) : I had just a paper published on the
definition of endothelitis. Instead of taking your time I'd
rather give you the reference : R. Sundmacher : Endothelitis
corneae. Begriffsbestimmung und klinische Abgrenzung. Klin.
Monatsbl. Augenheilk. 184, 163-167 (1984). I should only mention that there exist other types of viral endothelitis (e.g.
rubella endothelitis) that we observe endothelitis of unknown
origin (auto-antigen ??) and that even the Posner-Schlossman
syndrom may at least in part be brought about by a peculiar
type of endothelitis.
D.L. Easty (Bristol) : In endothelitis cases do you know that the
virus is replicating in the endothelium or do you suspect it?

R. Sundmacher (Freiburg) : I don't have proof, I suspect it.

D.L. Easty (Bristol) : Do you have evidence of that or are you just saying it ?

R. Sundmacher (Freiburg) : We did not investigate appropriate corneal buttons with the electron microscope, but we did aqueous taps, and we isolated herpes simplex virus quite regularly from cases with typical endothelitis. We cannot prove that the virus stemmed from the endothelium, but believe that it very probably does come from that source in these cases.

D.L. Easty (Bristol) : Have you tried taking endothelium off your transplants and culturing them separately ?

R. Sundmacher (Freiburg) : No, I haven't. Mostly, keratoplasties are done in rather bad cases where most of the endothelium had been lost preoperatively, some is damaged during the operation, and with the remaining cells the change seems little to find virus just in them.

P.C. Maudgal (Leuven) : Can we go to the next slides ? I'll skip the treatment part because we have already discussed it during the meeting. These are again two examples, perhaps Rainer can comment on them as to what type of keratitis it is ?

R. Sundmacher (Freiburg) : The one on your side is interstitial herpetic keratitis, the other one shows presumably chronic recurrent disciform keratitis with subsequent stromal scarring.

P.C. Maudgal (Leuven) : I feel relieved when you say that this scarring resulted from recurrent disciform keratitis. Yesterday, when I heard some speakers, I became afraid that I have been making wrong diagnosis all these years.
Next slides demonstrate two more examples.

R. Sundmacher (Freiburg) : Yes, this is excellent. You see the immune precipitates exactly behind the swollen disc - and only there ! This distribution is totally different from that in iritis.

P.C. Maudgal (Leuven) : In the next slides we find examples of postherpetic ulcers or indolent ulcers. When a patient presents with a longstanding corneal ulcer we carefully look for small dendritic extensions at the ulcer margin. Personally, if I find one of these dendritic extensions, I am sure it is an active herpes simplex infection. If the dendritic extensions are absent, and the ulcer has undermined edges, then it is an aseptic defect or indolent ulcer. Does anybody like to comment on this ?

R. Sundmacher (Freiburg) : I would like to stress that differential diagnosis becomes extremely difficult once you have stained the lesions because the dye makes it impossible to see the typical destruction pattern of the margins of the viral lesions.

P.C. Maudgal (Leuven) : Involvement of different ocular structures is seen in this slide. There is dendritic ulcer, stromal disease, and iritis. Pupil is distorted because of posterior synechia.

The last slide shows the problem of recurrence in keratoplasty patients. Management of these conditions has been discussed by several speakers during the meeting.

G.O. Waring (Atlanta) : It does seem a pity to pass over the treatment on one of the most difficult problems, whatever time it may be. You showed the indolent ulceration there, and that is one of the most difficult problems we have in herpes. Can we have 30 seconds or something for a comment ?

R. Sundmacher (Freiburg) : Sure, hours. I leave tomorrow.

G.O. Waring (Atlanta) : Dr. Keynon and his group have applied cyanoacrylate adhesives to the indolent defects, after all standard therapy had not worked. It has been found that it keeps the polys out, which probably are the source of the underlying stromal destruction. We only used it in a few cases. It has helped us a great deal, putting on a very thin layer of cyanoacrylate adhesive, and then putting on a soft contact lens. Have you any experience with that or are there other modes of managing these ?

P.C. Maudgal (Leuven) : I have no experience with cyanoacrylate adhesives in indolent ulcers. In different meetings I have seen the slides of eyes which had been treated by cyanoacrylate and laid on contact lenses. I really became afraid to use them because the slides demonstrated something different than what the speaker said.

During this meeting Dr. Thiel and Dr. Kok-van Alphen have told us that they found that the use of adhesives increases inflammation. Like them, we also sometimes use cryanoacrylate to plug the perforated cornea before keratoplasty. Our approach to the indolent ulcers is quite different. Perhaps you are aware of the "Yin-Yang" hypothesis where the role of cyclic-AMP and cyclic-GMP has been emphasized in the cell regulation (Goldberg et al. 1974). In alkali burned corneas, eyes treated by just putting a drop of water may do better than those eyes which do not receive any treatment. From these findings we reasoned that a hypothetic excess of an inhibitory enzyme could perhaps be dealt with by irrigating the eye frequently (Maudgal and Missotten : Superficial Keratitis, Monographs in Ophthalmology I, Dr. W. Junk Publishers, The Hague, 1980). So we started to wash these eyes copiously with Hartmann[R] (sodium lactate) solution every hour. We have not done any statistics of the data but almost all of our patients have done very well on this therapy. Sometimes, if eye washings are not effective, this happens often in marginal indolent ulcers and I believe immunological factors are playing a role there, then we perform a superficial keratectomy in the ulcer area and excision of the adjacent perilimbal conjunctiva.

R. Sundmacher (Freiburg) : Before you come to your closing remarks, I would like on behalf of all the participants to thank very warmly the local organizers, Drs. Maudgal and Missotten. Everybody attends a meeting with certain expectations. I must say that these expectations, at least mine, have widely been surpassed. Speaking in terms of "recurrences" of this symposium, it will be very hard for any organizer to meet the standards you have set here in terms of hospitality and efficiency. I would like to thank you both as well as your many collaborators who have made this meeting so pleasant. Thank you.

CLOSING REMARKS

P.C. Maudgal (Leuven) :

Traditionally, towards the end of a meeting the main events are re-emphasized, but I am not going to do that. We have heard some excellent lectures on the latest experimental and clinical research. I don't find it justifiable to repeat what eminent speakers have told themselves. It is my belief that all participants would have found answers to at least some of their questions, and all of you will go home with new ideas for future research. We had also the opportunity to discuss various approaches for the management of herpetic eye diseases which was very important for the clinicians among us. Looking back at two and a half days we have been together here, I have no doubt in saying that the meeting served its purpose and it was a very successful symposium. However, I wish we had some more time for the "General Discussion", as we had to skip repeatedly slides on herpes simplex virus infection and we had no time to discuss varicella-zoster virus and cytomegalovirus infections.

I want to thank you all who came from 18 different countries in such a large number to ensure the success of this meeting. My special thanks to all the speakers who presented the results of their painstaking work, and the chairmen who did an excellent job.

I shall be failing in my duty if I forget to express my gratitude to so many colleagues who have helped to run this meeting efficiently. The beautiful girls who handed over microphones to you and the projectionists behind are our residents. People doing secretarial work outside the hall also belong to our department. I have heard that participants have enjoyed and much appreciated the social program. Credit for this goes to Mrs. Missotten who arranged it, and I thank her for her efforts.

Maudgal, P.C. and Missotten, L., (eds.) Herpetic Eye Diseases.
© *1985, Dr W. Junk Publishers, Dordrecht/Boston/Lancaster. ISBN 978-94-010-8935-7*

440

Last but not the least, I am grateful to Professor L. Missotten
and Professor E. De Clercq. Both of them encouraged me to orga-
nise this meeting and they helped me and advised me whenever
I had difficulties.

Thank you all once more. Auf wiedersehn !

LIST OF PARTICIPANTS

ADAM Dieter, Dr. G. Mann Chem.-Pharm., Fabrik, Brunsbütteler
    Damm 165-173, P.O. Box 200456, D-1000 Berlin 20, W.-Germany
AHONEN Reijo, Dept. of Ophtalmology, Univ. of Helsinki, Haart-
    manink. 4C, SF-00290 Helsinki, Finland
AMEYE Christian, Eye Research Laboratory, Katholieke Universiteit
    Leuven, Capucienenvoer 7, 3000 Leuven, Belgium
APERS Roger, Amerikalei 75, 2000 Antwerpen, Belgium
ASBELL P.A., Mt.Sinai Medical Center, Annenberg 22-12,Fifth
    Avenue and 100th St., New-York NY 10029, USA
AZZOPARDI Anton, Univ. of Malta, "Shamrock" Flt. 1, Old Church
    Street,B'kara, Malta
BADANIOVA Dana, Te Couwelaarlei 29, 2100 Deurne, Belgium
BALZARINI Jan, Rega Institute for Medical Research, Katholieke
    Universiteit Leuven, Minderbroedersstraat 10, B-3000 Leuven,
    Belgium
BERNAERTS Ria, Rega Institute for Medical Research, Katholieke
    Universiteit Leuven, Minderbroedersstraat 10, B-3000 Leuven,
    Belgium
BEUNK H.J., Tramedico B.V., Postbus 192, 1380 AD Weesp, The
    Netherlands
BRABANT Leo, Gerechtstraat 1/101, 2800 Mechelen, Belgium
BRABANT Patrick, Mortelstraat 21, 9831 Deurle, Belgium
BUYCK Ann, Minderbroedersstr. 35/9, 3000 Leuven, Belgium
CARTER Clare, Univ. of Bristol, Dept. of Ophth.,The Medical
    School, University Walk, Bristol, U.K.
CENTIFANTO-FITZGERALD Ysolina, LSU Eye Center, 136 South Roman
    St., New-Orleans, Louisiana 70112, USA
CLAOUÉ Charles, Southampton Eye Hospital, Wilton Ave.,
    Southampton, Hampshire SO9 4XW, U.K.
CLAY C., Hôtel-Dieu, Service Ophtalmologie, Place du Parvis Notre
    Dame, 75004 Paris, France
COLIN Joseph, Centre Hospitalier Régional, Service d'Ophtalmologie,
    Avenue Foch, 29279 Brest Cedex, France
COLLA Brigitte, H. Geeststraat 8/5, 3000 Leuven, Belgium
COLLUM Louis M., Royal Victoria Eye and Ear Hospital, 54 Adelaïde
    Rd.,Dublin 2, Ireland
CRAWFORD Geoffrey J., Emory University, 2058 Palifox Dr. NE,
    Atlanta,Georgia 30307, USA
Cs. TÓTH László, Laarheidstr. 70, 1650 Beersel, Belgium
DATEMA Roelf, Astra Läkemedel AB, Dept. of Antiviral Chemo-
    therapy, 15185 Södertälje, Sweden
DAWSON Chandler R., F.I. Proctor Foundation, Univ. of California
    San Francisco, S-315, San Francisco, California 94143, USA
DE CLERCQ Erik, Rega Institute for Medical Research, Kath. Univ.-
    Leuven, Minderbroedersstr. 10, 3000 Leuven, Belgium
DE CLIPPELEIR Lucie, Tiensevest 156, 3000 Leuven, Belgium
DE CNODDER Béatrice, Ten Hovelaan 5/4, 3000 Leuven, Belgium

DECONINCK Hilde, Meilaan 82, 1200 Brussel, Belgium
DE KONING Erik W.J., Keizersgracht 290, 1016 EW Amsterdam, The Netherlands
DE LAEY Jean-Jacques, Dienst Oogheelkunde, Acad. Ziekenhuis Gent, De Pintelaan 135, 9000 Gent, Belgium
DEMEER Solange, Toekomststraat 33, 3500 Hasselt, Belgium
DEMOLS Emile, Vorstlaan 26 A, 1170 Brussel, Belgium
DE MUYNCK Marleen, Heilige Geeststr. 4/25, 3000 Leuven, Belgium
DENIS Josette, Hôtel-Dieu, Laboratoire du Service d'Ophtalmologie, Place du Parvis Notre Dame, 75004 Paris, France
DESGRANGES George, Rega Institute for Medical Research, Katholieke Univ. Leuven, Minderbroedersstraat 10, B-3000 Leuven, Belgium
DE SOMER Pieter, Kath.Univ.Leuven, Naamsestraat 22, 3000 Leuven, Belgium
DEVUYST Ann, Parklaan 8, 9000 Gent, Belgium
DIELTIENS May, Pelgrimstr. 1/13, 3000 Leuven, Belgium
DOERNER Thomas, Inter-Yeda Ltd, Kiryat Weizmann, Ness-Ziona 76110, Israel
DOMELA NIEUWENHUYS Onko, Oogheelkundige Kliniek, Acad. Ziekenhuis Groningen, Steenhouwerskade 78, Groningen, The Netherlands
DOMEN Francine, De Pintelaan 357, 9000 Gent, Belgium
DRALANDS Lieve, Dienst Oogziekten, U.Z. St. Rafaël, Capucienenvoer 7, 3000 Leuven, Belgium
EASTY David L., Dept. of Ophth., Bristol Eye Hospital, Lower Maudlin Str., Bristol BS1 2LX, U.K.
EPSTEIN Dan, Dept. of Ophth., Karolinska Hospital, 104 01 Stockholm, Sweden
FALCON Michael G., St. Thomas' Hospital, 4 The Orchard, London SE3 0QU, U.K.
FELLINGER Christa, Univ.Augenklinik, Auenbruggerplatz 4, A-8036 Graz,Austria
FIELD Hugh J., Dept. of Clinical Veterinary Medicine, Univ. of Cambridge, Madingsley Road, Cambridge CB3 OES, U.K.
FLOREN Ingrid, Dept. of Ophthalmology, University Hospital, 22185 Lund, Sweden
FOETS Beatrijs, Dienst Oogziekten, U.Z. St. Rafaël, Capucijnenvoer 7, 3000 Leuven, Belgium
FOSTER C. Stephen, Massachusetts Eye and Ear Infirmary, 243 Charles Street, Boston, MA 02114, USA
FRANCOIS Jules, Univ. of Ghent, Paul De Smet de Nayerplein 15, 9000 Gent, Belgium
GALLE Walburga, Platte-Lostraat 181, 3200 Leuven, Belgium
GEEROMS Bea, Kortrijkseweg 1, 9000 Ghent, Belgium
GEVERS Brigitte, Raoul Claesstraat 3/6, 3000 Leuven, Belgium
GOETHALS Marc, Schavei 63, 1900 Overijse, Belgium
GOFFIN Marleen, Boeimeerstraat 8, 2820 Bonheiden, Belgium
GORMLEY Robert J., 707 Pine Avenue, P.O. Box 812, Niagara Falls, NY 14302, USA
HARNEY Barbara, Bristol Eye Hospital, Lower Maudlin Street, Bristol BS1 2LX, U.K.
HAUSTRATE François, Harmoniestraat 33, 2018 Antwerpen, Belgium
HERBORT Carl P., Hôpital Ophtalmique Universitaire, 15 ave. de France, CH-1004 Lausanne, Switzerland

HOANG-XUAN Thanh, Hôtel-Dieu, Laboratoire d'Ophtalmologie, 1
  Place du Parvis notre Dame, 75004 Paris, France
HOLMBERG Åke S., Eye Department, Karolinska Hospital, 10401 Stock-
  holm, Sweden
HOUTHUYS Marie-Anne, Koning Albertlaan 31, 3320 Hoegaarden,
  Belgium
HOUTTEQUIET Ingrid, Leopoldstraat 36, 2800 Mechelen, Belgium
HUMMEL Klaus, c/o Merz + Co. GmbH & Co., Eckenheimer Landstr.
  100-104, D-6000 Frankfurt/Main, W.-Germany
HUNG Son On, St. Paul's Eye Hospital, Old Hall Street, Liverpool
  L3 9PF, U.K.
HYMAN Richard D., Pacific Medical Center, 2225 Port Chicago Hwy,
  Concord, Calif. 94520, USA
INGRAND Didier, Hopital Pitié Salpetrière, Sve. Virologie, 47
  Boulevard de l'Hôpital, 75013 Paris, France
ISENBORGHS Marc, Frilinglei 73, 2130 Brasschaat, Belgium
JAIN Inder S., Dept. of Ophth., Postgraduate institute of Medical
  Education and Research, Chandigarh-160012, India
JANSEN Guy, Antwerpsestg. 192, 2140 Westmalle, Belgium
JANSSENS Baudouin, Av. D. Yernaux 23, 1300 Wavre, Belgium
JANSSENS Myriam, P. Benoitlaan 59/8, 8200 Brugge, Belgium
JUEL-JENSEN Bent, Nuffield Dept. of Medicine, Univ. of Oxford,
  Radcliffe Infirmary, Oxford OX2 6HE, U.K.
JUNG Felicitas, Bremlaan 201, 1970 Wezembeek-Oppem, Belgium
KAECKENBEECK-COLSON Annette, 17 Drève des Chevreuils, 1640 Rhode
  Saint-Genèse, Belgium
KESTELOOT F., Oogziekten, U.Z. St.-Rafaël, Kapucijnenvoer 7,
  B-3000 Leuven, Belgium
KLOVEKORN Gunther, c/o Fa. Basotherm Gmbh. Leipzigstr. 26, 7950
  Biberach/Riss., W.-Germany
KNOEBEL Hans H., Marienkrankenhaus, Augenabteilung, Alfredstr.
  9, D-2000 Hamburg 76, W.-Germany
KOCH Monique, Kattendansstraat 122, 3500 Hasselt, Belgium
KOK-van ALPHEN Clara C., Diaconessenhuis Leiden, Warmonderweg
  12, 2341 KV Oegstgeest, The Netherlands

KORRA Ahmad E., Ophth. Dept., Faculty of Medicine, Univ. of
  Alexandria, 17 Raml Station Square, Alexandria, Egypt
KROLZIG Gabriele, Universitäts-Augenklinik Hamburg, Elb-
  chausse 156A, 2000 Hamburg 52, W.-Germany
LAGOUTTE Françoise, Hôpital des Enfants, 168 Cours de l'Argon-
  ne, 33077 Bordeaux, France
LAMBERTS Lieve, Nieuwstraat 35, 3180 Westerlo, Belgium
LANGOIS Martine, Laboratoire National de la Santé, Département
  d'Etudes des Maladies Virales, 8 Avenue Rockefeller, 69373
  Lyon Cedex 08, France
LE GLOATIEC Alain, Le Mercator, Rue de l'Industrie, Monaco
LERNOULD M.P., Château de la Fosse, Rue d'Alban, 12, 5870
  Mont St. Guibert, Belgium
LEYS Anita, Dienst Oogziekten, U.Z. St.Rafaël, Capucijnenvoer
  7, 3000 Leuven, Belgium
LEYS Magdalena, J. Hendrickxstraat 57, 2120 Schoten, Belgium
LEYS Monique, Rotterdam Oogziekenhuis, Schiedamsevest 180,
  3000 LM Rotterdam, The Netherlands

LIESEGANG Thomas J., Mayo Clinic, Dept. Ophthalmology,
Rochester, Minnesota 55905, USA
LIZON Isabelle, Hôtel-Dieu, Laboratoire d'Ophtalmologie, Place
du Parvis Notre Dame, 75004 Paris, France
LOWTH L.J, Suite 22, Thesis Court, Manuka, Canberra 2603,
Australia
MACKEN Louise, Baertlaan 29, 3009 Herent-Winksele, Belgium
MALAISE-STALS Jacqueline, Univ. de Liège, Clinique Ophtal-
mologique, Hôpital de Bavière, Boulevard de la Constitution
66, 4020 Liège, Belgium
MARECHAL-COURTOIS Christiane, Univ. de Liège, Clinique Ophtal-
mologique, Hôpital de Bavière, Boulevard de la Constitution
66, 4020 Liège, Belgium
MAUDGAL Prabhat C., Eye Research Laboratory and Ophthal-
mology Clinic, U.Z. St. Rafaël, Capucijnenvoer 7, 3000
Leuven, Belgium
McCREA J.A.S., Royal Victoria Hospital, Grosvenor Road, Belfast
BT12 6 BA, Northern Ireland
McGILL James I., The Eye Hospital, Wilton Avenue, Southampton
S09 4XW, U.K.
McGILLION Katharine A., The Wellcome Foundation Limited, 183
Euston Road, London NW1 2BP, U.K.
MERIWANI Sabah N., De Goddelijke Voorzienigheid Hospital,
Walramstr. 23, Sittard, The Netherlands
MEURS Petrus J., Kon.Nederlands Gasthuis voor Ooglijders, F.C.
Dondersstraat 65, 3572 JE Utrecht, The Netherlands
MIRIS Maria, Kapucijnenvoer 67/42, 3000 Leuven, Belgium
MISSOTTEN Luc, Dienst Oogziekten, U.Z. St. Rafaël, Kapucijnen-
voer 7, 3000 Leuven, Belgium
MONTEYNE Marie-Christine, Fonteinstraat 137/15, 3000 Leuven,
Belgium
MOREAU J.J.M., Lab. Delalande N.V., Middaglijnstraat 22, 1030
Brussel, Belgium
NELIS Joseph, Dr. Geensstraat 10, 3300 Tienen, Belgium
NENQUIN-KLAASSEN E., Ferrerlaan 114, 9000 Gent, Belgium
NEUMANN-HAEFELIN Dieter, Institut für Virologie, Zentrum für
Hygiene, Hermann- Herderstr. 11, D-7800 Freiburg, W.-
Germany
NIJS Ivo, Nijverheidslaan 23, 3650 Dilsen-Lanklaar, Belgium
NUYENS Michel, Hofkwartier 26, 2410 Herentals, Belgium
OH Jang O., Proctor Foundation, Rm S-315, University of Califor-
nia, San Francisco, CA 94143, USA
ÖHMAN Lena E., Dept. Ophth., University Hospital, 75185
Upsala, Sweden
ORSONI Jelka G., Institute of Ophth., University, 43100 Parma,
Italy
PALMISANO Lucia, Instituto di Ricerca Serono, Via Casilina 125,
00-176 Roma, Italy
PAPENDICK Uwe, Dept. of Clinical Research, Dr. Karl Thomae
GmbH, Postfach 1755, D-7950 Biberach/Riss, W.-Germany
PATHAK Ajay, Residentie Orion, Kikvorsstraat 867, 9000 Gent,
Belgium
PATTERSON Alan, St. Paul's Eye Hospital, Old Hall Street,
Liverpool L3 9PF, U.K.

PETRINI Orlando, Dispersa AG, Postfach 1086, CH-8401
    Winterthur, Switzerland
PIERRE Christine, Grote Steenweg 533, 2600 Berchem, Belgium
PLOVIER Maria, F. de Pillecijnlaan 22, 9160 Halle, Belgium
RADDA Thomas-Michaël, 1. Univ. Augenkliniek, Spitalgasse 2,
    1097 Wien, Austria
RAUS Peter, Tessenstraat 21/5R, 3000 Leuven, Belgium
REES Peter J., The Wellcome Research Laboratories, Beckenham,
    Kent, BR3 3BS, U.K.
REICH Margareta E., Univ.Augenklinik. Auenbruggerplatz 4,
    8036 Graz, Austria
RENAUDIE Michel, Laboratoires Wellcome, 159 rue Nationale,
    75640 Paris Cedex 13, France
ROMANO Amalia, M.& G . Goldschleger Eye Institute, Research
    Dept., Chaim Sheba Medical Center, Tel hashomer 52621
    RamatGan, Israël
ROMMEL Jos, Grote Markt 28, 8800 Roeselare, Belgium
RYCKAERT Sofie, S. Van Cauwenbergelaan 51, 9030 Wondelgem,
    Belgium
RYDBERG Mats V., Eye Dept., Region Hospital, S-70185 Örebro,
    Sweden
SCHAPIRA Serge, Boehringer Ingelheim N.V., 17 rue du Collège
    St. Michel, 1150 Brussels, Belgium
SCHMIDT Peter, Eye Dept., Centralsygehuset, DK-4700 Naestved,
    Denmark
SCHULTZ Richard O., Dept. of Ophth., Medical College of
    Winconsin, 8700 West Winconsin Ave., Milwaukee, Wisconsin
    53226, USA
SELS Martine, Wellcome, Industriezone III, 9440 Aalst, Belgium
SHEPHERD Ian, Dept. of Ophth., Royal Victoria Hospital, Gros-
    venorRoad, Belfast BT12 6BA, Northern Ireland
SHIELD M., Searle Research and Development, Division of G.D.-
    Searle & Co. Ltd., P.O. Box 53, Lane End Road, High
    Wycombe, Bucks HP 12 4HL, U.K.
SHIMELD Carolyn, Dept. of Ophth. Medical School, University
    Walk, Bristol BS8 1TH, U.K.
SMOLIN Gilbert, Proctor Foundation, 95 Kirkham Str., San
    Francisco, California 94122, USA
SPILEERS Werner, Heilige Geeststr. 82/6, 3000 Leuven, Belgium
STENEVI Ulf, Dept. of Ophth. University Hospital, S-22185 Lund,
    Sweden
STEVENSON Katharine E., Royal Berkshire Hospital Reading, 13,
    Milford Gardens, Oakmount park, Chandlers Ford, Hants,
    U.K.
STORMS Myriam, Oogziekten, U.Z. St-Rafaël, Kapucijnenvoer 7,
    B-3000 Leuven, Belgium
STULTING R.Doyle, Emory University, 1365 Clifton Road, NE
    Atlanta, GA 30322, USA
SUNDMACHER Rainer, University Eye Clinic, Killianstr., D-7800
    Freiburg, W.-Germany
SVENSSON Thorbjörn, Gaddaborgsvägen 40, S-81800 Valbo, Sweden
SWINNEN Titia, Guido Gezellestraat 30, 3290 Diest, Belgium
THIEL Hans-Jürgen, University Eye Hospital, Schleichstr. 12,
    D-7400 Tübingen, W.-Germany

THIJS Marie-Therese, Boomstraat 71, 2680 Bornem, Belgium
THOMSON Joyce M., The Wellcome Foundation Limited, 183 Euston
   Road, London NW1 2BP, U.K.
TOMPAY Balint, Ave. Faisans 17, 6110 Montigny le Tilleul,Belgium
TULLO Andrew B., Manchester Royal Eye Hospital, Oxford Road,
   Manchester M13 9WK U.K.
TYE Allan A., Elizabeth House, 231 North Terrace, Adelaide, South
   Australia, Australia 5000
VALVEKENS Frank, De Bayotstraat 26, 3000 Leuven, Belgium
VAN ASSCHE Emilienne, Blijde Inkomststraat 2, 3000 Leuven, Belgium
VAN DAMME Boudewijn, Labo Histo-en Cytochemie, U.Z. St. Rafaël,
   Minderbroedersstraat 12, 3000 Leuven, Belgium
VAN BIJSTERVELD O.P., Kon.Nederlands Gasthuis voor Ooglijders,
   F.C. Dondersstraat 65, Utrecht, The Netherlands
VAN DEN BERGH Anneleen, Provinciestraat 120, 2018 Antwerpen,
   Belgium
VAN DEN BERGHE Fabienne, Markt 39, 9900 Eeklo, Belgium
VANDEN BORRE Ann, Dienst Oogziekten, Katholieke Universiteit
   Leuven, Belgium
VAN GANSWIJK Renée, Academisch Ziekenhuis Leiden, Afdeling oog-
   heelkunde, Rijnsburgerweg, 2333 AA Leiden, The Netherlands
VAN GERVEN Ilse, Heilige Geeststraat 8/5, B-3000 Leuven, Belgium
VAN GINDERDEUREN Rita, Marcel Habetslaan 1, B-3600 Genk, Belgium
VAN HAESENDONCK Eduarda, Eye Research Laboratory, Kath. Univ.
   Leuven, Capucijnenvoer 7, B-3000 Leuven, Belgium
VAN HERCK Marleen, Tervuursestraat 99/41, B-3000 Leuven, Belgium
VAN HOECKE Christian, Wellcome, Industriezone III, 9440 Aalst,
   Belgium
VAN HYFTE R., Dienst oogziekten, U.Z. St.-Rafaël, Kapucijnenvoer
   7, B-3000 Leuven, Belgium
VAN KERCKHOVEN Michel, Grote Steenweg 465, 2600 Berchem, Belgium
VAN LOENEN Gerrit, Monterspad 34, 1383 DJ Weesp, The Netherlands
VAN TORNOUT Ingrid, Lammekenslaan 10, 8300 Knokke, Belgium
VANTRAPPEN Lut, Capucienenvoer 7, 3000 Leuven, Belgium
VAN VOOREN Henri, Grote markt 18, 2800 Mechelen, Belgium
VAN WING Francine, Weststraat 33, 8800 Roeselare, Belgium
VEKEMAN Ingrid, Azalealaan 6, 1740 Ternat, Belgium
VERBRUGGEN Alfons, Holsbeeksesteenweg 90, 3010 Wilsele, Belgium
VERBRUGGEN Walter, Antwerpsestraat 59/4, 2650 Boom, Belgium
VERSLUYS Suzel, Ev.Krankenhaus Essen-Werden, Gerard Haupt-
   mannstrasse 15, 4030 Ratingen, W.-Germany
VEUGELEN Danny, Dienst Oogziekten, U.Z. St.-Rafaël, Kapucijnen-
   voer 7, B-3000 Leuven, Belgium
VICTORIA-TRONCOSO V., Désiré Mercierlaan 136, 9219 Gentbrugge,
   Belgium
VIZA Dimitri, Faculté de médecine, 15 rue de l'Ecole de médecine,
   75006 Paris, France
VÖLKER-DIEBEN H.J.M., ., Diaconessenhuis, Houtlaan 55, 2333 AA
   Leiden, The Netherlands
VRIJGHEM Jérôme, Groot-Overlaar 222, 3300 Tienen, Belgium
WAPPLER Heinz, Kantonsspital St.-Gallen, Dept. of Ophth.,
   Rorschacherstrasse, 9000 St.-Gallen, Switzerland
WARING George O., Emory University, 1365 Clifton Road, Atlanta,
   Ga 30322, U.S.A.

WEEKERS Jean-Francois, Clinique Ophthalmologique, Hôpital de
    Bavière, 66 Boulevard de la Constitution, 4000 Liège, Belgium
WEIDLE Egon G., University Eye Hospital, Schleichstr. 12, D-7400
    Tübingen, W.-Germany
WETS Bernadette, Woluwedal 12/41, 1940 St. Stevens Woluwe, Belgium
WINTER Rolf, Univ. Augenklinik Hamburg, Martinistrasse 52, D-2000
    Hamburg 20, W.-Germany
WISTRAND Per J., University Hospital Eye Clinic, S-75014 Upsala,
    Sweden
WRIGHT Peter, Moorfields Eye Hospital, Institute of Ophth., City
    Road,London ECIV 2PD, U.K.